Lucinda G. Miller, PharmD, BCPS
Wallace J. Murray, PhD
Editors

Herbal Medicinals
A Clinician's Guide

Pre-publication
REVIEWS,
COMMENTARIES,
EVALUATIONS . . .

"The use of herbal medicines has skyrocketed in the last decade. Pharmacists and other practitioners must be aware of the positive and negative effects of herbal medicines to provide care for the general population. Dr. Lucinda Miller and Dr. Wallace Murray have provided the necessary information for practitioners to guide the use of these products for specific indications. In addition, the authors have used the case vignette to demonstrate the efficacy and toxicity of these 'untested' entities. Considering the public's desire to use herbal medicines, practitioners would be wise to be familiar with the various entities and *Herbal Medicinals: A Clinician's Guide* serves as an excellent reference."

Karen Theesen, PharmD, BCPP
Associate Professor
of Pharmacy Practice,
Creighton University,
Omaha, NE

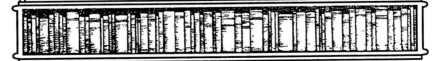

More pre-publication
REVIEWS, COMMENTARIES, EVALUATIONS . . .

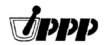

Pharmaceutical Products Press
An Imprint of The Haworth Press, Inc.

Herbal Medicinals
A Clinician's Guide

PHARMACEUTICAL PRODUCTS PRESS
Pharmaceutical Sciences
Mickey C. Smith, PhD
Executive Editor

New, Recent, and Forthcoming Titles:

Pharmaceutical Marketing: Strategy and Cases by Mickey C. Smith

International Pharmaceutical Services: The Drug Industry and Pharmacy Practice in Twenty-Three Major Countries of the World edited by Richard N. Spivey, Albert I. Wertheimer, and T. Donald Rucker

A Social History of the Minor Tranquilizers: The Quest for Small Comfort in the Age of Anxiety by Mickey C. Smith

Marketing Pharmaceutical Services: Patron Loyalty, Satisfaction, and Preferences edited by Harry A. Smith and Joel Coons

Nicotine Replacement: A Critical Evaluation edited by Ovide F. Pomerleau and Cynthia S. Pomerleau

Herbs of Choice: The Therapeutic Use of Phytomedicinals by Varro E. Tyler

Interpersonal Communication in Pharmaceutical Care by Helen Meldrum

Searching for Magic Bullets: Orphan Drugs, Consumer Activism, and Pharmaceutical Development by Lisa Ruby Basara and Michael Montagne

The Honest Herbal by Varro E. Tyler

Understanding the Pill: A Consumer's Guide to Oral Contraceptives by Greg Juhn

Pharmaceutical Chartbook, Second Edition edited by Abraham G. Hartzema and C. Daniel Mullins

The Handbook of Psychiatric Drug Therapy for Children and Adolescents by Karen A. Theesen

Children, Medicines, and Culture edited by Patricia J. Bush, Deanna J. Trakas, Emilio J. Sanz, Rolf L. Wirsing, Tuula Vaskilampi, and Alan Prout

Social and Behavioral Aspects of Pharmaceutical Care edited by Mickey C. Smith and Albert I. Wertheimer

Studies in Pharmaceutical Economics edited by Mickey C. Smith

Drugs of Natural Origin: Economic and Policy Aspects of Discovery, Development, and Marketing by Anthony Artuso

Medical Writing in Drug Development: A Practical Guide for Pharmaceutical Research by Robert J. Bonk

Improving the Quality of the Medication Use Process: Error Prevention and Reducing Adverse Drug Events edited by Alan Escovitz, Dev S. Pathak, and Philip J. Schneider

Access to Experimental Drugs in Terminal Illness: Ethical Issues by Udo Schuklenk

Herbal Medicinals: A Clinician's Guide by Lucinda Miller and Wallace J. Murray

Tyler's Herbs of Choice: The Therapeutic Use of Phytomedicinals by James Robbers and Varro E. Tyler

Herbal Medicinals
A Clinician's Guide

Lucinda G. Miller, PharmD, BCPS
Wallace J. Murray, PhD
Editors

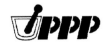

Pharmaceutical Products Press
An Imprint of The Haworth Press, Inc.
New York • London

Published by

Pharmaceutical Products Press®, an imprint of The Haworth Press, Inc., 10 Alice Street, Binghamton, NY 13904-1580

Cover design by Marylouise E. Doyle.

Library of Congress Cataloging-in-Publication Data

Herbal medicinals : a clinician's guide / Lucinda G. Miller, Wallace J. Murray, editors.
　　p.　cm.
Includes bibliographical references and index.
ISBN 0-7890-0467-4 (alk. paper).
1. Herbs—Therapeutic use. 2. Functional foods. I. Miller, Lucinda G. II. Murray, Wallace J.
[DNLM: 1. Medicine, Herbal. 2. Drugs, Chinese Herbal. 3. Drug Interactions. QV 767 H5345 1998]
RM666.H33H465 1998
615'.321—dc21
DNLM/DLC
for Library of Congress
98-12043
CIP

LM gratefully acknowledges the love and support
of her husband and daughters,
making this work possible.

CONTENTS

Chapter 8. Herbal Medications, Nutraceuticals, and Hypertension 135
Lucinda G. Miller, PharmD, BCPS
Louis A. Kazal Jr., MD

Chapter 9. Nutraceuticals for Management of Dyslipidemia and Atherosclerosis 163
Paul W. Jungnickel, PhD

Chapter 10. Asthma: A Review of Diagnostic, Pharmacotherapeutic, and Herbal Issues 189
John G. Prichard, MD
Lucinda G. Miller, PharmD, BCPS

ABOUT THE EDITORS

Lucinda G. Miller, PharmD, BCPS, is Professor and Vice Chairman of the pharmacy practice department of a prominent health sciences center in the Southwest. Previously, she was Assistant Professor in the Department of Family Practice at Baylor College of Medicine in Houston, Texas, where she received the Moise Teaching Award (outstanding family medicine faculty teaching award) in 1991. A board-certified pharmacotherapy specialist, she, along with Dr. Wallace J. Murray, began a course titled "Herbal Medicinals" at the University of Nebraska Medical Center in 1997. Dr. Miller has served on the Regional Advisory Council to the National Library of Medicine and has authored over eighty journal articles and book chapters.

Wallace J. Murray, PhD, is Associate Professor in the Department of Pharmaceutical Sciences in the College of Pharmacy at the University of Nebraska Medical Center, Omaha, Nebraska, where he is also a mentor for the Pharmacological Sciences Training Program. He is a consultant to the Battelle Institute and the U.S. Army Medical Research Institute for Infectious Diseases. A distinguished professor in the pharmacy field, Dr. Murray has received several teaching awards, grants, and contracts, and is a member of several professional organizations. He is the author of over fifty journal articles and several book chapters.

CONTRIBUTORS

Jan V. Beckwith, PharmD, is Assistant Professor, Idaho Drug Information Center, Idaho State University, Pocatello, Idaho.

Mark Blumenthal is Executive Director, American Botanical Council, Austin, Texas.

Teri L. Gabel, PharmD, BCPP, is Associate Professor, Department of Pharmacy Practice, College of Pharmacy, University of Nebraska Medical Center, Omaha, Nebraska.

Stephen Gillespie, PhD, is Associate Professor, Department of Pharmaceutical Sciences, College of Pharmacy, University of Wyoming, Laramie, Wyoming.

William R. Hamilton, PharmD, is Assistant Professor, Department of Pharmacy Practice, School of Pharmacy and Allied Health Professions, Omaha, Nebraska.

M. E. Blair Holbein, PhD, BCPS, BCAP, is Clinical Pharmacologist, Department of Internal Medicine, Presbyterian Hospital of Dallas, Dallas, Texas.

Marsha Cline Holleman, MD, MPH, is Medical Director, Houston Recovery Campus, and visiting Associate Professor, University of Texas Health Center—Houston School of Medicine, Houston, Texas.

Loren D. Israelsen, JD, is an associate of LDI Group, Salt Lake City, Utah.

Paul W. Jungnickel, PhD, is Associate Dean, School of Pharmacy, Auburn University, Auburn, Alabama.

Louis A. Kazal Jr., MD, is Medical Director, Navajo Health Foundation, Sage Memorial Hospital, Ganado, Arizona.

Larry Kincheloe, MD, FACOG, is Chairman, Department of Obstetrics and Gynecologist, Central Oklahoma Medical Group, Oklahoma City, Oklahoma.

James P. Knochel, MD, is Chairman, Department of Internal Medicine, Presbyterian Hospital of Dallas, Dallas, Texas.

Timothy R. McGuire, PharmD, is Associate Professor, Department of Pharmacy Practice, College of Pharmacy, University of Nebraska Medical Center, Omaha, Nebraska.

John G. Prichard, MD, is Director, Internal Medicine, Ventura County Medical Center, Ventura, California.

Sidney J. Stohs, PhD, is Professor and Dean, School of Pharmacy and Allied Health Professions, Omaha, Nebraska.

Foreword

One of the foremost factors increasing the complexity of medical practice is the rapidly expanding number of prescriptions. Add to these the accelerating acceptance of various forms of alternative medicine, most of them employing herbs of some form. The potential for drug interaction increases exponentially, especially when we add over-the-counter medications.

To my knowledge, this is the only book that addresses the role that herbs play in everyday medical care and the potential for adverse reactions when mixed with prescription drugs. The practicing physician can use it frequently to guide patients, such as those with diabetes whose blood sugar is poorly controlled, to avoid herbs that could be interfering with their medication. Until now, few physicians have thought of asking their patients about herbs they might be using. This book emphasizes the importance of including such questions in our everyday care of patients, especially those with chronic disease who are taking multiple medications, and cautioning them against the use of herbs that are potentially dangerous.

The goal of this book, as stated in the first chapter, is "to support safe and effective concomitant use of alternative and conventional medicines to achieve optimal patient outcomes." This is achieved and the book is a valuable addition to the armamentarium of the primary care physician.

Robert E. Rakel, MD
Professor, Department of Family
and Community Medicine,
Baylor College of Medicine,
Houston, Texas

NOTICE TO READER

Chapter 1

Herbal Medications
Interface with Conventional Medicine:
An Overview

Lucinda G. Miller, PharmD, BCPS

With nearly one-third of Americans engaging in alternative medicine practices, the potential for interactions with conventional medicines exists.[1] Yet, the majority of patients are reluctant to reveal their use of alternative medicine to their conventional health care providers. In fact, in the above-cited study, 70 percent of the individuals indicated they did not mention their use of alternative medicine to their personal physicians.[1] Most individuals such as these are well educated and have more than a median income.[2] Yet, communication suffered because they believed conventional health care providers would scoff at their use of alternative practices. It is time for conventional providers to acknowledge the use of alternative medicine and whether they approve or disapprove of such use, they need to be cognizant of known or potential issues in concomitant use.

It is the intent of this book to address known and potential interactions between conventional and alternative medicines through case-based vignettes. Additionally, herbal approaches that will create an adverse milieu for conventional medicine to optimize health will also be addressed. With this knowledge of the most serious consequences of these interactions, clinicians can directly ask patients about herbal remedy use much as they would question patients about over-the-counter medications in an effort to avert adverse drug interactions. In many cases, if a patient is taking a certain medication it should trigger the clinician to inquire of specific herb use, not only because of a potential interaction but because of the way the herb will affect the disease state for which the medication is being prescribed. Empowered with this knowledge, clinicians will better be able to serve their patients.

Each of the chapters will address in case-based format the pharmacology of the herb, potential and known interactions, adverse herbal side effects and effects on the disease state that may affect medication efficacy. The intent of this book is not to defame the use of herbal medications just as it is not Duke's intent to defame conventional pharmacologicals through his book *Meyler's Side Effects of Drugs.*[3] Rather, the intent of this book is to support safe and effective concomitant use of alternative and conventional medicines to achieve optimal patient outcomes. It is recognized that herbal medicine provides the underpinning for several orthodox medicines such as colchicine, digoxin, morphine, and vinca alkaloids. To assume herbal medications are safe and nontoxic because they are "natural" and can be obtained without a prescription is a potentially harmful illusion that belies the efficacy and potency of certain herbal remedies. Responsible use of herbal medications requires an interface with conventional medicine when the condition exceeds the maximal efficacy of the herbal remedies. To use them concomitantly requires an expertise seldom encountered in either faction today. It is hoped that this textbook will help bridge that gap.

DEFINITIONS

Before wading through the herbal literature, definitions must be understood. *Herbal medicinals* are those products derived from plant parts that elicit a pharmacologic effect. The herb is generally administered as a whole and is not fragmented or synthesized. The Food and Drug Administration prefers the term *botanical.*[4] *Nutraceuticals* are products that also possess a pharmacologic effect but are based on nutrients that exceed the boundaries of what are considered herbal medicinals. These nutrients, which may be synthesized, include minerals, vitamins, and cations (e.g., chromium, which has found use in diabetes mellitus).

Another term commonly encountered in this genre of literature is *phytopharmaceuticals.* These too are plant-based medicines but have been standardized on pharmacologically active constituents.[5] *Phytotherapy,* which uses phytopharmaceuticals to address disease, is the bridge in the European medical world between herbal folklore and modern clinical medicine.[6] In France, the term *vegetal drugs* is used, also referred to as *vegetable drugs,* which are plant materials used for medicinal purposes.[7] *Conventional medicines* refer to allopathic medicines in the mainstream armamentarium of Western medicine.

Many herbal products refer to their contents as either standardized or wildcrafted. Many European phytopharmaceuticals are standardized extracts of echinacea, valerian, saw palmetto, and gingko.[8] *Standardized* here refers to a particular marker chemical or active constituent.[8] *Wildcrafted,* however, denotes herbs gathered from the wild and not under cultivation. Hence, constituents and potency may vary widely depending on growing conditions and geographic region.

HOMEOPATHY VERSUS HERBAL REMEDIES

Paramount in this discussion is to distinguish between herbal remedies and homeopathic remedies. It is not unusual for both the public and health care professionals to consider the two entities as synonymous when in fact they are very different. Both entities employ plants, which is where the confusion starts. Herbal remedies contain active chemicals derived from a plant part (e.g., leaves, roots), which exert a pharmacologic effect. Homeopathic remedies, however, contain amounts of herbs so minute as to be unmeasurable. Homeopathy proponents contend that sufficient molecular memory exists to exert a therapeutic effect. Some attribute homeopathic activity to succussion, which is kinetic energy conveyed to the substance by manually mediated shaking of the substance for a specified period.[9,10] Advocates believe concomitant ingestion of coffee, mint, and camphor offset the effects of homeopathic remedies and hence should be avoided. At the very least it can be said that homeopathy defies scientific methods of explanation but works for some patients. However, most health care professionals view homeopathy as relying on the placebo effect.[11] Clearly, a consensus has yet to be reached on this issue.

SAFETY AND EFFICACY ISSUES

Prerequisite knowledge for safety and efficacy must address quality. In some instances, the product may not contain the labeled herb. In a Canadian study, no North American feverfew product contained the 0.2 percent parthenolide believed to be required for effectiveness.[12] The composition and potency of ginseng varies according to the location where grown, the season when harvested, method of curing and age of the root. In one report, 60 percent of ginseng samples contained substandard quality ginseng and 25 percent did not contain any ginseng.[13] Standardization of contents has also been issue. When studied, total panaxoside ginseng concentrations for 24 products varied from 0.26 to 6.85 mg per 250 mg sample.[13,14] In other instances, the herbal quantity contained may be so small as to be inconsequential (e.g., homeopathic remedies). This degree of variance is unacceptable.

Mislabeling

The consequences of mislabeling of herbal medicinals can be disastrous. Mislabeled as *Scutellaria* (skullcap), *Teucrium* has been sold in North American herb stores.[15] *Teucrium chamaedrys,* also known as germander, contains noxious diterpenoid compounds, known hepatotoxins.[16] Sold as a remedy for anal pruritus and for weight loss, this herb has resulted in hepatitis with associated hepatocyte necrosis.[16] Typically, jaundice and marked increases in serum aminotransferase levels occur following three to eighteen weeks of germander use. After discontinuing use, jaundice will disappear within eight weeks, with complete recovery within 1.5 to 6 months.[17] However, one nine-week-old patient was not as fortunate. This child experienced veno-occlusive disease following ingestion of an herbal tea that was obtained at a pharmacy and that contained pyrrolizidine alkaloid-rich *Senecio longilobus.*[18]

Plantain has been adulterated with digitalis. Referred to as the "Chomper incident," a Massachusetts woman was hospitalized after consuming a product called Chomper promoted as an herbal laxative and cleansing agent. The advisory released by the FDA describes the woman as experiencing abnormal heart rate with heart block.[19] Upon examination, the plantain was found to contain lanatosides, confirming digitalis adulteration.[20] It is theorized that inexperienced herb collectors mistook foxglove *(Digitalis lanata)* for plantain. This case further exemplifies the public toll when herbs are not sufficiently standardized and subjected to the same quality assurance measures expected of allopathic drugs.

Fatal outcomes have also followed use of some Chinese herbal remedies. Four non-Chinese adults ingested Chinese herbal remedies advocated for arthritis and back pain.[21] While all patients were afforded relief from their original ailments, they also incurred devastating side effects. All four patients experienced an explosive onset of an illness diagnosed as bacteremia. Two patients developed extensive necrotizing perirectal cellulitis with septic shock. One patient died. For those surviving, bone marrow recovery occurred within 11 to 20 days. Upon assay, the Chinese herbal products contained unlabeled antipyrine and phenylbutazone, agents known to cause agranulocytosis.[21]

These reports, in dramatic fashion, exemplify the need to regard herbal remedies as drugs with potencies that can cause desired as well as undesired effects. They further nest the notion that regulation and accountability should be imposed on manufacturers of herbal remedies. Chapter 17, "The History of Herbs in the United States," will address the heretofore contentious nature of herb regulation in the United States, explaining why at present we have no regulatory body protecting the public safety. This chapter represents the view of the American Botanical Council and not that of the FDA. However, as the reader progresses through this book, one will increasingly appreciate the need for such a regulatory body.

INDICATION PLURALISM

Seldom is an herb indicated for a singular indication but rather is indicated for several divergent uses, referred to here as indication pluralism. Ginseng is used as an adaptogen, immunostimulant, and as a tonic for tiredness, over-exertion, neurasthenia, hypotension, general and nervous weakness, mild depression, and to assist in giving birth.[22] It has also been advocated for anemia, arteriosclerosis, diabetes, edema, ulcers, and as an aphrodisiac.[23] Garlic is used for its antimicrobial action, antihyperlipidemic activity, fibrino-lytic effect, and for hypertension.[22] Garlic is allegedly useful to ward off vampires, demons, witches, and as an aphrodisiac.[23] Garlic has also been used to increase smooth muscle intestinal tone with an increase in peristalsis expected but with inhibition of such movements at large doses.[23] Ginkgo is advocated for intermittent claudication, Raynaud's disease, dizziness, memory loss, emotional lability, diabetic angiopathy, varicose conditions, post-thrombotic syndrome, and leg ulcers, due to its vasodilatory actions.[22] Ginkgo has also been touted as effective for asthma, tinnitus, and depres-sion.[23] Hence, in this cursory overview, ginseng, garlic, and ginkgo are advocated for fifteen, seven, and twelve indications, respectively. In contrast, most Western allopathic medicines are indicated for one to two indications (e.g., amitriptyline for depression and polymyalgia rheumatica).

Such indication pluralism as evidenced for many herbal medicinals may speak to their great usefulness. However, in the absence of supporting scien-tific literature, such pluralism detracts from the herb's credibility according to Western medicine. Whether all these indications will be validated by the rigor of scientific investigation has yet to be determined. Most likely, some but not all indications will be validated. Until this issue is completely addressed, the clinician is cautioned to view such claims skeptically but to remain open-minded as some claims may eventually be proven correct. This is an issue on which Eastern and Western medicine are in opposition. Western medicine prefers the "magic bullet" of a singular synthesized entity useful for one indication. Eastern medicine recognizes that a tonic, by stimulating a particu-lar system such as the immune system, may have varied interrelated benefi-cial effects that supersede a limited "magic bullet." A bridge allowing the two schools of thought to intersect in some fashion is needed if our patients are to benefit from the advances of both groups.

CONCLUSION

Much is not yet known regarding the pharmacology of herbal remedies. Anecdotal reports constitute the bulk of what is presently known regarding these entities and potential drug-herb interactions. In many instances the clinician is left with a knowledge of the disease states, known drug pharmacology, and only limited scientific documentation of herb pharmacology when trying to determine if a drug-herb-disease state interaction occurred. It is the intent of this book to help the clinician sort through that limited documentation when trying to arrive at a reasonable evaluation of potential drug-herb interactions.

The nature of herbal remedies, specifically the lack of standardization and possible adulteration, precludes controlled scientific investigation. Additionally, some herbal remedies contain nonherbal products such as arsenic and lead (e.g., "kushtay"). Undeclared conventional medicines (e.g, prednisolone, nonsteroidal anti-inflammatory drugs, and paracetamol) have been found in herbal products.[24] However, some European phytomedicines claim to be standardized extracts of echinacea, valerian, saw palmetto, and gingko.[8] Once widespread standardization without adulteration has been achieved, controlled studies of sufficient scientific rigor are needed.

As the clinician uses this textbook, it should be noted that it is not intended to be all-inclusive. Not every herb is addressed herein. The reader is advised to consult other compendiums as needed but to use this textbook as an initial guide to major interactions between herbalism and conventional medicine and as a guide to how to address the situation.

It is not the intent of this textbook to replace the clinician but rather to serve as a tool for the practitioner. Neither is it the intent of this book to sabotage use of herbal medications. Rather, herbal medicinals should be afforded the same respect as conventional medicines, recognizing that indiscriminate prescribing of either can result in harm.[25] Only individuals well-versed in herbal medicines should supervise their use. Of the 250,000 to 300,000 plant species, only 5,000 have been studied exhaustively for possible medical application; hence, our medicinal future is bright if the integrity of these plants and their growing conditions can be maintained.[26]

REFERENCES

1. Eisenberg D, Kessler RC, Foster C, Norlock FE, Calkins Dr, Delbancto TL. Unconventional medicine in the United States: Prevalence, costs and patterns of use. *N Engl J Med* 1993;328:246-352.

2. DeSmet PAGM. An introduction to herbal pharmacoepidemiology. *J Ethnopharmacol* 1993;39:197-208.

3. Dukes, MN (Ed.). *Meyler's side effects of drugs: An encyclopedia of adverse reactions and interactions,* twelfth edition, Elsevier, New York, 1992.

4. Hoffman FA, Leaders FE. Botanical (herbal) medicine in health care: A review from a regulatory perspective. *Pharm New* 1996;3:23-25.

5. Brown DJ. Phytotherapy: Herbal medicine meets clinical science. *NARD J* 1996:41-50.

6. Schilcher H. The significance of phytotherapy in Europe. *Zeitschrift Phytother* 1993;14:132-139.

7. Artiges A. What are the legal requirements for the use of phytopharmaceutical drugs in France? *J Ethnopharmacol* 1991;32:231-234.

8. Brevoort P. Botanical (herbal) medicine in the United States. *Pharm News* 1996;3:26-28.

9. Young TM. Nuclear magnetic resonance studies of succussed solutions. *J Am Institute Homeopathy* 1975;68:8-17.

10. Scofield AM. Experimental research in homeopathy: A critical review. *Br Homeopathic J* 1984;73:211-226.

11. Tyler VE. Herbal medicine is not homeopathy. *J Am Pharm Assoc* 1996; NS36;37.

12. Groenewegen WA, Heptinstall S. Feverfew. *Lancet* 1986;I:44-45.

13. Liberti LE, DerMarderosian A. Evaluation of commercial ginseng products. *J Pharmaceutical Sci* 1978;67:1487-1489.

14. Ziglar W. Ginseng products may not contain ginseng. *Whole Foods* 1979; 2(4):48-53.

15. Anonymous. Scullcap substitution. *HerbalGram* 1985;2:3.

16. Huxtable RJ. The myth of beneficent nature: The risk of herbal preparations. *Ann Intern Med* 1992;117:165-166.

17. Larrey D, Vial T, Pauwels A, et al. Hepatitis after germander (*Teucrium chamaedrys*) administration: Another instance of herbal medicine hepatotoxicity. *Ann Intern Med* 1992;117:129-132.

18. Stuppner H, Sperl W, Gassner I, Vogel W. Verwechslung von Tussligo farfara mit Petasites hybridus—ein aktueller fall von Pyrrolizidinalkaloid-Intoxikation. *Sci Pharm (Wein)* 1992;60:160-161.

19. Food and Drug Administration. FDA warns against dietary supplement products that may contain digitalis mislabeled as plantain, *Federal Register,* June 12, 1997.

20. Blumenthal, M. Industry alert: Plantain adulterated with digitalis. *HerbalGram* 1997;40:28-29.

21. Reis CA, Sahud MA. Agranulocytosis caused by Chinese herbal medicine: Dangers of medications containing aminopyrine and phenylbutazone. *JAMA* 1975; 231:352-355.

22. Weiss RF. Degenerative heart disease, arteriosclerosis, angina pectoris. In: Weiss RF (Ed.). *Herbal Medicine.* Hippokrates Verlag, Stuttgart, Germany, 1988: 162-183.

23. Tyler VE. *The honest herbal: A sensible guide to the use of herbs and related remedies,* third edition, The Haworth Press, Binghamton, NY, 1993.

24. Karaunanithy R, Sumita KP. Undeclared drugs in Chinese antirheumatoid medicine. *Int J Pharm Pract* 1991;1:117-119.

25. Thompson WAR. Herbs that heal. *J Royal Coll Gen Pract* 1976;26:365-370.

26. Abelson PH. Medicine from plants. *Science* 1990:247:513.

Chapter 2

Renal Implications
of Herbal Remedies

M. E. Blair Holbein, PhD, BCPS, BCAP
James P. Knochel, MD

OVERVIEW

The use of "herbal" or alternative medications is increasing.[1] While the etiology of this phenomenon is probably multifactorial, part of the trend is the increased availability of information published in the lay press such as books, electronic dissemination as in "infomercials," advertisements on radio and television, and posting of sites on the Internet. This is complicated by the 1994 Dietary Supplement Health and Education Act, which increased the availability of such preparations and gives implied sanction by the formation of the Office of Alternative Medicine of the National Institutes of Health.

The ramifications of using such preparations are twofold. First, people may choose to self-medicate for ailments related to kidney function and these preparations may or may not be efficacious. This use of alternative approaches may delay or prevent utilization of proven standard approaches. Second, unintended effects may occur. The difference between choices of standard Western medical practices and alternative herbal medications lies in the mandated requirement for demonstrated safety and efficacy of licensed pharmaceuticals in most of the industrialized countries. Very little information about the efficacy and safety of herbal preparations is equivalent to the criteria we demand for acknowledged pharmaceutical preparations. Adequately controlled randomized, double-blinded clinical trials published in peer-reviewed medical journals are nonexistent for essentially all of the herbal remedies. Safety issues surface as case reports in the literature rather than observed incidence in clinical trials. Moreover, many publications with

---

§ Indicates information taken from abstracts in English of Chinese or Japanese language reference.

studies of herbal preparations are in non-English publications that do not have wide distribution. (Studies in non-English publications are evaluated from the English translation of the abstract and are indicated by "§".) Thus, most of the discussion in this chapter will be focused mostly on safety issues since minimal efficacy data is available.

Renal effects of herbal preparations can be beneficial or harmful. Beneficial effects would include diuresis, protection of the kidney from effects of nephrotoxic agents, prevention or amelioration of renal lithiasis, and amelioration of renal failure. Harmful effects include polyuria causing dehydration, acute kidney failure or chronic renal insufficiency, and stone formation. Renal failure can produce secondary electrolyte and metabolic disturbances.

Renal effects of herbal preparations or intentional plant ingestion would be expected to parallel standard pharmaceuticals. Medication-induced renal disease is predominantly acute renal failure; the majority of this is char-acterized as acute tubular necrosis (38 percent) or due to hemo-dynamic (prerenal) effects (37 percent). Glomerular/vascular de-rangement accounts for about 16 percent and postrenal (obstructive) causes account for about 5 percent.[2] In the absence of statistics for herbal preparations, the "medication model" at least provides a framework for reviewing case reports.

CASES

Case Number 1

A tourist is brought to the emergency room for evaluation of injuries sustained in a fall that includes a possible broken arm. The young woman is from Belgium. She is 28 years old. Pertinent findings in addition to her physical injury include a serum creatinine of 2.3 mg/dl and a modestly elevated blood pressure of 135/95 mm Hg. Her current medications include prednisone 5 mg every other day and enalapril 25 mg daily. Her medical history reveals that her renal insufficiency is due to ingestion of Chinese herbs dispensed at a weight-loss clinic in Belgium. She takes corticosteroids in an effort to prevent further loss of renal function. She mentions that she is concerned about the long-term consequences of the injury to her kidney. What is the evidence for nephrotoxicity of herbal preparations? Are there studies of the sequelae and natural history of such toxicity?

Radix Aristolochia Fangchi

Perhaps the best documented nephrotoxicity associated with herbal preparations occurred between 1991 and 1992 in Belgium. Young women who had taken "slimming treatments" from a clinic experienced rapidly progressive renal failure. The major histologic lesion was extensive interstitial fibrosis with atrophy and loss of the tubules.[3] The treatments had included an herbal mix that contained cascara powder, acetazolamide, belladonna extract, Hou Po *(Cortex Magnolia officinalis)*, Han Fang Ji *(Radix stephania tetrandra).*[4] Some researchers have postulated that the medication in fact did not contain Han Fang Ji, as had been intended, but possibly had been mistakenly formulated with Guang Fan Ji *(Radix Aristolochia Fangchi).*[5] Accordingly, the toxic component was reportedly aristolochic acid.[6] One study of the Belgian patients demonstrated a beneficial effect of corticosteroids on the progression of renal failure.[7] These investigators also report that of 81 individuals in the Belgium Registry, 30 have renal failure, 12 have stable moderate impairment, and 39 have progressive renal loss.[7] Aristolochic acid has been shown to produce adducts with DNA[8] and the identification of DNA damage in the kidneys of patients with the syndrome may have implications for the subsequent development of cancers in these individuals.[9] Based on apparently similar histopathology it has been suggested that the same toxic principle might have been causative in a similar event, Balkan endemic nephropathy.[10] Nephrotoxicity due to *Aristolochia pistolochia* has also been reported.[11]

Other herbal preparations have been documented to have toxicity to the kidney. These include some preparations that were intended to have effects specific to the kidney and some are advocated for these uses.

Aconitum carmichaeli, Aconitum kusnezoffli,
Tripterygium wilfordii

Study description. Mice were treated with decoction (1, 5, 10 mg herb /25 g wt) for four days. The higher doses produced histologic tissue damage to the liver and the kidney.[12]

Crotalaria juncea Seeds

Study description. The effect of an ethanolic extract of *Crotalaria juncea* Lin. (Leguminosea) seeds was tested in adult rats (200 mg/kg). There were histologic changes in the liver, adrenals, and spleen. The kidney showed degeneration and exfoliation of renal tubular cells.[13]

Unspecified Preparation

Study description. A single well-documented case of adult Fanconi syndrome that was induced by the ingestion of a crude mixture of Chinese medications is described. The patient had renal glycosuria, hypokalemia, hypophosphatemia, metabolic acidosis, a low threshold of tubular bicarbonate excretion, and generalized aminoaciduria. The syndrome abated with discontinuation of the mixture and reappeared with rechallenge.[14] A case of interstitial nephritis induced by herbal medicines has also been reported.[15]

Artemisia absinthium (Wormwood Plant)

Study description. A single case report describes a 31-year-old man who ingested about 10 ml of wormwood oil. He had a seizure that resulted in rhabdomyolysis and subsequent acute renal failure. A liqueur made from the wormwood plant, absinthe, has been long-recognized as neurotoxic and is banned in Europe and the United States. The wormwood oil was obtained in this case via electronic commerce from a purveyor of essential oils. The renal failure was secondary to the other effects of the wormwood oil.[16]

Epidemiology

There are also a small number of studies looking at the incidence of renal toxicity attributable to a variety of herbal preparations.

Study description. Forty consecutive cases of acute tubular necrosis were studied in Nigeria. Traditional herbal remedies were the most commonly identified precipitating factor (37.5 percent). Most patients were anuric at presentation. One death was associated with nephrotoxicity from the herbal preparations.[17]

Study description. Over a four-year-period at Baragwanath Hospital, Johannesburg, South Africa, 91 cases of renal failure due to use of herbal preparations were reported.[18]

Case Number 2

A 70-year-old woman comes to clinic for routine monitoring of her antihypertensive medications. It is noted that she has a slight increase in blood pressure and her serum electrolytes show a drop in potassium to 2.9 mEq/l. You question her about her compliance with her medications and diet. She insists that she has been compliant. Further questioning reveals that her granddaughter, who is in Europe for the summer, had sent her a box of her favorite candy, licorice. Are there any metabolic/electrolyte disturbances induced by effects of herbal preparations on the kidney?

Glycyrrhiza glabra

Glycyrrhiza is found in some preparations of licorice prepared outside the United States and is present in sufficient quantities to produce pharmacologic effect. In the United States, it is found in herbal preparations, moistened chewing tobaccos (e.g., Beech Nut and Red Man), in some liqueurs (anise), and cough preparations.[19] *Glycyrrhiza* is well-recognized for a mineralocorticoid effect (aldosterone) on the kidney. *Glycyrrhiza* inhibits 11-β-hydroxysteroid dehydrogenase, the enzyme that prevents cortisol from acting like a mineralocorticoid at the aldosterone receptor site. When 11-β-OH dehydrogenase is inhibited, cortisol behaves exactly like aldosterone. Problems in electrolyte balance (especially hypokalemia) and blood pressure homeostasis can occur.[20] Even relatively modest intake (50-100 g daily intake studied in 30 patients) can produce significant elevations of blood pressure and a potentially severe hypokalemia. A significant change in the cortisol/cortisone ratio was also reported.[21] These effects are generally modest but a number of cases of fatal licorice-induced hypokalemic rhabdomyolysis and renal failure have been reported.[22] Most patients present with classical findings of primary aldosteronism except their plasma aldosterone values are abnormally low rather than elevated.

Other Agents with Effects on Electrolytes and Minerals

Perillae frutescens, Zizyphys vulgaris, Magnolia officinalis, Scutellaria baicalensis

Study description. Other agents reportedly have demonstrated 11-β-hydroxysteroid dehydrogenase inhibition including *Perillae frutescens, Zizyphys vulgaris, Magnolia officinalis,* and *Scutellaria baicalensis.*[23] It is unknown if these too will have the same propensity to cause electrolyte and fluid abnormalities. Note that primary injury to the kidney resulting in acute or chronic kidney failure will also produce secondary metabolic/electrolyte effects.

Case Number 3

A 54-year-old man comes to the emergent care clinic complaining of nausea, vague upper abdominal discomfort, and weakness. He last saw his primary care physician two months ago prior to his trip to Hong Kong on business. He states that he was healthy at that time and there were no unusual results from his laboratory studies. He takes ramipril (Altace) daily for his essential hypertension. His serum creatinine is found to be markedly elevated at 2.6 mg/dl; stool guaiac is positive. On further questioning he states that he hurt his back on his trip and that he had obtained an herbal preparation in Hong Kong for his back pain, Cow's Head brand of Tung Shueh. He has continued to take it because it has significantly eased his back pain.[24] What compounds have been identified in herbal preparations?

The occurrence of nephrotoxicity attributable to the inclusion of adulterants and contaminants nonherbal as well as herbal has also been documented. The adulterant use of nonsteroidal anti-inflammatory compounds can produce adverse events including nephrotoxicity and gastrointestinal irritation that is identical to that seen with intentional use. Documented instances include Cow's Head brand of Tung Shueh, which has been shown to contain 3.86 mg indomethacin, 16 mg mefenamic acid, 7.94 mg diclofenac, and 0.73 mg of diazepam per tablet.[25] If taken as labeled the total daily dose of nonsteroidals would be 50 mg indomethacin, 200 mg mefenamic acid, and 100 mg diclofenac. The presence of these prescription medications was not indicated in the labeling so that patients who have been instructed to avoid such agents would be unaware of their ingestion.

Other Studies of Documented Adulterants and Contaminants

Study description. The presence of phenylbutazone in Jamu resulted in drug eruptions which may be severe.[26]

Study description. Chinese herbal medications of five patients with complications including massive gastrointestinal bleeding were analyzed. All contained unlabeled mefenamic acid and diazepam.[27]

Study description. A case report of a single patient with acute interstitial nephritis secondary to ingestion of a Chinese herbal medicine adulterated with mefenamic acid.[28]

Study description. The presence of diazepam in Tung Shueh likewise has presented serious problems when tested for in an employer's drug screen.[27]

Study description. Heavy metal contaminants have been identified. Mercury has been found in cinnabar and calomel, which are ingredients in Chinese patent medicines available in the open market.[29]

Case Number 4

A 56-year-old Hawaiian man of Chinese descent with chronic renal failure states that he is taking an herbal preparation prescribed by a traditional Chinese practitioner. The product contains Chinese rhubarb. Will this product help his renal failure? What are the side effects?

Studies Examining Palliative Effects on the Kidney

Rheum rhaponticum (Chinese Rhubarb)

Study description. §Rheum is a cathartic that was tested for an effect on the progression of uremia. In a prospective clinical trial rheum was compared with captopril (Capoten) in patients with elevated serum creatinine and a combination group receiving both. Regression analysis of the change in 1/serum creatinine versus time showed delayed progression of renal failure in the rheum ($\pm$ captopril) treated group. There was an accompanying increase in serum albumin. The investigators also studied 56 nephrectomized rats treated with rheum and compared to untreated. They observed a decreased O_2 consumption in the remnant kidney, lessened azotemia, increased albumin and transferrin, and decreased blood cholesterol and triglycerides.[30]

Study description. A controlled study of chronic renal failure in a rat model of subtotal nephrectomy showed rhubarb extract had no effect on the systemic hypertension, but significant effect on proteinuria and severity of glomerulosclerosis in the remnant kidney.[31]

Study description. A Chinese clinical trial compared Rheum E with and without captopril in 30 patients with chronic renal failure. A dietary therapy-only group served as a control. The treatment group showed a slower progression of renal failure and the Rheum groups showed better rise in serum albumin.[32]

Other agents

Juzen-Taiho-to

Study description. §The effects of oral administration of Juzen-taiho-to on the adverse effects and efficacy of cis-diammine dichloroplatinum (CDDP) were studied in male mice. Following two weeks of antecedent oral dosing of Juzen-taiho-to, the LD50 for CDDP was increased. The effectiveness of CDDP in a model of murine bladder tumor was enhanced and survival was significantly prolonged with herb treatment.[33]

Study description. A similar study using fractionated compounds likewise showed a protective effect on CDDP-induced toxicity by two different fractions.[34]

Epimedium sagittatum

Study description. §Study of chronic renal insufficiency induced in Wistar rats showed a significant decrease in BUN and serum creatinine. The histologic studies showed an inhibition of hypertrophy of glomeruli, decreased deposition of IgG, C3, fibrin, and fibronectin along the glomerular capillary walls.[35]

Jin Gui Shen Qi, Liu Wei Di Huang

Study description. §In a clinical trial of patients receiving radiotherapy or chemotherapy for small cell lung cancer, groups were randomized to receive Jin Gui Shen Qi or Liu Wei Di Huang or no herbal therapy. The herb-receiving groups had a significantly greater response rate to the anti-tumor therapy and a significantly longer survival.[36]

Man Shen Ling

Study description. §A Chinese herbal preparation that contains Astragalu and Rehmannia was studied. A study of 100 cases of chronic nephritis showed an improvement in proteinuria, hematuria, renal function, edema, anemia, and anorexia compared to a control group. No adverse effects were noted. An animal model of chronic nephritis showed immunosuppressive effects analogous to cyclophosphamide. Histology showed anti-inflammatory effects without toxic, mutagenic, teratogenic, or carcinogenic effects.[37]

Packera candidissima rheum, Senecio candidissimus Greene

Study description. Hepatotoxic pyrrolizidine alkaloids were identified in both *Packera candidissima* (rheum) and *Senecio candidissimus* (Greene). These herbs are used in certain cultural groups in Northern Mexico and the Hispanic population in the Southwestern United States for the treatment of kidney ailments.[38]

Rhizome Wheat Starch

Study description. Thirty patients with chronic renal failure were placed on a dietetic therapy with rhizome wheat starch. The authors of this study reported a statistically significant improvement in the BUN and serum creatinine and an increase in albumin.[39]

Sairei-to (Chai Ling Tang)

Study description. Fifty-nine children with steroid-dependent nephrotic syndrome were studied. Thirty-seven were given sairei-to in addition to corticosteroids. Thirty-two children received cyclosporin plus corticosteroid and served as controls. The results were similar between the two groups.[40]

Study description. §Sairei-to is thought to improve proteinuria in minimal change nephrotic syndrome. A study of immune-modulatory effects of sairei-to in a rat model of nephrotoxic nephritis used controls, sairei-to, methylprednisolone, and the combination of the two agents. All treatment groups had decreased proteinuria. Histology revealed significant improvement in treated groups with suppression of glomerular inflammation.[41]

Vandellia cordifolia

Study description. In studies of the effect of *Vandellia cordifolia* administered orally and intraperitoneally, the authors reported a diuretic effect in normal rats. In rabbits there was a decrease in glomerular filtration rate and renal blood flow in both normal and glycerin-induced insufficient kidneys. Both Na and K reabsorption were inhibited and there was a hypertensive effect. In folk medicine, *Vandellia* is advocated for nephritis and uremia.[42]

Green Tea Leaf (Camellia sinensis L.)

Study description. Rats were fed diets containing 3 percent green or black tea leaf powder. Treated animals were protected from tert-butyl hydroperoxide-induced lipid peroxidation of kidney tissues.[43]

Magnesium Lithospermate B (Dan Shen)

Study description. A series of investigations showed that oral administration of magnesium lithospermate B to rats produced significant increases in glomerular filtration rate, renal plasma flow, and renal blood flow. These actions are thought to be due to activation of kallikrein and promotion of prostaglandin E2.[44,45,46]

Clerodendron trichotomum

Study description. An extract of *Clerodendron trichotomum* by both oral and intravenous administration was studied for effect on rats and dogs. The herbal extract prevented and acutely reversed the increase in blood pressure in spontaneously hypertensive rats and was without effect on normotensive rats. Intravenous administration produced renal vasodilation and increase urine flow and urinary sodium excretion.[47]

Ginkgo biloba Extract

Study description. Anti-inflammatory effects have been demonstrated with terpene components of ginkgo biloba, namely ginkgolide BN 52021, which appears to have specific antagonist effects on platelet activating factor (PAF) when tested in animal models. PAF plays a role in immune-mediated renal disease as well as asthma, anaphylaxis, and other immunologically mediated diseases.[48]

The question arises whether there is reason to believe that there is any beneficial effect of herbs advocated for palliative properties on the kidneys. There is in fact some very preliminary evidence that there are some potentially interesting compounds that have not been exploited pharmacologically. Unfortunately, most of the published studies are far less stringent than are required for acceptance of standard pharmaceutical preparations. Some of the animal studies likewise point to a possible utility. But clinical trials and standard toxicologic studies are lacking. Some of the compounds may be innocuous enough to permit a laissez-faire approach, especially if there is reason to feel that the patient would be emotionally impacted or the clinician/patient relationship impaired by adherence to more stringent criteria.

Case Number 5

A 64-year-old woman in your ambulatory clinic who has a history of passing several renal stones wants to take "natural" medications both to avoid further stone formation and to induce diuresis for "swollen feet." What options are available? Are they effective?

Herbs Advocated for Treatment or Prevention of Renal Stones

Arctium lappa, Arctostaphylos uva ursi, Equisetum arvense, Lithospermum officinale, Silene saxifragua, Taraxacum officinale, Verbena officinalis

Study description. In studies of female Wistar rats the utility of seven different herbal therapies for urolithiasis (*Lithospermum officinale, Taraxacum officinale, Equisetum arvense, Arctostaphylos uva ursi, Arctium lappa, Silene saxifragua*) was estimated to be less effective than the recognized benefit of less toxic alternatives.[49]

Choreito, Urajirogashi

Study description. Male Wistar rats were used for a model of urolithiasis to study pyruvate versus herbal medicines choreito (an herbal preparation) and urajirogashi. Both herbal preparations were inferior to pyruvate in preventing urolithiasis but did have some modest effect in increasing oxalate and magnesium excretion and increasing urine volume.[50]

Study description. A study of kagosou and choreito, which contains Takusya, showed no effect. Takusya showed some benefit.[51]

Crataeva nurvala Bark

Study description. Calcium oxalate lithiasis is diminished in rats given a decoction of *Crataeva nurvala* bark.[52]

Herbs Advocated for Diuresis

Kyushin (Toad Venom)

Study description. A study of kyushin (KY-2, KY-R) in guinea pigs and rabbits showed a significant increase in urinary volume.[53]

Bredemeyera floribunda Willd. Polygalaceae

Study description. A crude extract of the roots of *Bredemeyera floribunda* Willd. Polygalaceae, a Brazilian folk medicine, was administered intravenously to rats (0.05 mg/min/100 g). There was an increase in urine flow, glomerular filtration rate, fractional water and sodium excretion, potassium excretion, and solute clearance. In "antidiuresis" rats the extract also increased reabsorption of water in the collecting duct and in water diuresis animals the extract increased free water clearance. The effect is dose-dependent and produces hypotension. Higher doses produce bradycardia and eventually death. The investigators suggest a detergent-like action with the glomerulus and possible effect on the Na^+–K^+ ATPase countertransport system.[54, 55]

Vandellia cordifolia

Study description. Investigators studied renal effects in rats and rabbits of *Vandellia cordifolia,* a wild herb used in Taiwanese folk remedies for nephritis, uremia, furuncle, and carbuncle. There was a decrease in GFR and RBF in normal animals but no effect in insufficient kidneys in rabbits. It produced diuresis and inhibited sodium and potassium reabsorption.[56]

As with most of the studies of utility of herbal preparations, there is a paucity of reliable data on the utility of any of these agents for legitimate therapeutic needs. Certainly none has any demonstrated advantage in terms of efficacy or safety when compared to standard pharmaceutical preparations.

Herbs Advocated for Diuretic Effects
Shown to Be Without Effect

Aeru lanata,[57] *Portulaca pilosa,* and *Achyrocline satureioides,*[58] herbs advocated for renal effects, were unstudied.

The USDA maintains a compendium of herbal products and active ingredients that is available at their Web site. The list includes herbal products that have been promoted for use in kidney diseases. The list is not meant to be an endorsement but a reference. The list as of 1997 is included as an appendix to this chapter.

MEDICINAL AND PHARMACEUTICAL CHEMISTRY ASPECTS

Historical pharmacognosy holds the origins of modern clinical pharmacology. Today's pharmacopeia contains many pure extracts and chemical analogues of products with foundations in herbal remedies (e.g., digoxin and vincristine). We are even now introducing medicines from natural products (taxol). Some herbal remedies seem to have promise and are certainly worth further exploration. However, the well-documented renal toxicity associated with selected agents is cause for concern. It is often assumed by the lay public that herbal preparations are unlikely to be toxic. This is clearly not the case. Herbal preparation-induced acute renal necrosis and chronic renal failure belie the assumed innocuous nature of these preparations. Substantial morbidities such as chronic renal failure, dialysis, or renal transplant and even death have been seen with herbal products. Since these herbal preparations are not single chemical entities no active or toxic component can be subjected to standardized tests of efficacy and safety. Without this information none of these preparations can be used with the same assurances that we have come to expect from standard pharmaceuticals.

DISCUSSION

Even for those practitioners with little familiarity with the phytochemical basis of pharmacology, the plausibility of significant pharmacologic effects of herbal preparations is understood. Unfortunately, very little has been done to clarify the utility and dangers of these medicaments. The paucity of solid clinical data should not prejudice the practitioner to assume that these products are either innocuous or ineffective. Unfortunately, there is too little information to allow recommendation of any of the reviewed substances at this time. Some compounds do show promise, but clearly require much more study and elucidation of mechanisms to be useful. Some effects observed are produced more reliably and predictably by well-established pharmaceutical agents. Many more compounds seem innocuous, but are without benefit as well. Conversely, there is very convincing information about toxicity, such as Aristolochia-induced renal failure. Other compounds may be nephrotoxic, but are not so well documented. (See Table 2.1 for a summary of aspects.)

Placing these observations in perspective, when hospital admissions were examined in Hong Kong, a region with a mix of traditional Chinese and Western medicine, investigators found medical admissions to hospitals attributed to adverse reactions to Chinese herbal remedies were very low (0.2 percent).[59] While this rate seems modest by Western standards, it does not account for admissions due to conditions inadequately treated by traditional Chinese medication that might have been adequately treated using Western medicines.

With the wide availability of herbal preparations, practitioners must be aware of their use by patients with the inevitable sequelae of unpredictable toxicity or efficacy and the unknown impact of underutilization of standard therapies. The total impact of alternative therapies is unknown.

TABLE 2.1. Medicinal and Pharmaceutical Chemistry Aspects Summary

Taxonomic name	Common name	Comments	Evidence for efficacy	Evidence for toxicity
Radix Aristolochia Fangchi	Guang Fan Ji	acute interstitial nephritis		A
Aristolochia pistolochia		nephrotoxicity		C
Aconitum carmichaeli, Aconitum kusnezofili		nephrotoxicity, hepatotoxicity		C
Tripterygium wilfordii		nephrotoxicity, hepatotoxicity		C
Crotalaria juncea		acute tubular nephritis		C
Glycyrrhiza glabra		pseudohyperaldosteronism		A
Perillae frutescens		pseudohyperaldosteronism		D
Zizyphys vulgaris		pseudohyperaldosteronism		D
Magnolia officinalis		pseudohyperaldosteronism		D
Scutellaria baicalensis		pseudohyperaldosteronism		D
	Tung Shueh	adulterated with nonsteroidal anti-inflammatory agents		A
mercury	cinnabar, calomel	contaminant		D
	Juzen-taiho-to	nephroprotection—chemotherapy	D	

TABLE 2.1 *(continued)*

Taxonomic name	Common name	Comments	Evidence for efficacy	Evidence for toxicity
Epimedium sagittatum		improved renal failure	D	
	Jin Gui Shen Qi	nephroprotection—chemotherapy	D	
	Liu Wei Di Huang	nephroprotection—chemotherapy	D	
	Man Shen Ling (Astragalu, Rehmannia)	improved chronic renal failure	C	
Packera candidissima rheum		advocated for kidney, hepatotoxic	E	
Senecio candidissimus Greene		advocated for kidney, hepatotoxic	E	
Rheum rhaponticum	Chinese rhubarb	improved chronic renal failure	C	
	rhizome wheat starch	improved chronic renal failure	D	
	Sairei-to, Chai Ling Tang	nephrotic syndrome	B	
Vandellia cordifolia		improved chronic renal failure	C	

Camellia sinensis L.	Green tea leaf	prevent lipid peroxides	D
Magnesium lithospermate B	Dan Shen	improved chronic renal failure	C
Clerodendron trichotomum		improved chronic renal failure, treat hypertension	D
Ginkgo biloba		improved chronic renal failure, anti-inflammatory	C
Arctium lappa		urolithiasis, minimally effective	C
Arctostaphylos uva ursi		urolithiasis, minimally effective	C
Equisetum arvense		urolithiasis, minimally effective	C
Lithospermum officinale		urolithiasis, minimally effective	C
Silene saxifragua		urolithiasis, minimally effective	C
Taraxacum officinale		urolithiasis, minimally effective	C
	Choreito, Urajirogashi	urolithiasis, minimally effective	D

TABLE 2.1 *(continued)*

Taxonomic name	Common name	Comments	Evidence for efficacy	Evidence for toxicity
	Crataeva nurvala bark	oxalate lithiasis	D	
	Yushin (toad venom)	mild diuretic	D	
Bredemeyera floribunda Willd. (Polygalaceae)		mild diuretic, cardiovascular toxicity	D	D
Vandellia cordifolia		decreased GFR, diuretic	D	
Aeru lanata		without diuretic effect		
Portulaca pilosa		without diuretic effect		
Achyrocline satureioides		without diuretic effect		

Notes:

A = demonstrated in adequately controlled clinical trial or well-documented clinical effect.

B = demonstrated in adequately controlled animal studies, possibly reliable.

C = reported in clinical trials of undetermined or marginal quality, but suggestive of effect.

D = reported in clinical trials of undetermined quality; poorly documented case reports, inferred effect.

E = minimal information.

blank = no data or not applicable.

* Combination products given common names without attribution of effects to a single component.

APPENDIX

Plants Used for the Kidney per USDA Database[60]

Abrus precatorius (Fabaceae)
Acacia sieberana (Fabaceae)
Acaena sanguisorbae (Rosaceae)
Achillea millefolium (Asteraceae)
Alchemilla arvensis (Rosaceae)
Alisma plantago (Alismataceae)
Allium porrum (Liliaceae)
Allium sativum (Liliaceae)
Amaranthus bidentata (Amaranthaceae)
Ammi visnaga (Apiaceae)
Annona muricata (Annonaceae)
Apocynum androsaemifolium (Apocynaceae)
Aquilaria agallocha (Thymelaeaceae)
Argemone mexicana (Papaveraceae)
Argemone platyceras (Papaveraceae)
Arundo kakao (Poaceae)
Ascyrum hyppericoides (Clusiaceae)
Asimina reticulata (Annonaceae)
Asparagus officinalis (Liliaceae)
Asparagus plumosus (Liliaceae)
Asplenium ceterach (Aspleniaceae)
Azorella caespitosa (Apiaceae)

Bixa orellana (Bixaceae)
Borreria latifolia (Rubiaceae)

Cacalia decomposita (Asteraceae)
Calendula officinalis (Asteraceae)
Canavalia ensiformis (Fabaceae)
Capsella bursa-pastoris (Brassicaceae)
Cassia covesii (Fabaceae)
Cassia occidentalis (Fabaceae)
Cassia tora (Fabaceae)
Castanea sativa (Fagaceae)
Cenchrus palmeri (Poaceae)
Chimaphila umbellata (Ericaceae)
Cibotium barometz (Dicksoniaceae)
Cimicifuga racemosa (Ranunculaceae)

Cinnamomum verum (Lauraceae)
Cissampelos pareira (Menispermaceae)
Citrullus lanatus (Cucurbitaceae)
Citrus acida (Rutaceae)
Clematis vitalba (Ranunculaceae)
Clerodendrum triphyllum (Verbenaceae)
Clinopodium laevigatum (Lamiaceae)
Cnidium monnieri (Apiaceae)
Cochlospermum vitifolium (Bixaceae)
Coffea arabica (Rubiaceae)
Coprosma australis (Rubiaceae)
Croton incanus (Euphorbiaceae)
Croton leucophyllus (Euphorbiaceae)
Cudrania triloba (Moraceae)
Cupressus sempervirens (Cupressaceae)
Curculigo orchioides (Liliaceae)
Cuscuta japonica (Cuscutaceae)
Cynodon dactylon (Poaceae)

Dactyloctenium aegyptium (Poaceae)
Daucus carota (Apiaceae)
Desmodium cajanifolia (Fabaceae)
Diospyros virginiana (Ebenaceae)
Dipsacus japonicus (Dipsacaceae)
Disciphania calocarpa (Menispermaceae)
Drynaria fortunei (Polypodiaceae)

Eclipta prostrata (Asteraceae)
Ehretia tinifolia (Boraginaceae)
Equisetum arvense (Equisetaceae)
Equisetum bogotense (Equisetaceae)
Erigeron canadensis (Asteraceae)
Eryngium aquaticum (Apiaceae)
Eryngium heterophyllum (Apiaceae)
Eryngium yuccifolium (Apiaceae)
Eucommia ulmoides (Eucommiaceae)
Euphorbia pekinensis (Euphorbiaceae)
Exacum lawii (Gentianaceae)
Eysenhardtia adenostylis (Fabaceae)
Eysenhardtia polystachya (Fabaceae)
Eysenhardtia texana (Fabaceae)

Fabiana imbricata (Solanaceae)
Foeniculum vulgare (Apiaceae)
Fragaria virginiana (Rosaceae)

Gardenia jasminoides (Rubiaceae)
Glechoma hederaceum (Lamiaceae)
Glehnia littoralis (Apiaceae)
Glycine hispida (Fabaceae)
Grindelia squarrosa (Asteraceae)
Guazuma ulmifolia (Sterculiaceae)
Gunnera perpensa (Gunneraceae)
Gynura sarmentosa (Asteraceae)

Haplopappus fremontii (Asteraceae)
Hibiscus furcatus (Malvaceae)
Hydrangea arborescens (Hydrangeaceae)
Hydrocotyle umbellata (Apiaceae)
Hymenaea courbaril (Fabaceae)
Hypericum perforatum (Clusiaceae)
Hyssopus officinalis (Lamiaceae)

Ipomoea batatas (Convolvulaceae)
Ipomoea stans (Convolvulaceae)

Jatropha urens (Euphorbiaceae)
Juglans regia (Juglandaceae)
Juglans sieboldiana (Juglandaceae)
Juniperus communis (Cupressaceae)
Juniperus horizontalis (Cupressaceae)

Kigelia africana (Bignoniaceae)
Krameria ixina (Krameriaceae)

Lagenandra ovata (Araceae)
Lamium album (Lamiaceae)
Lespedeza cuneata (Fabaceae)
Lithospermum officinale (Boraginaceae)
Lycium chinense (Solanaceae)

Mahonia repens (Berberidaceae)
Marah oregana (Cucurbitaceae)

Marrubium vulgare (Lamiaceae)
Momordica charantia (Cucurbitaceae)
Morinda citrifolia (Rubiaceae)
Morus bombycis (Moraceae)
Murraya koenigii (Rutaceae)
Mussaenda raiatensis (Rubiaceae)
Nasturtium officinale (Brassicaceae)

Ocimum basilicum (Lamiaceae)
Ophiopogon japonicum (Liliaceae)
Opuntia ficus-indica (Cactaceae)
Orobanche sp (Orobanchaceae)
Orthosiphon aristatus (Lamiaceae)
Orthosiphon spiralis (Lamiaceae)
Orthosiphon stamineus (Lamiaceae)

Panax schinseng (Araliaceae)
Peperomia reflexa (Piperaceae)
Petroselinum crispum (Apiaceae)
Phyllanthus niruri (Euphorbiaceae)
Phyllanthus rosellus (Euphorbiaceae)
Phytolacca esculenta (Phytolaccaceae)
Picea mariana (Pinaceae)
Picea sitchnsis (Pinaceae)
Pimpinella anisum (Apiaceae)
Pinus palustris (Pinaceae)
Piper cubeba (Piperaceae)
Piper excelsum (Piperaceae)
Piper longum (Piperaceae)
Piper methystichum (Piperaceae)
Piper umbellatum (Piperaceae)
Pithecellobium unguis-cati (Fabaceae)
Pityrogramma calomelanos (Adiantaceae)
Plantago asiatica (Plantaginaceae)
Plantago major (Plantaginaceae)
Plantago ovata (Plantaginaceae)
Pleurophora pungens (Lythraceae)
Polygonum amplexicaule (Polygonaceae)
Polygonum aviculare (Polygonaceae)
Polygonum hydropiper (Polygonaceae)
Polygonum multiflorum (Polygonaceae)

Polypodium barometz (Polypodiaceae)
Polypodium maritimum (Polypodiaceae)
Pomaderris elliptica (Rhamnaceae)
Populus balsamifera (Salicaceae)
Portulaca oleracea (Portulacaceae)
Portulaca quadrifida (Portulacaceae)
Potentilla anserina (Rosaceae)
Potentilla fruticosa (Rosaceae)
Psoralea corylifolia (Fabaceae)
Psoralea pubescens (Fabaceae)
Pterocarpus pallidus (Fabaceae)
Puya gummifera (Bromeliaceae)

Randia cinerea (Rubiaceae)
Randia echinocarpa (Rubiaceae)
Ranunculus scleratus (Ranunculaceae)
Rehmannia glutinosa (Scrophulariaceae)
Rhododendron fortunei (Ericaceae)
Rhus aromatica (Anacardiaceae)
Ribes americanum (Grossulariaceae)
Rosa laevigata (Rosaceae)
Rubia tinctorum (Rubiaceae)
Rudbeckia laciniata (Asteraceae)

Salmalia malabarica (Bombacaceae)
Salvia coccinea (Lamiaceae)
Salvia macrophylla (Lamiaceae)
Sapindus saponaria (Sapindaceae)
Sarracenia flava (Sarraceniaceae)
Sassafras albidum (Lauraceae)
Scaphium scaphigerum (Sterculiaceae)
Schkuhria pinnata (Asteraceae)
Scoparia dulcis (Scrophulariaceae)
Selaginella lepidophylla (Selaginellaceae)
Selinum monnieri (Apiaceae)
Senecio aureus (Asteraceae)
Senecio bellidifolius (Asteraceae)
Sesamum indicum (Pedaliaceae)
Setaria viridis (Poaceae)

Smilax aristolochiaefolia (Smilacaceae)
Smilax moranensis (Smilacaceae)
Solanum mammosum (Solanaceae)
Solanum melongena (Solanaceae)
Solanum nigrum (Solanaceae)
Solanum nodum (Solanaceae)
Spathodea campanulata (Bignoniaceae)
Spergularia rubra (Caryophyllaceae)
Stachys officinalis (Lamiaceae)
Symplocos tinctoria (Symplocaceae)

Taraxacum officinale (Asteraceae)
Tarchonanthus camphoratus (Asteraceae)
Tephrosia piscatoria (Fabaceae)
Tephrosia purpurea (Fabaceae)
Theobroma cacao (Sterculiaceae)
Tiarella cordifolia (Saxifragaceae)
Tribulus alatus (Zygophyllaceae)
Trigonella foenum-graecum (Fabaceae)
Triumfetta semitriloba (Tiliaceae)
Tropaeolum majus (Tropaeolaceae)
Tropaeolum minus (Tropaeolaceae)
Tropaeolum peregrinum (Tropaeolaceae)
Turnera diffusa (Turneraceae)

Ulmus americana (Ulmaceae)

Vaccinium globulare (Ericaceae)
Vigna angularis (Fabaceae)
Vigna unguiculata (Fabaceae)

Xanthium strumarium (Asteraceae)

Zanthoxylum piperitum (Rutaceae)
Zizania aquatica (Poaceae)
Zizania caduciflora (Poaceae)

REFERENCES

§ Indicates information taken from abstracts in English of Chinese or Japanese language reference.

1. Marwick C. Growing use of medicinal botanicals forces assessment by drug regulators (news). *JAMA* 1995;273:607-609.
2. Abraham PA and Matzke GR. Drug-induced renal disease. In DiPiro JT, Talbert RL, Hayes PE, Yee GC, Posey LM. *Pharmacotherapy: A pathophysiologic approach.* Elsevier, New York, 1989, 543-558.
3. Depierreux M, Van Damme B, Vander Houte K, Vanherweghem JL. Pathologic aspects of a newly described nephropathy related to the prolonged use of Chinese herbs. *Am J Kidney Dis* 1994;24:172-180.
4. Vanherweghem JL, Depierreux M, Tielemans C, Abramowicz D, Dratw M, Jadoul M, Richard C, Banderveld D, Berbeelen D, Ban Haelen-Fastre R, Van Haelen M. Rapidly progressive interstitial renal fibrosis in young women: Association with slimming regimen including Chinese herbs. *Lancet* 1993;341:387-391.
5. Vanherweghem JL. A new form of nephropathy secondary to the absorption of Chinese herbs. *Bulletin et Memoires de l'Adacemie Royale de Medecine de Belgique* 1994;149:128-35.
6. Vanhaelen M, Vanhaelen-Fastre'R, But P, Vanherweghem JL. Identification of aristolochic acid in Chinese herbs. *Lancet* 1994;343:174.
7. Banherweghem JL, Abramowicz D, Tielemans C, Deierreux M. Effects of steroids on the progression of renal failure in chronic interstitial renal fibrosis: A pilot study in Chinese herbs nephropathy. *Am J Kidney Dis* 1996;27:209-215.
8. Schmeiser HH, Bieler CA, Wiesler M, VanYperssele de Strihou C, Cosyns JP. Detection of DNA adducts formed by aristolochic acid in renal tissue from patients with Chinese herbs nephropathy. *Cancer Res* 1996;56:2025-2028.
9. Vanherweghem JL, Tielemans C, Simon J, Depierreux M. Chinese herbs nephropathy and renal pelvic carcinoma. *Nephro, Dialy, Transpl* 1995;10:270-273.
10. Cosyns JP, Jadoul M, Squifflet JP, DePlaen JF, Ferluga D, Van Ypersele de Strihou C. Chinese herbs nephropathy: A clue to Balkan endemic nephropathy? *Kidney Intern* 1994;45:1680-1688.
11. Pena JM, Borras M, Ramos J, Montoliu J. Rapidly progressive interstitial renal fibrosis due to chronic intake of a herb *(Aristolochia pistolochia)* infusion. *Nephrol Dial Transplant* 1996;11:1359-1360.
12. Chan WY, Ng TB, Lu JL, Cao YX, Wang MZ, Liu WK. Effects of decoction prepared from *Aconitum carmichaeli, Aconitum kusnezoffii* and *Tripterygium wilfordii* on serum lactate dehydrogenase activity. *Hum Exp Tox* 1995;4:489-493.
13. Prakash AO, Dehadrai S, Jonathan S. Toxicological studies on the ethanolic extract of *Crotalaria juncea* seeds in rats. *J Ethnopharm* 1995;45;167-176.
14. Izumotani T, Ishimurea A, Tsumura K, Goto K, Nishizawa Y, Morii H. An adult case of Fanconi syndrome due to a mixture of Chinese crude drugs. *Nephron* 1993;65:137-140.

15. Miura H, Nakayama M, Sato T. A case of acute interstitial nephritis induced by herb medicines. *Jpn J Med* 1982;21:192-196.

16. Weisbord SD, Soule JB, Kimmel PL. Poison on line—Acute renal failure caused by oil of wormwood purchased through the Internet. *N Engl J Med* 1997; 337:825-827.

17. Kadiri S, Ogunlesi A, Osinfade K, Akinkugebe OO. *Afr J Medicine Med Sci* 1992;21:91-96.

18. Gold CH. Acute renal failure from herbal and patent remedies in Blacks. *Clin Nephrol* 1980;14:128-134.

19. Blachley JD, Knochel JP. Tobacco chewer's hypokalemia: Licorice revisited. *N Engl J Med* 1980;302:784-785.

20. Schambelan M. Licorice ingestion and blood pressure regulating hormones. *Steroids* 1994;59:127-130.

21. Sigurijonsdottir HA, Jagnarsson J, Franzson L, Sigurdsson G. Is blood pressure commonly raised by moderate consumption of liquorice? *J Hum Hypertens* 1995;9:348.

22. Saito T, Tsuboi Y, Fujisawa G, Sakuma N, Honda K, Okada K, Saito K, Ishikawa S, Saito T. An autopsy case of licorice-induced hypokalemic rhabdomyolysis associated with acute renal failure: Special reference to profound calcium deposition in skeletal and cardiac muscle. *Nippon Jinzo Gakkai Shi* 1994;36:1308-1314.

23. Homma M, Oka K, Niitsuma T, Itoh H. A novel 11 beta-hydroxysteroid dehydrogenase inhibitor contained in saiboku-to, a herbal remedy for steroid-dependent bronchial asthma. *J Pharma Pharmacol* 1994;46:305-309.

24. Case adapted from: Anderson LA. Concern regarding herbal toxicities: Case reports and counseling tips. *Ann Pharmacother* 1996;30:79-80.

25. Flore AE. Contamination of urine with diazepam and mefenamic acid from an Oriental remedy. *J Occup Med* 1991;33:1168-1169.

26. Miura H, Nakayama M, Sato T. A case of acute interstitial nephritis induced by herb medicines. *Jan J Med* 1982;21:192-196.

27. Gertner E, Marshall PS, Filandrinos D, Potek AS, Smith TM. Complications resulting from the use of Chinese herbal medications containing undeclared prescription drugs. *Arthritis Rheum* 1995;38:614-617.

28. Abt AB, Oh JY, Huntington RA, Burkhart KK. Chinese herbal medicine induced acute renal failure. *Archives Int Med* 1995;155:211-212.

29. Kang-Yum E, Oransky SH. Chinese patent medicine as a potential source of mercury poisoning. *Vet Hum Toxicol* 1992;34:235-238.

30. Li LS, Liu ZH. Clinical and experimental studies of rheum on preventing progression of chronic renal failure. *Chung Hsi I Chieh Ho Tsa Chih* 1991;11:392-396.

31. Zhang G, Nahas AM. The effect of rhubarb extract on experimental renal fibrosis. *Nephrol Dial Transplant* 1996;11:186-190.

32. Zhang JH, Li LS, Zhang M. Clinical effects of rheum and captopril on preventing progression of chronic renal failure. *Chin Med J* 1990;788-793.

33. §Ebisuno S, Hirano A, Kyoku I, Ohkawa T, Iijima O, Fujii Y, Hosoya E. Basal studies on combination of Chinese medicine in cancer chemotherapy protec-

tive effects on the toxic side effects of CDDP and antitumor effects with CDDP on murine bladder tumor (MBT-2). *Nippon Gan Chiryo Gakkai Shi* 1989;24:1305-1312.

34. Kiyohara H, Matsumoto T, Komatsu Y, Yamada H. Protective effect of oral administration of apectic polysaccharide fraction from a Kanpo (Japanese herbal) medicine "Juzen-Taiho-To" on adverse effects of cis-diaminedichloroplatinum. *Plant Med* 1995;61:531-534.

35. Cheng QL, Chen XM, Shi SZ. Effects of *Epimedium sagittatum* on immunopathology and extracellular matrices in rats with chronic renal insufficiency. *Chung Hua Nei Ko Tsa Chih* 1994;33:83-86.

36. Liu XY, Ang, NQ. Effect of liu wei di huyang or jin gui shen qi decoction as an adjuvant treatment in small cell lung cancer. *Chung Hsi I Chieh Ho Tsa Chih* 1990;10:720-722.

37. Su ZZ, He YY, Chen G. Clinical and experimental study of effects of manshen-ling oral liquid in the treatment of 100 cases of chronic nephritis. *Chuyng Kuo Chung Hsi I Chieh Ho Tsa Chih* 1993;13:269-272.

38. Bah M, Bye R, Pereda-Miranda R. Hepatotoxic pyrrolizidine alkaloids in the Mexican medicinal plant candidissima (Asteraceae: Senecioneae). *J Ethnopharmacol* 1994;43:19-30.

39. Feng Y. Study on rhizome wheat starch diet therapy in chronic renal failure patients. *Chung Hua Hu Li Tsa Chih* 1994;29:707-710.

40. Liu XY. Therapeutic effect of chai-ling-tang (sairei-to) on the steroiddependent nephrotic syndrome in children. *Am J Chin Med* 1995:23;255-260.

41. §Nagata M, Kawaguchi H, Komatsu Y, Hattori M, Itoh K. The effects of sairei-to on nephrotoxic serum nephritis in rats—possible effects on intraglomerular cell mediated immunity. *Nippon Jinzo Gakkai Shi* 1989;31:713-721.

42. Tsai HY, Chiang RT, Tan TW, Chenm HC. The effects of *Vandellia cordifolia* on renal functions and arterial blood pressure. *Am J Chin Med* 1989;17:203-210.

43. Sano M, Takahashi Y, Yoshino K, Shimoi K, Nakamura Y, Tomita I, Oguni I, Konomoto H. *Biological & Pharmaceutical Bulletin* 1995;18:1006-1008.

44. Yokozawa T, Lee TW, Chung HY, Oura H, Nonaka G, Nishioka I. Renal responses to magnesium lithospermate B. *J Pharmacy & Pharmacol* 1990;42: 712-715.

45. Yokozawa T, Chung HY, Lee TW, Oura H, Nonaka G, Nishioka I. Magnesium lithospermate B improves renal function via the kallikrein-prostaglandin system in rats with renal failure. *Jap J Nephrol* 1990;32:893-898.

46. Yokozawa T, Oura H, Lee TW, Nonaka G, Nishioka I. Augmentation of renal response by magnesium lithospermate B. *Nephron* 1991;57:78-83.

47. Lu GW, Miura K, Yukimura T, Yamamoto K. Effects of extract from *Clerodendron trichotomum* on blood pressure and renal function in rats and dogs. *J Ethnopharmacology* 1994;42:77-82.

48. Braquet P, Hosford D. Ethnopharmacology and the development of natural PAF antagonist as therapeutic agents. *J Ethnopharmacol* 1991;32:135-139.

49. Grases F, Melero G, Costa-Bauza A, Prieto R. Urolithiasis and phytotherapy. *Int Urol Nephrol* 1994;26:507-511.

50. Ogawa Y, Morzumi M, Tanaka T, Yamaguchi K. A comparison between effects of pyruvate and herb medicines in preventing experimental oxalate urolithiasis in rats. *Hinyokika Kiyo* 1986;32:1127-1133.

51. Koide T, Yamaguchi S, Utsunomiya M, Yoshioka T, Sugiyama K. The inhibitory effect of kampou extracts on in vitro calcium oxalate crystallization and in vivo stone formation in an animal model. *Int J Urol* 1995;2:81-86.

52. Varalakshmi P, Shamila Y, Latha E. Effect of *Crataeva nurvala* in experimental urolithiasis. *J Ethnopharmacol* 1990;28:313-321.

53. Shoji M, Oguni Y, Sato H, Morishita S, Ito C, Higuchi M, Sakanashi M. Pharmacological actions of "kyushin," a drug containing toad venom (2): Effects on urinary volume and electrolyte excretion. *Am J Chin Med* 1993;21:17-31.

54. Bevevino LH, Aires MM. Effect of crude extract of roots of *Bredemeyera floribunda* Willd. II. Effect on glomerular filtration rate and renal tubular function of rats. *J Ethnopharmacol* 1994;43:203-207.

55. Bevevino LH, Vieira FS, Casola AC, Sanioto SM. Effect of crude extract of roots of *Bredemeyera floribunda* Willd. I. Effect on arterial blood pressure and renal excretion in the rat. *J Ethnopharmacol* 1994;43:197-201.

56. Tsai HY, Chiang RT, Tan TW, Chenm GC. The effects of *Vandellia cordifolia* on renal functions and arterial blood pressure. *Am J Chinese Medicine* 1989;17:203-210.

57. Goonaratna C, Thabrew I, Wijewardena K. Does *Aerua lanata* have diuretic properties? *Indian J Physiol Pharmacol* 1993;37:135-137.

58. Rocha MJ, Fulgencio SF, Rabetti AC, Nicolau M, Poli A, Simoes CM, Ribeiro-do-Valle RM. Effects of hydroalcoholic extracts of *Portulaca pilosa* and *Achyrocline satureioides* on urinary sodium and potassium excretion. *J Ethnopharmacol* 1994;43:179-183.

59. Chan TY, Chan ANY, Critchley JA. Hospital admissions due to adverse reactions to Chinese herbal medicine. *J Tropical Medicine & Hygiene* 1992;296-298.

60. Phytochemical Database-USDA-ARS-NGRL Stephen M. Beckstrom-Sternberg and James A. Duke, http://www.ars-grin.gov/cgi-bin/duke/ethnobotuse.pl.

Chapter 3

Hepatic Effects of Herbal Remedies

William R. Hamilton, PharmD
Sidney J. Stohs, PhD

INTRODUCTION

As the largest gland of the body, the liver filters waste products, detoxifies poisons and other foreign chemicals via microsomal enzyme systems, stores extra blood and vitamins, dismantles proteins into amino acids, assembles proteins as albumin, recycles iron from old blood cells, and produces bile to digest fats.[1] Bile is a vital body fluid, and herbal remedies are commonly used throughout the world to restore proper bile flow. Rest, good nutrition, and cleansing are frequent treatment recommendations for patients with liver dysfunctions.[2] Treatment may involve fasting or special restricted diets, followed by an herbal or natural product to cleanse or "flush" the liver, as, for example, a combination of olive oil, lemon juice, garlic, and cayenne.

The classification of liver diseases is difficult because the etiology and pathogenic mechanisms involved are obscure in many instances. As a consequence, a morphologic classification of liver disease is sometimes used.[3] Using a morphologic classification, liver diseases can be divided into parenchymal, hepatobiliary, and vascular types. Parenchymal liver diseases may be due to hepatitis (viral, drug, or toxin induced), cirrhosis, infiltrations, space-occupying lesions, and functional disorders associated with jaundice. Most common causes of cirrhosis are associated with viral hepatitis and alcoholic liver disease, with a smaller percentage of cases stemming from documented intoxication with industrial chemicals, poisons, or drugs. Various infiltrations leading to parenchymal liver disease are associated with glycogen, fat, amyloid, lymphoma, leukemia, and granuloma. Space-occupying lesions include abscesses (pyogenic, amoebic), cysts, hepatomas, and metastatic tumors. Functional disorders of the liver associated with jaundice include cholestasis of pregnancy, benign recurrent cholestasis, and various disorders such as Gilbert's syndrome.

Hepatobiliary forms of liver disease are associated with extrahepatic biliary obstruction as produced by stones, strictures, or tumors as well as cholangitis. Vascular liver diseases are associated with chronic passive congestion and cardiac cirrhosis, hepatic and portal vein thromboses, pylephlebitis, and arteriovenous malformation.[3]

Environmental, societal, and pathological influences frequently stress hepatic function. Numerous dietary factors, drugs, viruses, and other foreign chemicals challenge the liver. Despite significant capacity for regeneration and tolerance of these compounds, the liver when stressed over prolonged periods responds with inflammation, cirrhosis, and decreased function leading to jaundice and possibly death.[1,3,4] Alcohol consumption is a societal example of self-induced hepatotoxicity. Short of a liver transplant, relatively few options are available for treatment of liver diseases.

Corticosteroids have been shown to reduce overall morbidity of alcoholic hepatitis patients.[4] Carithers and colleagues[5] demonstrated a reduced short-term mortality using methylprednisolone in very sick patients. Mortality in the treatment group was 6 percent compared to 35 percent in the placebo group.

Treatment of chronic viral hepatitis includes exercise as tolerated, avoidance of potentially hepatotoxic drugs, and a healthy diet. Interferon is now the treatment of choice for patients with chronic hepatitis B, C, and D infections. However, only a small proportion of patients respond favorably to therapies such as corticosteroids and interferons. Furthermore, fewer patients have lasting response and even fewer are cured. Thus, a need exists for more effective, more widely applicable, and less costly therapies for chronic forms of hepatitis.[6]

Various herbal products have been anecdotally used throughout history to treat liver diseases. However, exceedingly few well-controlled studies have been conducted to substantiate that various products are efficacious in the treatment of liver disease. In recent years, numerous animal studies have been conducted which confirm that a number of herbal products are capable of providing significant protection against various toxins and can enhance liver function. Liver-protecting substances can be grouped into several categories:[7]

- Antioxidants   milk thistle, ginkgo, capillaris
- Stabilizing agents   milk thistle, garlic
- Choleretics   artichoke, capillaris, garlic
- Sulfur sources   milk thistle, dandelion, cabbage, garlic
- Enzyme-inducing agents schizandra, cabbage

This chapter provides several case studies involving patients with liver diseases including alcoholic cirrhosis, drug-induced hepatitis, hepatitis secondary to blood transfusion, and hepatocellular carcinoma. Various treatment options including herbal and natural products will be considered in each case. Furthermore, herbs used for treating various hepatic disorders are summarized in table form. In most cases, reports of efficacy are anecdotal with few well-controlled studies having been conducted.

CASE STUDIES

Patient Number 1: Silybum marianum for Alcoholic Cirrhosis

> TC is a 58-year-old male with a history of alcohol abuse. He is experiencing weight loss, digestive disturbances including loss of appetite, and right upper quadrant pain. Ascites are present but not severe. Laboratory values include elevated serum alanine aminotransferase (ALT) 72 IU/liter (nl 8-46), aspartate aminotransferase (AST) 58 IU/liter (nl 7-46), and alkaline phosphatase (ALP) 134 IU/liter (nl 25-100).

Traditional management of cirrhosis is largely symptomatic,[8] with therapy being tailored to the severity of the symptoms. Fluid and electrolyte balance may need adjustment. Antiemetics may be given for nausea, while analgesics are administered for pain after evaluating risk of further gastrointestinal injury. Vitamin therapy includes thiamine 50 to 100 mg per day and vitamin K 10 mg subcutaneously daily for three or more days if the prothrombin time is elevated.

The flavonoid silibinin, the main compound extracted from the milk thistle (*Silybum marianum*, L. Gartneri), has been shown to have hepatoprotective properties in acute and chronic liver injury. Silymarin is the collective name for the flavolignans silibinin (silybin), silidianin, and silichristin (silychristin), which are extracted from milk thistle, *S. marianum*. Synonyms include Mary thistle, St. Mary thistle, marian thistle, lady's thistle, and holy thistle.[9]

Therapeutic benefit for the use of milk thistle products is supported by a double-blind, prospective, randomized study involving 170 patients with cirrhosis.[10] In this study, 87 patients received 140 mg silymarin three times daily, while 83 patients received a placebo. Following a mean observation period of 41 months, 24 patients in the treatment group had died, with 18 deaths being related to liver disease. The four-year survival of the treatment group was 58 percent ± 9 percent. In the placebo group, 37 patients had died, with 31 deaths related to liver disease. Four-year survival in the placebo group was 39 percent ± 9 percent (p = 0.036). Analysis of subgroups indicated that treatment was effective in patients with alcoholic cirrhosis (p < 0.01). No side effects of silymarin treatment were observed.

In patient TC, optimal benefit will be achieved if he is able to stop his alcohol consumption and consume a balanced and nutritious diet. Regardless of the success of abstinence, TC should be started on silymarin 200 mg of concentrated extract (140 mg of silymarin)[11] taken as two capsules three times daily.[12] The parameters used to assess a beneficial effect of the drug on the progression of chronic liver disease appear to be unreliable. In the study group, follow-up transaminases, serum albumin, and serum bilirubin revealed no differences between the two study groups.[10] Mortality was used in this study to measure effectiveness of therapy. Clinical improvement (fatigue, jaundice, ascites, etc.) can be used to estimate the benefit of continuing therapy. During this study, patients were followed for a minimum of two years with a mean observation period of 41 months. Based on the lack of adverse effects associated with daily silymarin administration, and the high incidence of mortality associated with chronic liver disease, continuous long-term use of silymarin may be warranted.

The mechanisms of action of silymarin are incompletely understood. The effect of silymarin appears to be the prevention of metabolic or toxic effects of alcohol on the liver. Alcohol is metabolized to more reactive products that deplete antioxidants such as glutathione and produce tissue-damaging effects. It may also reduce the degree of collagen deposition in the liver and therefore the extent of circulatory changes in the liver and the portal system.[10] Silymarin not only prevents the depletion of glutathione (GSH) induced by alcohol and other liver toxins, its antioxidant activity helps prevent liver damage. It also has the ability to stimulate liver protein synthesis.[13] Selective inhibition of leukotriene formation by Kupffer cells can at least partially account for the hepatoprotective properties of silibinin.[14]

Lipid peroxidation is an indicator of oxidative tissue damage due to the formation of free radicals and reactive oxygen species in response to xenobiotics such as alcohol and drugs, which induce liver damage. Palasciano and colleagues[15] measured serum levels of malondialdehyde (a major product of the oxidation of polyunsaturated fatty acids) and normal indices of hepatocellular function. In a double-blind, placebo-controlled clinical trial, these investigators demonstrated that the most positive results were obtained when the hepatotoxin was discontinued and silymarin was given in doses of 800 mg per day in two divided doses. Although the indices of hepatocellular damage were improved with silymarin treatment, the difference between the treated groups and placebo was not statistically significant.[15]

In a study by Scheiber and Izogen,[16] silymarin treatment was shown to produce measurable improvement in hepatic changes associated with chronic cirrhosis. In another study, 10 patients with histologically confirmed alcoholic liver steatosis were treated for three months with 200 mg silymarin three times daily. Results showed definite improvement of liver cell function and histologic pattern of liver steatosis.[17]

A review of 46 human studies conducted prior to 1990 is presented in *Milk Thistle, The Liver Herb* by Hobbs.[18] Investigations lasted from 81 hours to four years. A total of 5,732 patients were included with a range per study of 6 to over 2,000 patients. Several studies were double-blinded and placebo-controlled. Alcoholism, hepatitis B, cirrhosis, amanita poisoning, and exposure to toluene and xylene were among the diagnoses investigated. These studies generally indicated positive outcomes from the use of silymarin.

Numerous studies in rodents have shown that silymarin protects against glutathione depletion, lipid peroxidation, and oxidative tissue damage induced experimentally by various chemicals. For example, silymarin protects against liver lesions induced by carbon tetrachloride,[19,20,21] tert-butyl-hydroperoxide,[20,21,22] microcystin-LR,[23,24] phenylhydrazine,[25] lindane,[26] benzo(a)pyrene,[27] phalloidin,[28] the carcinogen 12-O-tetradecanoylphorbol-13-acetate,[29] bromobenzene,[30] acetaminophen,[31] ethanol, isoniazid, and rifampicin.[32] Thus, silymarin has been shown to provide protection against the toxicity of a wide range of carcinogens and hepatotoxins.

In summary, current evidence indicates that protection against liver damage by silymarin is due to prevention of free radical damage, decreased formation of damaging leukotrienes, and stimulation of the production of new liver cells. Although well-controlled, supporting human studies are limited, the double-blind study[10] involving 170 patients with cirrhosis suggests that mortality of patients with cirrhosis is reduced by treatment with silymarin. This effect was more pronounced in alcoholic cirrhosis. Adverse effects have generally been absent in human studies.[33] The superiority of silymarin over other chemoprotectants has been demonstrated.[20] Finally, numerous studies in animals have demonstrated that silymarin is effective in preventing toxicity and liver damage associated with various toxins, pesticides, and halogenated cyclic hydrocarbons.[19-32]

Patient Number 2: Garlic and Acetaminophen Toxicity— Drug-Induced Hepatitis

RF has been taking 6 grams of acetaminophen daily for several weeks. As a consequence, he is presenting with nausea, vomiting, liver tenderness, and low blood pressure (110/46).

Acetaminophen is one of the most commonly used drugs which, if taken in large amounts, is capable of inducing hepatitis. Acetaminophen is metabolized to oxidized, highly reactive metabolites that are normally detoxified by reacting with the sulfhydryl group of glutathione. This conjugated product is less toxic and readily excreted. When acute or chronic high doses of acetaminophen deplete glutathione, the metabolites bind covalently to various macromolecules in hepatocytes, leading to necrosis. Increases in serum AST and ALT indicate the extent of necrosis in the liver.[34] Primary treatment of acetaminophen toxicity involves discontinuation of the acetaminophen. N-Acetylcysteine is usually given to supply sulfhydryl groups in acute overdoses.[35]

Animal studies indicate the protective effects of garlic and related organosulfur compounds on acetaminophen-induced hepatotoxicity. In a study by Wang and colleagues,[36] fresh garlic homogenates were administered to Swiss-Webster mice two hours prior to, or immediately after acetaminophen treatment (0.2 g/kg). Acetaminophen-induced hepatotoxicity was essentially prevented by the garlic, as indicated by serum levels of alanine aminotransferase and lactate dehydrogenase and by liver histopathology. The amount of oxidized metabolites of acetaminophen excreted in the urine was also significantly decreased by the fresh garlic homogenate. An S-allyl structure appears to be a common feature for most sulfides to inhibit cytochrome P-450 2E1-dependent activity and to display good protective activities.

In another animal study, the combination of PMC (dimethyl-4,4'-dimethoxy-5,6,5',6'-dimethylene dioxybiphenyl-2,2'-dicarboxylate) and garlic oil in preventing hepatic injury in rats and mice from carbon tetrachloride exposure was investigated.[37] The results demonstrated that this combination effectively suppressed carbon tetrachloride-induced hepatotoxicity. Garlic oil alone was effective in preventing alterations in triglyceride and cholesterol metabolism and also prevented allyl alcohol-induced hepatotoxicity.

Investigations on the hepatoprotective activity of six sulphur-containing components of garlic including allicin have shown that most of these compounds are capable of protecting against carbon tetrachloride-induced cytotoxicity.[38] Garlic has been shown to protect against the hepatotoxicity of heavy metals including cadmium, methylmercury, and phenylmercury in rats.[39] Garlic also prevents aflatoxin B1-induced hepatocellular carcinomas in the toad *Bufo regularis*.[40] Furthermore, garlic provides protection against the hepatic histopathological effects of large doses of collagen and arachidonic acid in rabbits.[41] Thus, various studies in animals have demonstrated that garlic exhibits hepatoprotective effects against chemically diverse hepatotoxins.

Caldwell[42] has provided anecdotal evidence for the therapeutic efficacy of garlic in a report involving a patient with severe hepatopulmonary syndrome who failed somatostatin therapy and declined liver transplantation. This patient began using powdered garlic *(Allium sativum)* at a dose of four teaspoonfuls once or twice daily. Improvement was noted four months after starting this therapy. She experienced partial palliation of her symptoms and some objective signs of improvement over 18 months of continuous self-medication.

In summary, animal studies and anecdotal human reports indicate a positive role for garlic in treatment of mild cases of acetaminophen-induced hepatotoxicity and hepatotoxicity induced by a variety of other toxins. It appears unlikely that funding will be provided for major prospective studies involving garlic in humans due to the unpatentability of garlic. The accepted treatment using N-acetylcysteine currently appears more appropriate considering the level of research, the standardization of the product, and the seriousness of the complications associated with acetaminophen toxicity.

Patient Number 3: Coenzyme Q10—
Increased Liver Enzymes Secondary
to Lovastatin Therapy

PF has been taking lovastatin (Mevacor, Merck) 20 mg daily for two years and continues to have elevated liver enzymes, where the ALT is 44 µ/L (nl 7-24), and the AST is 38 µ/L (nl 8-20 µ/L). Is there an herbal product that will provide some control of his apparent hepatotoxic reaction to the lovastatin?

Lovastatin is a cholesterol-lowering drug which may produce oxidative stress by reducing levels of the endogenous antioxidant coenzyme Q10 (CoQ10) in humans[43] and animals.[44,45] Hepatotoxicity is an adverse effect associated with the use of lovastatin and other 3-hydroxy-3-methylglutaryl-coenzyme A (HMG-CoA) reductase inhibitors, as exemplified by hepatic necrosis, hepatitis, and elevated liver enzymes.[46] Approximately 11 percent of patients taking lovastatin experience some elevation of liver enzymes.[47]

Walravens and colleagues[48] describe a single case report where the daily administration of 30 mg coenzyme Q10 eliminated the myopathy associated with the daily use of lovastatin. After five months of coenzyme Q10 therapy and no lovastatin, the lovastatin was restarted at a dose of 10 mg five or six times a week. Phosphokinase levels increased slightly to 800 U/l, but cramping did not recur. Coenzyme Q10 (ubiquinone) is available as a nutritional supplement, and may be useful in preventing the hepatotoxicity associated with lovastatin.

Loop and colleagues[49] examined the effects of lovastatin and ethanol on various factors in rat livers including coenzyme Q10 and vitamin E levels.

Ethanol, either separately or in combination with lovastatin, diminished liver stores of coenzyme Q10 by almost 40 percent. Furthermore, both lovastatin and ethanol significantly deceased alpha-tocopherol (vitamin E) concentrations, an effect largely overcome by coenzyme Q10 administration. As expected, lovastatin had no effect on coenzyme Q10 levels in animals supplemented with this antioxidant.

Another study demonstrated protection against lipid peroxidative damage to rat liver by diets that included coenzyme Q10 (and other antioxidants).[50] They concluded that "protection by multiple antioxidants against lipid peroxidation may translate to prevention of peroxidative damage to human tissue, a factor in human disease."

The safety and efficacy of administering coenzyme Q10 have been studied by Langsjoen and colleagues[51] in 424 patients with various forms of cardiovascular disease over an eight-year period. Doses of coenzyme Q10 ranged from 75 to 600 mg per day by mouth, averaging 242 mg per day. No apparent side effects from treatment with coenzyme Q10, other than a single case of transient nausea, were reported. A statistically significant improvement in myocardial function was documented using echocardiography as demonstrated by left ventricular wall thickness, mitral valve inflow slope, and fractional shortening. Furthermore, 43 percent of the patients receiving coenzyme Q10 stopped using between one and three of the one to five drugs being used at the start of the study. Six percent of the patients required the addition of one drug.[51] Discontinuation of cardiac medications should be done only with the direct supervision of a physician.

In an earlier study using 100 mg per day of coenzyme Q10, Langsjoen and colleagues[52] demonstrated a significantly improved cardiac function and a pronounced increase in survival in conjunction with coenzyme Q10 therapy. The survival rates were 75 percent during the 46-month study for the 137 patients treated with coenzyme Q10. This group included 43 patients with ejection fractions below 40 percent. This was compared to a 36-month survival rate of 25 percent for 182 patients with ejection fractions below 46 percent on conventional therapy without coenzyme Q10. "The improved cardiac function and pronounced increase of survival show that therapy with coenzyme Q10 is remarkably beneficial due to correction of coenzyme Q10 deficiency in mechanisms of bioenergetics."[52]

In summary, animal research and human studies indicate a positive benefit of coenzyme Q10 supplementation. Toxicity appears to be minimal in patients with doses as high as 600 mg/kg. Doses of 100 mg per day have been suggested in one outcome study,[52] although a scientifically established dose for humans remains to be determined.

Patient Number 4: Phyllanthus Species Used to Treat Hepatitis

VB is a 34-year-old woman who received a blood transfusion following an automobile accident. She now presents with a flulike syndrome, loss of appetite, gastrointestinal complaints, and a headache. The symptoms have persisted for several weeks. Urinalysis shows a dark urine and stools are chalky. Jaundice is not apparent. Subsequent studies suggested that VB is suffering from hepatitis, presumably as a result of receiving a transfusion contaminated with hepatitis B virus.

Extracts of *Phyllanthus* species have been shown to exhibit antihepatotoxic activity.[53,54,55,56] Blumberg and associates[57] demonstrated that extracts of *Phyllanthus amarus* (Chen-Chu Ts'ao, pearl grass) inhibited woodchuck hepatitis virus. When human carriers of hepatitis B virus were treated orally for one month with the extract of *Phyllanthus,* the virus disappeared in approximately 60 percent of the carriers, and was not detectable during the observation period.

An extract of *Phyllanthus amarus* can suppress expression of hepatitis B surface antigen in human hepatoma cells.[58] Thus, phyllanthus may be a safe and effective means of treating hepatitis B virus.

Several contradictory studies have also been reported with respect to the effectiveness of *Phyllanthus amarus* on hepatitis B virus. A study by Munshi and colleagues[59] involving the use of 114 ducks infected with duck hepatitis B virus demonstrated that alcoholic extracts of *P. amarus* and *P. maderaspatensis* exhibited no definitive antiviral properties in the treated ducks. The reason for the discrepancy is not known, but may be due to the origin of the plant material, the extraction procedure, plant species variation, or virus sensitivity and susceptibility.

Another study compared three species of the *Phyllanthus* genus to treat chronic hepatitis B in human subjects.[60] *Phyllanthus urinaria* (gathered in Henan Province, China) produced a substantial clearance of the hepatitis B e-antigen as well as the appearance of antibodies to that antigen. The Chinese preparation was administered at a dose of 0.3 g three times daily for one month. Thereafter, the dose was increased to 0.6 g three times daily for one month, followed by 0.9 g three times daily during the third month. An Indian preparation was administered at a consistent dose of 0.5 g three times daily for three months. Further studies may clarify a difference in the specific principles of the herb.[60]

This case provides an example of the complications associated with the use of herbal products. Studies to be compared may not have used the same product or may have prepared the product differently, leading to conflicting results. At this time it appears that *Phyllanthus amarus* should be used cautiously and may be of limited benefit unless subsequent studies provide evidence of consistent positive results.

Patient Number 5: Sho-Saiko-to for Chemoprevention of Hepatocellular Carcinoma

KR is a 57-year-old female with a diagnosis of cirrhosis of the liver. She has eliminated an eleven-year habit of alcohol consumption. She is negative for hepatitis B surface antigen (HbsAg). Serum bilirubin is 2 mg/dl (nl, 0.2 to 1.0 mg/dl) and serum albumin is 3.1 g/dl (nl, 3.8 to 5.0 g/dl). Ultrasonography and serum assay of alpha-fetoprotein (AFP) are negative. Is there an herbal preparation indicated for chemoprevention of hepatocellular carcinoma, since approximately 80 percent of patients who develop hepatocellular carcinoma have underlying cirrhosis?

Yano and colleagues[61] state that Sho-saiko-to (TJ-9, Xino-chai-hu-tang) "is the most popular herbal medicine in Japan and is used in the treatment of various chronic liver diseases." It is a Japanese modified, traditional herbal medicine that consists of crude ingredients extracted from seven herbs including *Bupleurum* root, *Pinellia* tuber, *Scutellaria* root, jujube root, ginseng root, licorice (glycyrrhiza) root, and ginger rhizome.

Due to the widespread use of this herbal product, a prospective, randomized, nonblind controlled study was performed to evaluate the preventive effect of Sho-saiko-to on hepatocellular carcinomas (HCC).[62] Two hundred sixty patients with cirrhosis were included in the study. Patients in the Sho-saiko-to group received 7.5 g of the drug daily in addition to conventional drugs that were not specified in the article. The conventional drugs were also given to the control group. All patients were monitored for six months. This study demonstrated a reduction in the incidence of HCC in the trial group (23 percent incidence in the trial group versus 34 percent in the control group [$p = 0.071$]). In a subgroup of patients without hepatitis B surface antigen (HbsAg), the incidence of cancer development was significantly lower ($p = 0.024$) in the trial group (22 percent incidence in the trial group versus 39 percent in the control group). The overall survival rate was higher for the trial group (75 percent) compared to the control group (61 percent) ($p = 0.053$). Again the subgroup without HbsAg achieved statistical significance with respect to survival ($p = 0.043$—76 percent survival for the trial group versus 60 percent for the control group).[62]

Several possible mechanisms exist with respect to the pharmacological and cytoprotective effects of Sho-saiko-to. Yano and colleagues[61] demonstrated that the water-soluble ingredients (solution did not contain high levels of flavonoids) of this herbal medicine inhibit the proliferation of a human hepatocellular carcinoma cell line and a cholangiocarcinoma cell line in a concentration-dependent manner by inducing apoptosis and arresting at the G-0/G-1 phase. Furthermore, the drug suppressed proliferation of the carcinoma cell lines more strongly than did each of the major ingredients. Furthermore, Sho-saiko-to induces tumor necrosis factor alpha (TNF-α) and granulocyte colony-stimulating factor (GCSF) in vitro in peripheral blood monocytes from patients with liver cirrhosis accompanied by hepatocellular carcinoma.[63] Earlier studies by these same investigators demonstrated that this herbal drug enhanced cytokine production in cultured peripheral mononuclear cells from patients with cirrhosis.[64] These results suggest that the drug's clinical efficacy may involve enhancement of the immunological functions of the body.

In addition to its ability to modulate the immune system, Sho-saiko-to has been shown to protect the liver from injury by free radicals, which occur in an ischemic state during endotoxemia.[65] In studies involving the use of mice treated with endotoxin, Sho-saiko-to was shown to decrease endotoxin-induced lipid peroxide levels and xanthine oxidase activity while enhancing superoxide dismutase and glutathione peroxidase activities. These results suggest that Sho-saiko-to exerted effects that prevented endotoxin-induced formation of reactive oxygen species and oxidative tissue damage.

In summary, these studies indicate clinical benefit for patients with cirrhosis and/or hepatocellular carcinoma associated with the use of the herbal mixture known as Sho-saiko-to. The dose of Sho-saiko-to in the prospective study[62] was 7.5 g per day in addition to the conventional drugs given to the patients.

A summary of herbs that may have hepatic effects is presented in Table 3.1.

DANDELION

The historical medicinal use of dandelion *(Taraxacum officinale,* Pu Gong Ying) dates back to the tenth and eleventh centuries.[70] Some references[13,71] state that dandelion exhibits properties such as enhancement of bile flow (cholekinetic), improvement in liver congestion, choleretic activity, and use in treating hepatitis. Clinical use of dandelion is officially recognized in Britain, France, and Germany.[72]

Although dandelion does possess a slight laxative effect and the leaves may have a mild diuretic effect, V. Tyler states that the "culinary applications far outweigh any medicinal uses for this common plant."[73] Furthermore, the *Lawrence Review of Natural Products*[74] concludes that no pharmacological

TABLE 3.1. Herbs Used for Hepatic Therapy

Herb (supplement)	Therapeutic indication	Recommended dose	Animal studies	Anecdotal evidence	Controlled human studies
Milk thistle (Silybum marianum)	hepatoprotectant	800 to 1200 mg per day in two or three divided doses	+	+	+
Schisandra (Schizandra) Schisandra chinensis	hepatoprotectant	none indicated safety and efficacy have not been established	+	+	–
Garlic (Allium sativum) Stinking rose, treacle, nectar of the gods, camphor of the poor man's treacle	antioxidant	varies with product	+	+	–
Lipoic acid [66,67,68] (not an herb)	liver detoxifier, antioxidant, hepatoprotectant	50 to 200 mg per day	+	+	–
Phyllanthus amarus	Hepatitis B	0.3 to 0.9 gm three times a day	±	±	–
Artichoke (Cynara scolymus)	strong choleretic, hepatoprotectant	none indicated	+	+	–

Coenzyme Q10 (co-factor) Ubiquinone	heart disease, hepatoprotectant	100 mg daily	+	+	−
Sho-saiko-to (TJ-9)	cancer—preventive	7.5 g per day	+	+	+
Dandelion (*Taraxacum officinale*) piss-in-bed, lion's tooth, Pu Gong Ting, blow ball-bitterwort, wild endive, etc.	Cholagogue (stimulates flow of bile from gallbladder) lithotriptic (dissolves kidney and bladder stones)[69]	Tea, tincture, salad	−	+	−*
Turmeric (*Curcuma longa*)	jaundice and hepatitis (bile stimulating)	300 mg three times daily	±	+	−

Notes:
+ implies reasonable studies or reports (not exhaustive)
− implies lack of studies or reports
± implies mixed information or limited studies
* see specific discussion of dandelion

activity has been documented for dandelion. It is tempting to impart therapeutic ability to readily available weeds. To date, the therapeutic efficacy of dandelion has not been substantiated.

CURCUMA LONGA

Curcuma longa or curcumin is a component of the spice turmeric. Animal studies have demonstrated curcumin's ability to inhibit iron-catalyzed lipid peroxidation,[75] strongly inhibit cytochrome P450 and glutathione S-transferase,[76] and decrease inflammation by lowering the production of reactive oxygen species in macrophages. Furthermore, it exhibits anticarcinogenesis and chemoprevention activities.[77] Soni, Rajan, and Kuttan[78] demonstrated the positive effect of curcumin in reversing the liver damage produced by feeding aflatoxin B1 to ducklings. Curcumin has been shown to lower lipid peroxidation in plasma and urine, probably secondary to its hypocholesterolemic, antioxidant, and free radical scavenger properties.[79,80] Thus, animal models appear to imply a positive health benefit to the liver. Unfortunately, curcumin is far less active orally than after parenteral administration,[81] and no human studies have been published to confirm these benefits in humans.

HERBAL SYSTEMS
AND COMBINATION PRODUCTS

Several products are available as combinations of various herbs based on historical usage and traditional medical systems. Sho-saiko-to was previously discussed. Some of these combination products are based on traditional Chinese and Ayurvedic medicine. In addition, numerous other combination products to treat liver diseases and disorders are available in health food stores and herbal remedy shops.

Traditional Chinese medicine uses combinations of herbs to treat diseases. Herbal use is divided into two groups: empirical and traditional. Empirical herbal medicine is usually practiced by individuals without formal training. Secret formulas may be handed down from generation to generation within a family. Traditional Chinese medicine (TCM) is considered a science and is taught by doctors or teachers. Although based on theories that are part of Chinese philosophy, testing has occurred through hundreds of years of experience.[82] TCM recognizes five bodily systems, each of which is associated with one of the five primary elements in nature. Internal organs are thought to be connected to external parts of the body that they affect.

According to TCM, the liver's main function is to regulate the flow of "Qi (chi)" or "life energy." Treatment attempts to cure blockage, stagnation, or overstimulation of chi.[83] Chen, Yang, and Liang[84] evaluated a program for diagnosing Liver-Qi Deficiency Syndrome (LQDS) based on the TCM theory and clinical practice. Four experimental groups were compared to determine the value of using clinical evaluations such as lactate dehydrogenase (LDH) and albumin to diagnose LQDS. While it is difficult to evaluate the results, this type of study is being used to document a correlation between clinical medicine and traditional Chinese medicine.

The healing techniques and preventive methods of Ayurveda include "herbal food supplements to help us access our body's innate healing intelligence, strengthen the immune system and bring balance to mind and body . . ."[85] Ayurveda evolved in India as a medical system that promotes longevity through knowledge of natural rhythms.[86] Ayurvedic herbs are classified according to dozens of factors. Heyn[87] suggests the following herbs to strengthen the liver:

- Amalki (*Emblica officinalis* Gaertn.—Euphorbiaceae)
- Kutaki or Katuka (*Picrorhiza kurroa* Royle et Benth.—Scrophulariaceae)
- Aloe (*Aloe barbadensis* Mill.—Liliaceae)

However, as with other herbal products purported to be useful for various liver disorders, well-defined, controlled clinical studies are not available to support or refute the use of these products. Health food stores usually stock brands of herbal formulas that are promoted as an aid to liver function. They combine several herbs, vitamins, and other ingredients. Some examples and their compositions follow:

Liver Plus—InnerLights

Composed of lecithin (soya), calcium phosphate dibasic, choline bitatrate, inositol, betaine HCl, kelp, whole desiccated bovine liver, stearic acid, niacinamide, wild yam root, dandelion root, zinc amino acid chelate, niacin, magnesium amino acid chelate, pyridoxine HCl, cyanocobalamin, calcium sulfate, calcium sulfate, magnesium phosphates, sodium sulfate, and silicate oxide. Dose: Two capsules with each meal.

Hepato-Pure Liver Formula—Planetary Formulas

Combination of Chinese and Ayurvedic ingredients including bupleurum, wild yam root, Oregon grape root, lycli berry, cyperus, dandelion root and extract, dong quai, peony alba, ginger root, fennel seed, green citrus peel, milk thistle seed extract, dong quai extract. Dose: Two capsules two or three times daily between meals.

Other examples include Organ Toner and Clear Stream from New Moon Extracts, and Liv-R-Action from Nature's Plus. Liverall, made by Schiff, is an example of a dried liver product. It contains 660 mg Argentinean beef liver dried at a low temperature.

Dr. Terry Willard's[88] Liver Formula includes the following ingredients: milk thistle extract (GP 80 percent silymarin) *(Silybum marianum)*, dandelion root *(Taraxacum officinale)*, ginger root *(Zingiber officinalis)*, burdock root *(Arctium lappa)*, parsley root *(Petroselinum sativum)*, and black radish *(Raphanus sativus nigra)*.

Review of the literature failed to identify scientific outcome studies supporting the use of the above combination products. Herbalists with years of experience and training generally develop combinations to complement their personal philosophies in some cases. These combinations may become commercial products.

Various protocols to improve liver function and general health call for "cleansing" the liver system using a combination of fasting, a cleansing diet, and specific herbal combinations. The concept of cleaning an organ that is designed as a filter and detoxifier is appealing.[72,88] Other than the intuitive concept based on traditional systems, review of the literature produced no investigations of the benefits or risks of a "liver flush." The concept that herbal products can flush the liver and cleanse the body is widely stated in pamphlets and literature available in herbal shops and health food stores. Support for these concepts is usually anecdotal. No well-documented, controlled studies exist that either support or refute these concepts.

Historical usage of herbal products for hepatic treatment or support includes numerous possibly beneficial herbs. A review of available literature is presented in Table 3.2. Standard general references used were *The Lawrence Review of Natural Products, The Honest Herbal* by V. Tyler, and individual publications researched using WinSpirs® data retrieval system. The German Commission E monographs translation is not available at this time but would also serve as a standard of clinical applications referenced by scientific studies.

TABLE 3.2. Other Herbal Products That Have Limited Support for Usage but Are Employed as Hepatic Treatment Options

Herb	Common Names	Literature Support*	Reference
Barberry	Oregon grape, berberis, jaundice berry, and others	none found	*Lawrence Review of Natural Products* July 1991
Black radish		none found	none found
Boldo (*Peumus boldus* Mol.)	Boldine, Chilean tree	effective antioxidant, mainly for liver ailments	*Pharmacol Res.* 1994[89]
Burdock	Great burdock, gobo	none found	*Lawrence Review of Natural Products* July 1991 and *The Honest Herbal* 3rd Ed. p. 63
Calandine		none found	none found
Catechin (isolated from *Uncaria gambier*)		none found	none found
Cheonanthus		none found	none found
Echinacea	American coneflower, snakeroot, black susan, hedgehog, and others	none found	*Lawrence Review of Natural Products* May 1995 and *HerbalGram*[90]

TABLE 3.2 (continued)

Herb	Common Names	Literature Support*	Reference
Fennel	carosella, garden fennel, wild fennel, and others	none found	*Lawrence Review of Natural Products* August 1994
Goldenseal	hydrastis	none found	*The Honest Herbal* 3rd Ed. p. 175
Hops	European hops, common hops, lupulin	none found	*Lawrence Review of Natural Products* May 1991 and *The Honest Herbal* 3rd Ed. p. 175
Yeast (*Saccharomyces cerevisiae*)		yeast raised levels of cytochrome P-450, which may increase or decrease the toxicity of a chemical or drug	*HerbalGram* May 23, 1988[91]
Horsetail	souring rush, bottle brush, scouring rush, shave grass	none found	*Lawrence Review of Natural Products* October 1991 and *The Honest Herbal* 3rd Ed. p. 179
Irish moss		none found	none found

Licorice (Glycyrrhiza glabra)		potential toxicity associated with excessive consumption	Lawrence Review of Natural Products June 1989
Marijuana (Cannabis sativa)	banji, hemp, grass, and many others	none found	Lawrence Review of Natural Products August 1990
Rose hips		none found	Lawrence Review of Natural Products September 1991 and The Honest Herbal 3rd Ed. p.263
Suma	dried root of a tropical plant native to the Amazon rain forests (not related to ginseng)	historical usage only, no safety studies, no published studies	The Honest Herbal 3rd Ed. p.303
Thyme		none found	none found
Wahoo		none found	none found
Yellow Dock (Rumex crispus)	curly dock	astringent and laxative properties	The Honest Herbal 3rd Ed. p. 325

Note:
* "none found" indicates literature was unavailable for review or the source referenced does not indicate any use for hepatic therapy.

SUMMARY

Exposure to dietary factors, environmental factors, drugs, other foreign chemicals, and viruses challenges the liver, resulting in hepatobiliary, vascular, and parenchymal diseases as well as space-filling lesions. Historically, various herbal products have been used anecdotally to treat diverse liver diseases. Unfortunately, very few well-controlled human, clinical studies have been conducted to either substantiate or refute claims of efficacy with respect to various products in the treatment of liver disorders and diseases. However, in recent years, a growing number of animal studies have been conducted which confirm that a number of herbal products are capable of enhancing liver function and providing protection against various toxins, cancer, and viral diseases.

The most effective herbal and natural products in treating liver diseases are summarized in Table 3.3, while other products that have been reported to be effective against liver disorders but for which little supporting evidence is available are summarized in Table 3.2. Case studies have been presented demonstrating the use of milk thistle (silymarin) in treating cirrhosis, garlic in treating acetaminophen toxicity, coenzyme Q10 in treating toxicity associated with HMGCoA reductase inhibitors, phyllanthus in treating hepatitis, and Sho-saiko-to in the prevention of hepatocellular carcinoma. Although numerous products are touted to flush the liver and cleanse the body, no well-documented controlled, clinical studies exist that either support or refute these concepts.

TABLE 3.3. Summary Table

Condition	Herb (nutritional supplement)	Mechanism of action (proposed)	Suggested dose
Cirrhosis	Milk thistle (Silymarin concentrated extract)	prevention of some metabolic effects, reduce degree of collagen deposition, stimulate liver protein synthesis, inhibition of leukotriene formation, prevention of free radical damage	420 mg to 800 mg per day in two or three divided doses
Acetaminophen toxicity	Garlic (and related organosulfur compounds)	inhibition of lipid peroxidation by scavenging free radical metabolites	
Elevated liver enzymes secondary to HMGCoA enzyme reductase inhibitors	Coenzyme Q10	antioxidant, protection against lipid peroxidation	100 mg per day (established dose for humans questioned)
Hepatitis	*Phyllanthus amarus* (pearl grass)		variation in studies secondary to differences in specific principles
Hepatocellular carcinoma (preventative)	Sho-saiko-to	promotion of liver regeneration, inhibition of abnormal cellular growth	7.5 g per day in addition to the conventional drugs

REFERENCES

1. Arias IM, Boyer JL, Fausto N, Jakoby WB, Schachter D, Shafritz BA, *The Liver: Biology and Pathobiology,* Third Edition, Raven Press, New York (1994).

2. Hobbs C, *Natural Liver Therapy: Herbs and Other Natural Remedies for a Healthy Liver,* Third Edition, Botanica Press, Santa Cruz, CA (1993).

3. Wilson JD, Braunwald E, Isselbacher KJ, Petersdorf RG, Martin JB, Fauci AS, Root RK, *Harrison's Principles of Internal Medicine,* Twelfth Edition, McGraw-Hill, New York (1991), pp. 1301-1358.

4. Dipiro JT, Talbert RL, Yee GC, Matzke GR, Wells BG, Posey LM, *Pharmacotherapy: A Pathophysiologic Approach,* Third Edition, Appleton and Lange, Stamford, CT (1997), p. 791.

5. Carithers RL, Herlong HF, Diehl AM, Shaw EW, Combes B, Fallon Hj, "Methyprednisolone therapy in patients with severe alcoholic hepatitis: A randomized multicenter trial." *Ann Intern Med,* 1989;110:685-690.

6. Dipiro JT, Talbert RL, Yee GC, Matzke GR, Wells BG, Posey LM, *Pharmacotherapy: A Pathophysiologic Approach,* Third Edition, Appleton and Lange, Stamford, CT (1997), pp. 839-840.

7. Hobbs C, *Foundations of Health: The Liver and Digestive Herbal,* Botanica Press, Capitola CA (1992), p. 124.

8. Herfindal ET, Gourley DR, Hart LL, *Clinical Pharmacy and Therapeutics,* Fifth Edition, Williams and Wilkins, Philadelphia (1992), p. 465.

9. Leung AY, Foster S, *Encyclopedia of Common Natural Ingredients Used in Food, Drugs, and Cosmetics,* Second Edition, John Wiley and Sons, Inc., New York (1996), p. 366.

10. Ferenci P, Dragosics B, Dittrich H, Frank H, Benda L, Lochs H, et al., "Randomized controlled trial of silymarin treatment in patients with cirrhosis of the liver." *J Hepatol,* 9(1), 105-113 (1989).

11. Tyler VE, *The Honest Herbal,* Third Edition, The Haworth Press, Binghamton, NY (1992), p. 210.

12. Balch JF, Balch PA, *Prescription for Nutritional Healing,* Avery Publishing Group Inc., Garden City, NY (1990), p. 139.

13. Murray MT, Pissorno JE, *Encylopedia of Natural Medicine,* Prima Publishing, Rocklin, CA (1991), p. 83.

14. Dehmlow C, Erhard J, de-Groot H, "Inhibition of Kupffer cell functions as an explanation for the hepatoprotective properties of silibinin." *Hepatology,* 23(4), 749-754 (1996).

15. Palasciano G, Portincasa P, Palmieri V, Ciani D, Vendemiale G, Altomare E, "The effect of silymarin on plasma levels of malondialdehyde in patients receiving long-term treatment with psychotropic drugs." *Curr Therap Res,* 55(5), 537-545 (1994).

16. Scheiber V, Wohlzogen I, Analysis of a certain type of 2 × 3 tables, exemplified by biopsy findings in a controlled clinical trial. *Int J Clin Pharmacol Biopharm* 1978;16(11):533-535.

17. Canini F, Bartolucci L, Cristallini E, Gradoli C, Rossi A, Ribacchi R, Valori C, "The use of silymarin in the management of the alcoholic fatty liver." *Clin Ter,* 114(4), 307-314 (1985)

18. Hobbs C, *Milk Thistle: The Liver Herb,* Second Edition, Botanica Press, Santa Cruz, CA (1992), pp. 14-24.

19. Muriel P, Mourele M, "The role of membrane composition in ATPase activities on cirrhotic rat liver: Effect of silymarin." *J Appl Toxicol,* 10(4), 281-284 (1990).

20. Koul IB, Kapil A, "Evaluation of the liver protective potential of piperine, an active principle of black and long peppers." *Planta Med,* 59(5), 413-417 (1993).

21. Kapil A, Koul IB, Banerjee SK, Gupta BD, "Antihepatotoxic effects of major diterpenoid constituents of *Andrographis paniculata.*" *Biochem Pharmacol,* 46(1), 182-185 (1993).

22. Joyeux M, Rolland A, Fleurentin J, Mortier F, Dorfman P, "tert-Butyl hydroperoxide-induced injury in isolated rat hepatocytes: A model for studying anti-hepatotoxic crude drugs." *Planta Med,* 56(2), 171-174 (1990).

23. Mereish KA, Solow R, "Effect of antihepatotoxic agents against microcystin-LR toxicity in cultured rat hepatocytes." *Pharm Res,* March 7, 256-259 (1990).

24. Hermansky SJ, Stohs SJ, Eldeen ZM, Roche VF, Mereish KA, "Evaluation of potential chemoprotectants against microcystin-LR hepatotoxicity in mice." *J Appl Toxicol,* 11(1), 65-73 (1991).

25. Valenzuela A, Guerra R, "Protective effect of the flavonoid silybin dihemisuccinate on the toxicity of phenylhydrazine on rat liver." *FEBS-Lett,* 181(2), 291-294 (Feb 25, 1985).

26. Szpunar K, Gorecki P, Wroncinski T, Iwaszkiewicz J, "Effect of silymarin on hepatotoxic action of lindane." *Herba Pol,* 22(2), 167-171 (1976).

27. Meiss R, Heinrich U, Robenek H, Themann H, "Effect of silybin on hepatic cell membranes after damage by polycyclic aromatic hydrocarbons (PAH)." *Agents-Actions,* 12(1-2), 254-257 (1982).

28. Tuchweber B, Sieck R, Trost W, "Prevention of silybin of phalloidin-induced acute hepatotoxicity." *Toxicol Appl Pharmacol,* 51(2), 265-275 (1979).

29. Agarwal R, Katiyar SK, Lundgren DW, Mukhtar H, "Inhibitory effect of sillymarin, an anti-hepatotoxic flavonoid, on 12-0-tetradecanoylphorbol-13-acetate-induced epidermal ornithine decarboxylase activity and mRNA in SENCAR mice." *Carcinogenesis,* 15(6), 1099-1103 (1994).

30. Paya M, Ferrandiz ML, Sanz MJ, Alcaraz MJ, "Effects of phenolic compounds on bromobenzene-mediated hepatotoxicity in mice." *Xenobiotica,* 23(3), 327-333 (1993).

31. Campos R, Garrido A, Guerra R, Valenzuela A, "Silybin dihemisuccinate protects against glutathione depletion and lipid peroxidation induced by acetaminophen on rat liver." *Planta Med,* 55(5), 417-419 (1989).

32. Ortenberg EA, Zhikhareva AI, Byshevskii A, "Impairment of lipid metabolism in the liver and its correction after exposure to ethanol and antitubercular agents." *Vopr Med Khim,* 31(6), 24-27 (November-December 1985).

33. Olin BR, Dombek CE, Hulbert MK, Liberti L, "Milk thistle." *The Lawrence Review of Natural Products* (March 1988), p. 2.

34. Herfindal ET, Gourley DR, Hart LL, *Clinical Pharmacy and Therapeutics,* Fifth Edition, Williams and Wilkins, Philadelphia (1992), pp. 458-459.

35. Herfindal, ET, Gourley, DR, Hart, LL, *Clinical Pharmacy and Therapeutics,* Fifth Edition, Williams and Wilkins, Philadelphia (1992), p. 57.

36. Wang EJ, Li Y, Lin M, Chen L, Stein AP, Reuhl KR, Yang CS, "Protective effects of garlic and related organosulfur compounds on acetaminophen-induced hepatoxicity in mice." *Toxicol and Appl Pharmacol* 136(1), 146-154 (1996).

37. Kim SG, Nam SY, Chung HC, Hong SY, Jung KH, "Enhanced effectiveness of dimethyl-4,4″-dimethoxy-5,6,5′,6′-dimethylene dioxyphenyl-2,2′-dicarboxylate in combination with garlic oil against experimental hepatic injury in rats and mice." *J Pharm Pharmacol,* 47(8), 678-682 (1995).

38. Nakagawa S, Yoshida S, Hirao Y, Kasuga S, Fuwa T, "Cytoprotective activity of components of garlic, ginseng and ciuwjia on hepatocyte injury induced by carbon tetrachloride in vitro." *Hiroshima J Med Sci,* 34(3), 303-309 (1985).

39. Cha CW, "A study on the effect of garlic to the heavy metal poisoning of a rat." *J Korean Med Sci,* 2(4), 213-224 (1987).

40. el-Mofty MM, Sakr SA, Essawy A, Abdel-Gawad HS, "Preventive action of garlic on aflatoxin B1-induced carcinogenesis in the toad *Bufo regularis." Nutr Cancer,* 21(1), 95-100 (1994).

41. Alnaqeeb MA, Ali M, Thonson M, Khater SH, Gomes SA, al-Hassan JM, "Histopathological evidence of protective action of garlic against collagen and arachidonic acid toxicity in rabbits." *Prostaglandins Leukot Essent Fatty Acids,* 46(4), 301-306 (1992).

42. Caldwell SH, Jeffers LJ, Narula OS, Laang EA, Reddy KR, Schiff ER, "Ancient remedies revisited: Does *Allium sativum* (garlic) palliate the hepatopulmonary syndrome?" *J Clin Gastroenterol,* 15(3), 248-250 (1992).

43. Folkers K, Langsjoen P, Willis R, Richardson P, Xia LJ, Ye CQ, Tamagawa H, "Lovastatin decreases coenzyme Q levels in humans." *Proc Natl Acad Sci USA,* 87(22), 8931-8934 (1990).

44. Satoh K, Yamato A, Nakai T, Hoshi K, Ichihara K, "Effects of 3-hydroxy-3-methylglutryl coenzyme A reductase inhibitors on mitochondrial respiration in ischaemic dog hearts." *Br J Pharmacol,* 116(2), 1894-1898 (1995).

45. Loop RA, Anthony M, Willis RA, Folkers K, "Effects of ethanol, lovastatin and coenzyme Q10 treatment on antioxidants and TBA reactive material in liver of rats." *Mol Aspects Med,* 15 suppl, s195-206 (1994).

46. Farmer JA, Gotto AM Jr, "Currently available hypolipidaemic drugs and future therapeutic developments." *Baillieres Clin Endocrinol Metab,* 9(4), 825-847 (1995).

47. Sewester CS, Olin BR, Hebel SK, Hagemann RC (eds.), *Facts and Comparisons,* St. Louis, MO, p. 171s.

48. Walravens PA, Greene C, Frerman FE, "Lovastatin, isoprenes, and myopathy." *Lancet,* 2 (November 4, 1989), 1097-1098.

49. Loop RA, Anthony M, Willis RA, Folkers K, "Effects of ethanol, lovastatin and coenzyme Q10 treatment on antioxidants and TBA reactive material in liver of rats." *Mol Aspects Med,* 15 suppl., 195-206 (1994).

50. Chen H, Tappel A, "Protection by multiple antioxidants against lipid peroxidation in rat liver homogenate." *Lipids,* 31(1), 47-50 (1996).

51. Langsjoen H, Langsjoen P, Langsjoen P, Willis R, Folkers K, "Usefulness of coenzyme Q10 in clinical cardiology: A long-term study." *Mol Aspects Med,* 115 suppl., s165-175 (1994).

52. Langjoen PH, Folkers K, Lyson K, Muratsu K, Lyson T, Langsjoen P, "Pronounced increase of survival of patients with cardiomyopathy when treated with coenzyme Q_{10} and conventional therapy." *Int J Tissue React,* 12(3), 163-168 (1990).

53. Syamasundar KV, Singh B, Thakur RS, Husain A, Kiso Y, Hikino H, "Antihepatotoxic principles of *Phyllanthus niruri* herbs." *J Ethnopharmacol,* 14(1), 41-44 (1985).

54. Reddy BP, Murthy VN, Venkateshwarlu V, Kokate CK, Rambhau D, "Antihepatotoxic activity of *Phyllanthus niruri, Tinospora cordifolia* and *Ricinus communis.*" *Indian Drugs,* 30(7), 338-341 (1993).

55. Prakash A, Satyan KS, Wahi SP, Singh RP, "Comparative hepatoprotective activity of three species, *P. urinaria, P. niruri* and *P. simplex,* on carbon tetrachloride induced liver injury in the rat." *Phytother Res,* 9(8), 594-596 (1995).

56. Gulati RK, Agarwal S, Agrawal SS, "Hepatoprotective studies on *Phyllanthus emblica* Linn. and quercetin." *Indian J Exp Biol,* 33(4), 261-268 (1995).

57. Blumberg BS, Milman I, Venkateswaran PS, Thyagarajan SP, "Hepatitis B virus and hepatocellular carcinoma treatment of HBV carriers with *Phyllanthus amarus.*" *Cancer Detect Prev,* 14(2), 195-201 (1989).

58. Yeh SF, Hong CY, Huang YL, Liu TY, Choo KB, Chou CK, "Effect of an extract from *Phyllanthus amarus* on hepatitis B surface antigen gene expression in human hepatoma cells." *Antiviral Res,* 20(3), 185-192 (1993).

59. Munshi A, Mehrotra R, Ramesh R, Panda SK, "Evaluation of anti-hepadnavirus activity of *Phyllanthus amarus* and *Phyllanthus maderaspatensis* in duck hepatitis B virus carrier Pekin ducks." *J Med Virol,* 41(4), 275-281 (1993).

60. Wang M, Cheng H, Li Y, Meng L, Zhao G, Mai K, "Herbs of the genus *Phyllanthus* in the treatment of chronic hepatitis B: Observation with three preparations from different geographic sites." *J Lab Clin Med,* 126(4), 350-352 (1995).

61. Yano H, Mizoguchi A, Fukuda K, Haramaki M, Ogasawara S, Momosaki S, Kojiro M, "The herbal medicine Sho-saiko-to inhibits proliferation of cancer cell lines by inducing apoptosis and arrest at the G_0/G_1 phase." *Cancer Res,* 54(2), 448-454 (1994).

62. Oka H, Yamamoto S, Kuroki T, Harihara S, Marumo T, Kim SR, Monna T, Kobayashi K, Tango T, "Prospective study of chemoprevention of hepatocellular carcinoma with Sho-saiko-to (TJ-9)." *Cancer,* 76(5), 743-749 (1995).

63. Yamashiki M, Nishimura A, Nomoto M, Suzuki H, Kosaka Y, "Herbal medicine 'Sho-saiko-to' induces tumor necrosis factor-alpha and granulocyte colony-stimulating factor in vitro in peripheral blood mononuclear cells of patients with hepatocellular carcinoma." *J Gastroenterol Hepatol,* 11(2), 137-142 (1996).

64. Yamashiki M, Kosaka Y, Nishimura A, Okuda Y, Hamaguchi K, Kondo I, Ichida F, "The herbal medicine Sho-saiko-to improves cytokine production of peripheral blood mononuclear cells in patients with liver cirrhosis." *Curr Ther Res Clin Exp,* 54(1), 86-97 (1993).

65. Sakaguchi S, Tsutsumi E, Yokota K, "Preventive effects of a traditional Chinese medicine (Sho-saiko-to) against oxygen toxicity and membrane damage during endotoxemia." *Biol Pharm Bull,* 16(8), 782-786 (1993).

66. Whitaker J, "A 'universal antioxidant' that saves lives," *Health and Healing: Tomorrow's Healing Medicine Today,* 6(10), 1-2 (1996).

67. Scherban AN, Korkhov SI, Nazarov NV, Krivitskii NM, Kislukhin VV, Kopytov SV, Kholodov IG, "The use of a vitamin metabolite complex for correcting the disorders in systemic and organ hemodynamics during liver resection under conditions of acute blood loss." *Patol Fiziol Eksp Ter,* July-August (4), 28-29 (1990).

68. Ramakrishnan N, Wolfe WW, Catravas GN, "Radioprotection of hematopoietic tissues in mice by lipoic acid." *Radiat Res* 130(3), 360-365 (1992).

69. Weed SS, *Healing Wise,* Ash Tree Publishing, New York (1989), p. 141.

70. Hobbs C, *Foundations of Health: The Liver and Digestive Herbal,* Botanica Press, Capitola, CA (1992), p. 251.

71. Mowrey DB, *The Scientific Validation of Herbal Medicine,* Keats Publishing, Inc., New Canaan, CT (1986), p. 179.

72. Barney DP, *Clinical Applications of Herbal Medicine,* Woodland Publishing, Inc., Pleasant Grove, UT (1996), pp. 60-61.

73. Tyler VE, *The Honest Herbal,* Third Edition, The Haworth Press, Binghamton, NY (1992), p. 110.

74. DerMarderosian A (Ed.), "Dandelion." *The Lawrence Review of Natural Products,* Facts and Comparisons, St. Louis, MO (December, 1987).

75. Sreejayan N, Rao MN, "Curcuminoids as potent inhibitors of lipid peroxidation." *J Pharm Pharmacol,* 46(12), 1013-1016 (1994).

76. Oetari S, Sudibyo M, Commandeur JN, Samhoedi R, Vermeulen NP, "Effects of curcumin on cytochrome P450 and glutathione S-transferase activities in rat liver." *Biochem Pharmacol,* 51(1), 39-45 (1996).

77. Mukundan MA, Chacko MC, Annapurna VV, Krishnaswamy K, "Effect of turmeric and curcumin on BP-DNA adducts." *Carcinogenesis,* 14(3), 493-496 (1993).

78. Soni KB, Rajan A, Kuttan R, "Reversal of aflatoxin-induced liver damage by turmeric and curcumin." *Cancer Lett,* 66(2), 115-121 (1992).

79. Babu PS, Srinivasan K, "Influence of dietary curcumin and cholesterol on the progression of experimentally induced diabetes in albino rat." *Mol Cell Biochem,* 152(1), 13-21 (1995).

80. Reddy AC, Lokesh BR, "Effect of dietary turmeric *(Curcuma longa)* on iron-induced lipid peroxidation in the rat liver." *Food Chem Toxicol,* 32(3), 279-283 (1994).

81. Ammon HP, Wahl MA, "Pharmacology of Curcuma longa." *Planta Med,* 57(1), 1-7 (1991).

82. Dundass H, "When East meets West." *Can Pharm J,* 127 (April), 134-136, 141 (1994).

83. Wang X, "Understanding traditional chinese medicine." *Protocol Botanical Med,* 1(1), 11-12 (Summer, 1995).

84. Chen JX, Yang WY, Liang R, "Preliminary study on pathophysiology of liver-qi deficiency syndrome." *Chung Kuo Chung Hsi I Chieh Ho Tsa Chih,* 15(2), 67-70 (1995).

85. Anselmo P, Brooks JS, *Ayurvedic Secrets to Longevity and Total Health,* Prentice-Hall, Englewood Cliffs, NJ (1996), p. 1.

86. Gerson S, "Understanding Ayurveda." *Protocol Botanical Med,* 1(1) 13-17 (Summer, 1995).

87. Heyn B, *Ayurveda: The Indian Art of Natural Medicine and Life Extension,* Healing Arts Press, Rochester, VT (1990).

88. Willard T, *Herbs: Their Clinical Uses,* Wild Rose College of Natural Healing, Ltd., Calgary, Alberta, Canada (1996), pp. 29,118,180.

89. Speisky H, Cassels BK, "Boldo and Boldine: An emerging case of natural drug development." *Pharmacol Res,* 29(1), 1-12 (1994).

90. Hobbs C, Foster S, "Echinacea: A literature review." *HerbalGram,* Supplement #30 (1994).

91. Blumenthal M, McCaleb R, Johnston B, Close B, "Herbs may help metabolize toxins." *HerbalGram,* 17(3) (Summer, 1988).

Chapter 4

Herbal Medicines
for Colds and Flu

Wallace J. Murray, PhD

INTRODUCTION

Over 120 strains of virus are known to lead to a set of symptomatologies known as the "common cold," also called acute coryza, acute rhinitis, or catarrh. These highly contagious, acute infections are localized in the upper respiratory tract, and, depending on the severity, the symptoms can be any of the following. One of the first symptoms is nasal congestion and discharge accompanied by sneezing. The discharge is initially watery, but becomes thicker with time. Pharyngitis, an irritating, sometimes referred to as "tickling," sensation in a dry or sore throat, is another symptom. Since pharyngitis can be the result of more serious diseases such as streptococcal infection ("strep throat"), scarlet fever, tonsillitis, or measles, a physician's evaluation is recommended. Nasal discharge ("postnasal drip") and sore throat give rise to a cough, which is initially a dry cough, turning later to a productive cough. Laryngitis with hoarseness and loss of voice may also occur. Hot or warm sensations, characterized as a "low-grade fever," also occur in the common cold. A headache may be an accompanying symptom.[1,2,3,4]

The common cold is considered a less virulent infection than influenza or "flu," which is caused by a similar series of viruses. Higher fevers are seen with influenza. In addition to the symptoms of a cold, symptoms accompanying the flu may be malaise, joint and muscle aches and, sometimes, gastrointestinal disturbances.[3,4] Both the common cold and the flu are self-limiting diseases; they usually run their course in five to seven days. However, secondary bacterial diseases may cause complications, and some symptoms, such as a cough, may persist for weeks.[4]

Since cures for the common cold are nonexistent, treatment consists principally of relieving symptoms.[3,5] Table 4.1 summarizes the over-the-counter (OTC) and prescription drugs commonly used to treat the symptoms of colds and flu. Many drugs are combination products, and some of the active ingredients may not be in therapeutic doses and some may antagonize the action of others.[3] Recommended symptomatic treatment is to use one or more single products at the recommended dosage.[3]

HERBAL MEDICINES

The most effective herbal treatments for the symptoms of colds and flu are those used to treat coughs.[4] Most of these fall into the antitussive and expectorant categories.

Case Study: Coltsfoot

TF, a 24-year-old female, visits your pharmacy complaining that she has had the flu for the past few days, and now she has an itchy throat and has fits of coughing spells. She does not want to use any of the usual OTC medications because they "dry her out" and either make her very drowsy or very "nervous." In any case, when she uses them, she usually ends up feeling "icky." She says her grandmother has recommended the use of coltsfoot for her sore throat and cough. What do you say to her?

Discussion: Mucilaginous Antitussives

Coltsfoot has a long history of usage as an herbal antitussive.[4,6] The antitussive action of many herbals, such as coltsfoot, is due to their mucilage component. Mucilages are polysaccharides secreted by plant cells. Someone with a pharmacy or science background would refer to them as hydrophilic colloids; a nutritionist would categorize them as soluble fibers. In any case, in water they form a viscous gel. If used in a tea, herbals containing mucilages form a coating over the surface of the mucous membranes, thus preventing mechanical irritation and consequently the urge to cough.[4] Unfortunately, coltsfoot is an herbal that, in addition to its mucilage component, also contains pyrrolizidine alkaloids (PAs).[7,8,9]

Pyrrolizidine alkaloids are present in a number of plant species used in African, Caribbean, and South American countries as food sources or as medicinal "bush teas." Notable plant species with high levels of PAs include: *Crotolaria, Heliotropium,* and *Senecio.*[10] Hepatotoxicity associated with their

TABLE 4.1. Commonly Used Allopathic Medicines for the Relief of Cold and Flu Symptoms

Symptom	Agents usually used or recommended	Pharmacologic or therapeutic effects	Adverse effects and cautions
Nasal Discharge (Rhinorrhea)	Antihistamines (e.g., diphenhydramine, doxylamine, pyrilamine, chlorphenira-mine)	Anticholinergic effect (dry up nasal and pharyngeal secretions)	Sedation; paradoxical hyperac-tivity in children
Nasal Congestion	Sympathomimetics (topical nasal sprays include ephedrine, naphazoline, phenylephrine; oral products contain phenylephrine, phenylpropanolamine, pseudoephedrine)	α-Adrenergic agonists (vasoconstric-tion of nasal microvasculature of engorged nasal mucosa; drainage of sinuses and clearing of airways)	Tolerance developed to nasal sprays leading to rebound congestion, hypertension, restlessness, tachycardia, nausea, vomiting, anorexia
Cough (Nonproductive)	Antitussives (e.g., prescription narcotic agents such as codeine, hydrocodone; OTC such as dextromethorphan)	Depresses cough reflex in medulla	Narcotic agents are potentially addicting, sedating, and may cause constipation; Dextrome-thorphan sometimes causes GI distress
Cough (Productive)	Expectorants (e.g., guaifenesin, terpin hydrate, syrup of ipecac, KI)	Decreases sputum viscosity to facilitate expectoration	Evidence for efficacy not con-vincing; steam or cool mist may help liquify secretions

Table 4.1 (continued)

Symptom	Agents usually used or recommended	Pharmacologic or therapeutic effects	Adverse effects and cautions
Sore Throat (Pharyngitis) or Laryngitis	Warm saline gargles, anesthetics (e.g., solutions of benzocaine, phenol salts); demulcents (elm bark, tincture of benzoin, various lozenges); nonsugar candies	Soothes mucous membranes	None
Fever and Headache	Analgesics/antipyretics (e.g., acetaminophen, aspirin, ibuprofen)	Antipyretic effect of these agents not fully understood	Avoid aspirin in children (Reye's syndrome); aspirin may cause GI distress and has potential for hypersensitivity reactions

Source: Huls CS, Mullenix TA, Prince RA: "Upper Respiratory Infections." In *Clinical Pharmacy and Therapeutics,* Fifth Edition, Herfindal ET, Gourleyk DR, Hart LL, Eds., Williams & Wilkens, Baltimore, MD, 1992; Bryant BG, Lombardi TP: "Cold, Cough, and Allergy Products." In *Handbook of Nonprescription Drugs,* Ninth Edition, American Pharmaceutical Association, Washington, DC, 1990.

consumption is well documented and is attributed to their constituent pyrrolizidine alkaloids.[11,12] Pyrrolizidine alkaloids are divided into two categories based on the saturation of the nitrogen-containing heterocyclic nucleus. An unsaturated nucleus (found in borage, coltsfoot, comfrey, or life root) is considered toxic; a saturated nucleus (found in echinacea) is considered nontoxic. The levels of PAs in borage and coltsfoot are considered too low to be of clinical significance. However, the dangers associated with acute or chronic low-dose exposures have not been evaluated. Numerous animal studies have shown comfrey to be hepatotoxic, and two cases of human hepatotoxicity have been reported.[12,13]

Unsaturated (Toxic) Pyrrolizidine   Saturated (Non-toxic) Pyrrolizidine

The hepatotoxity of the PAs is hypothesized as being dependent on their metabolic conversion to a fully aromatized pyrrole derivative. Only the unsaturated PAs can undergo this conversion, accounting for their toxicity. The pyrroles thus formed are chemically reactive and serve as biological alkylating agents. This is depicted as follows:

$X, Y = SH_2, NH_2, OH$

Hepatotoxic Covalenty
Bound to Cellular Nucleophiles

The underlying toxicity of these compounds attack by cellular nucleophiles. These reactions are similar to those found in toxicity associated with acetaminophen overdose. In light of the PA content of coltsfoot, and the absence of adequate long-range studies, the use of coltsfoot should not be recommended.

Other herbals that contain mucilaginous polysaccharides include: iceland moss, marshmallow root, mullein flowers, plantain leaves, and slippery elm.[4,6] Teas and lozenges containing these herbals are available. Lozenges are the preferred dosage form as they provide a sustained release of mucilage to the back of the throat.

Expectorants

As colds or flu persist, irritation of the bronchioles occurs, resulting in an increase in the mucoprotein and mucopolysaccharide content of the secretions, creating a more viscous fluid (phlegm). This and other factors reduce the ability of the celia to move and reduce the ability of coughing to move the thickened secretions out. Expectorants reduce the viscosity of the secretions, allowing the secretions to move out with a "productive cough." Some herbals (e.g., ipecac and lobelia) are categorized as *nauseant-expectorants* as they contain alkaloids which, through reflex stimulation of the vomiting center mediated by the vagus nerve, cause an increase in bronchial secretions. The *volatile herbals* (e.g., peppermint, anise, fennel, horehound, eucalyptus leaves, thyme) exert a direct stimulating effect on the bronchial tree by means of local irritation. A third type of expectorant is called *surface-tension modifiers*. These herbals exert their effects through their saponin constituents. Supposedly, the saponins in these herbals reduce the surface tension of the secretions, enabling them to separate from the mucous membrane so that they can be removed by expectoration. Senega snakeroot is the only herbal recommended in this category.[4]

For patient TF, recommend a mucilaginous antitussive such as slippery elm and any of a number of lozenges that contain the volatile oils of peppermint (menthol), anise (anethol), or others.

IMMUNOSTIMULANTS

Case Study: Echinacea

DR, a male patient in his mid-forties, approaches you at your community pharmacy and says he is beginning to feel the achiness that he associates with the first stages of the flu. He further says he has been reading that echinacea can help to prevent or treat viral infections, and he wonders whether he should try it. He notes several dosage forms are available, and he asks what you recommend. What do you tell him?

Discussion

Echinacea had its origins of use in Euro-American medicine in Nebraska.[4] The settlers in the Central Plains adopted its use from the traditional medicine of Native Americans. A small but growing body of evidence is evolving to support echinacea's use as a wound healing agent (topical) and as an immunostimulant (internal).

Most evidence comes from studies of its effects in laboratory animals.[14,15,16] When ethanolic extracts are administered orally to rats, phagocytosis is enhanced significantly. In mice, ethanolic extracts induced generalized immunostimulation as assessed by increases in phagocytic, metabolic, and bactericidal activities of peritoneal macrophages. Echinacea increases phagocytosis and promotes the activity of the lymphocytes, resulting in the increased release of tumor necrosis factor (TNF).[4] The identity of the agents in echinacea responsible for these effects is under investigation and it may be that several principles acting in concert are responsible. A high molecular weight polysaccharide component and an alkamide fraction have been found to activate phagocytosis; another constituent, arabinogalactan, promotes release of TNF.[17]

The hyperbole associated with echinacea use makes it difficult to separate fact from fiction. Tyler appears to prefer the use of the hydroalcoholic extracts over the capsulated forms. There is anecdotal evidence that the immune response is associated with stimulation of the oral lymphatic system and suggests holding or swishing the hydroalcoholic extract in the mouth before swallowing. The extract has the double attraction of being useful for the healing of hard-to-heal, superficial wounds.[4,18]

Use of echinacea in patients with severe systemic infections such as tuberculosis, collagen diseases, and multiple sclerosis is to be avoided. Echinacea may interfere with immunosuppressive therapy. It is further recommended that echinacea use be restricted to ten days to two weeks and never over eight successive weeks. Echinacea possesses saturated pyrrolizidine alkaloids that are not believed to be toxic. In light of the lack of safety information and toxicity data, its use during pregnancy and lactation should be avoided.[4,6]

Vitamin C

In 1970, Nobel laureate Linus Pauling authored a controversial book that championed the ingestion of large amounts of vitamin C—doses 30 to 200 times that recommended by the National Research Council—to prevent and treat the common cold. Since that time, many have taken his ideas quite seriously. Pauling advocated taking between 2 and 9 g of vitamin C per day (RDA is 60 mg/d).[19]

Many studies have attempted to verify these claims. For example, in 1982 a study was done in which identical twins were given either 1 g of vitamin C (ascorbic acid) per day or they were given a sugar pill.[20] In this trial, the two groups' frequency of contracting a cold was almost identical, although it was reported that the duration of the cold was 19 percent shorter in the group receiving the ascorbic acid supplement. The study concluded that vitamin C may have a small effect on the duration of a cold. Similar studies have come to the same conclusion: taking vitamin C at a dose of around 1 g per day may have a slight effect in decreasing the severity of a cold.[20]

In none of the studies are the doses as high as those recommended by Pauling. He was of the opinion that doses had to be at least 2 g per day to have an effect. However, doses this large can have detrimental effects.[21] Specifically, the chemistry of the kidney and blood chemistry profiles may be altered. Effects noted with 1 to 3 g doses of vitamin C are interference with oral anticoagulant therapy; increases in serum concentrations on oral contraceptives; increased GI absorption of aspirin, iron, zinc, and calcium; decreased therapeutic response to tricyclic antidepressants; interference with several diagnostic tests such as Clinitest, Testape, and the Hemocult home-test kit.[22]

Zinc Lozenges

Clinical studies have shown that ionic zinc (Zn^{2+}) dissolved in the mouth significantly shortens the manifestations of the common cold.[23] The mechanism of action is unknown. Zinc ions are proposed to bind to the rhinovirus, thus preventing the virus from replicating.[24] Zinc works at the source of the common cold rather than treating the symptoms as decongestants, antihistamines, and other over-the-counter cold remedies do.

In their study, Mossad and colleagues concluded that volunteers given the zinc lozenges recovered from the common cold nearly twice as fast as those given a placebo. The study consisted of 100 participants instructed to suck on a zinc lozenge every two hours, starting within twenty-four hours of their first symptoms. Half the subjects were given Cold-Eeze and the other half were given a placebo that tasted like zinc. Those given the zinc recovered completely in a median of 4.4 days, compared with 7.6 days for the placebo group. Some side effects did occur during the study. Eighty percent of the participants complained about the taste, and 20 percent suffered nausea during the study.[23]

Zinc is required for inhibition of rhinoviral replication by preventing the formation of viral proteins. Elevated concentrations of zinc in and around the nasal cavity are proposed to help in the adhesion to binding sites on the rhinovirus surface, thereby preventing the virus from binding to the cells. Larger than normal concentrations of zinc are needed to prevent infection because zinc adheres to capillary walls also.[24]

According to the studies cited, zinc gluconate produces a significant reduction in the duration and severity of symptoms, even as much as four days. This effect is more noticeable when zinc lozenges are taken every two hours while awake for the duration of the cold. Also, a greater effect can be seen when treatment is begun within the first twenty-four hours of symptoms.

Some side effects can occur while consuming the zinc lozenges. A small percentage of the population may experience nausea from the zinc. Some people may not like the taste of zinc lozenges and refuse therapy because of it. (See Table 4.2 for a summary of herbal medicines for colds and flu.)

TABLE 4.2. Herbal Medicines for Colds and Flu

Herbal medicine	Use	Reported active constituents	Precautions and interactions	Usual dosing
Anise (*Pimpinella anisum*)	The volatile oil is reported to have expectorant action. Used in bronchial catarrh, pertussis, spasmodic cough	Volatile oils, especially anethol	Anethol, the principal constituent, is said to have sympathomimetic effects. Polymerized anethol is reportedly estrogenic. May cause contact dermatitis. Since reportedly an abortifacient and lactogenic, avoid use in pregnancy and lactation.	Oil: .05-.2 mL TID
Boneset (*Eupatorium perfoliatum*)	Antipyretic; influenza	Sesquiterpene lactones	A member of the Asteraceae family (e.g., chamomile, feverfew); individuals with hypersensitivity to this family should avoid its use.	Herb: 1-2 g QD
Coltsfoot (*Tussilago farfara*)	Antitussive, demulcent	Mucilages. Contains pyrrolizidine alkaloids.	Pyrrolizidine alkaloids are known hepatotoxicants. Has abortifacient effects; should not be taken during pregnancy and lactation.	Dried root/rhizome: 2.4 g in decoction TID
Echinacea (*Echinacea augustifolia*, *E. pallida*); Purple cornflower (*E. purpurea*) is a different species with similar properties.	Effectiveness proven for prophylaxis and treatment of cold and flu symptoms. Appears to work by stimulating phagocytosis.	Polysaccharides, polyacetylenes, and sesquiterpene esters are reported to increase phagocytosis.	Continuous use (> 6-8 weeks) may lead to immunosuppression; contraindicated in autoimmune diseases. Parenteral use not recommended (can cause chills, fever, nausea, vomiting, allergies).	Concentrations of chemical constituents in commercial products can vary. Maximum adult dose is 6-9 mL of expressed fresh juice or 1.5-7.5 mL of tincture or 2-5 g of dried root. Tincture is preferred as not all the active constituents are water soluble. Use no more than 6-8 weeks.

74

	Uses	Active Constituents	Cautions/Side Effects	Dosing
Feverfew (*Tanacetum parthenium*)	Used primarily for the prophylactic treatment of migraine (spasmolytic effect on cerebral vessels). Has been used to treat fevers and menstrual problems.	Parthenolide and other sesquiterpene lactones	Do not use during pregnancy (stimulates menstruation) or lactation or in children under 2 yrs. May have GI effects. Chewing fresh leaves can lead to mouth ulceration. May interact with anticoagulants to increase bleeding. Caution in individuals hypersensitive to Asteraceae family (see Echinacea).	Concentrations of active plant constituents in commercial products vary. Adult dose is 125 mg dried leaves (parthenolide content no less than 0.2%) QD or BID.
Horehound (*Marrubium vulgare*)	Controversial use as expectorant, antitussive, cough suppressant, digestive aid, appetite stimulant. Hypoglycemia shown in rabbits.	Volatile oils; marrubiin, a diterpene lactone	No side effects reported in humans. Large doses have produced cardiac irregularities.	Adult dose is 2 g (2 heaping tsps) of dried cut herb, in 240 mL of boiling water. Take 3-5 times per day (up to 0.75-1L per day).
Siberian Ginseng (*Eleutherococcus senticosus*); same family but not the same species as *Panax ginseng* (Korean ginseng) or *Panax quinquefolium* (American ginseng)	Injectable form being studied to increase levels of immunocompetent cells (T-cells). Use not supported by adequate clinical studies. Not proven to increase endurance.	Eleutherosides	No adverse reactions reported; toxicity reports attributed to adulterants. May produce aggressive behavior in animals.	Frequently mislabeled or adulterated. For this reason, use is not recommended.

TABLE 4.2 (continued)

Herbal medicine	Use	Reported active constituents	Precautions and interactions	Usual dosing
Slippery Elm (Ulmus rubra)	Acts as a demulcent and an emollient to treat sore throats, gastritis, colitis, gastric or duodenal ulcers.	Mucilaginous antitussive	Pollen can be an allergen. May cause contact dermatitis.	Adult dose is 0.5-2 g of powdered bark steeped in 10 parts hot water (5-20 mL). Lozenges also available. Liquid extract dose is 5 mL TID.
White Willow Salix purpurea, S. fragilis, S. daphnoides contain the most salicin; S. albas is also used.	Used as an analgesic and antipyretic. Salicin, the active component, is converted to salicylic acid; likely to provide subtherapeutic doses.	Salicin (A salicyate)	May show adverse reactions similar to salicylates. Not shown to affect platelet function or to interact with anticoagulants.	Concentrations of salicin and other salicylates in commercial products vary. Longer time of onset and longer duration of action than salicylic acid. Difficult to achieve therapeutic levels by using plant alone.

Source: Anderson LJ, Patriarca PA, Hierholzer JC, Noble GR, Viral respiratory illnesses, Med Clin N Am 67:1009-1030 (1983).

REFERENCES

1. Anderson LJ, Patriarca PA, Hierholzer JC, Noble GR: Viral respiratory illnesses. *Med Clin N Am 67*:1009-1030 (1983).

2. Tyrrell DAJ, Cohen S, Schlarb JE: Signs and symptoms in common colds. *Epidemiol Infect 111*:143-156 (1993).

3. Huls CS, Mullenix TA, Prince RA: "Upper Respiratory Infections." In *Clinical Pharmacy and Therapeutics*, Fifth Edition, Herfindal ET, Gourley DR, Hart LL, Eds., Williams & Wilkins, Baltimore, MD, 1992, pp. 132-142.

4. Tyler VE: *Herbs of Choice: The Therapeutic Use of Phytomedicinals*, The Haworth Press, Binghamton, NY, 1994.

5. Bryant BG and Lombardi TP: "Cough, Cold and Allergy Products." In *Handbook of Nonprescription Drugs*, Ninth Edition, American Pharmaceutical Association, Washington, DC, 1990.

6. Newall CA, Anderson LA, Phillipson JD: *Herbal Medicines: A Guide for Health-Care Professionals*, Pharmaceutical Press, London, 1996.

7. Borka L, Onshuus J: Senkirkine contents in the leaves of *Tussilago farfara* L. *Medd-Nor-Farm-Selsk 41*(3):165-168 (1979).

8. Sener B, Ergun F: Pyrrolizidine alkaloids from *Tussilago farfara* L. *Gazi Univ Eczacilik Fak Derg 10*(2):137-141 (1993).

9. Roder E, Wiedenfeld H, Jost EJ: Tussilagine—a new pyrrolizidine alkaloid from *Tussilago farfara Planta Med 41*:99-102 (1981).

10. Huxtable RJ: New aspects of the toxicology and pharmacology of pyrrolizidine alkaloids. *Pharmacol 10*:159-167 (1979).

11. McLean EK: The toxic actions of pyrrolizidine (Senecio) alkaloids. *Pharmacol Rev 22*:429-483 (1970).

12. Huxtable RJ, Luthy J, Zweifel U: Toxicity of comfrey-pepsin preparations. *New Engl J Med 315*:1095 (1986).

13. Ridker PM, McDermott WV: Comfrey herb tea and hepatic veno-occlusive disease. *Lancet i*:657-658 (1989).

14. Houghton PJ: Echinacea. *Pharm J 253*:342-343 (1994).

15. Hobbs C: Echinacea—a literature review. *HerbalGram No. 30*:33-47 (1994).

16. Miovich M, Ed.: *The Echinacea Handbook*, Eclectic Medical Publications, Portland, OR, 1989.

17. Stimpel M, Proksch A, Wagner H, Lohmann-Matthes ML: Macrophage activation and induction of macrophage cytotoxicity by purified polysaccharide fractions from the plant *Echinacea purpurea. Infection Immunity 46*:845-849 (1984).

18. Tyler VE: What pharmacists should know about herbal remedies. *American Pharmacy NS36*:29-35 (1996).

19. Beaton: Vitamin C and the common cold. *Can Med Assoc J 105*:355-357 (1971).

20. Carr AB, Einstein R, Lai LY, Martin NG, Starmer GA: Vitamin C and the common cold: Using identical twins as controls. *Med J Austral 2*: 411-412 (1982).

21. Barnes LA: Safety considerations with high ascorbic acid dosage. *Ann NY Acad Sci 258*:523-528 (1975).

22. Holbrook JM, McCarter DN: "General Nutrition." In *Clinical Pharmacy and Therapeutics*, Fifth Edition, Herfindal ET, Gourley DR, Hart LL, Eds., Williams & Wilkins, Baltimore, MD, 1992, pp. 74-87.

23. Mossad SB, Macknin ML, Medendorp SV, Mason P: Zinc gluconate lozenges for treating the common cold. a randomized, double-blind, placebo-controlled study. *Ann Int Med 125(2)*:81-88 (1996).

24. Novick SG, Godfrey JC, Godfrey NJ, Wilder, HR: How does zinc modify the common cold? Clinical observations and implications regarding mechanisms of action. *Med Hypoth 46(3)*:295-302 (March 1996).

Chapter 5

Herbal Medications
for Gastrointestinal Problems

Wallace J. Murray, PhD

INTRODUCTION

One of the more common uses of herbal medications is for various digestive system problems. This chapter reviews some herbal medicines used for the treatment of (1) nausea and vomiting resulting principally from motion sickness; (2) indigestion or "heartburn"; (3) diarrhea; and (4) constipation. Table 5.1 summarizes some of the common herbals and OTC preparations available for the treatment of these gastrointestinal (GI) ailments.[1-4]

TABLE 5.1. Herbals and OTC Medications for Various GI Ailments

Condition	Herbal	OTC
Nausea/vomiting	Ginger	Emetrol Dramamine
Indigestion/ heartburn	Licorice Deglycyrrhizinated licorice Peppermint	Tums/Rolaids Antacids Pepcid AC Tagamet Zantac
Diarrhea	Bilberry	Immodium AD
Constipation	Psyllium Senna/Cascara	Metamucil Dulcolax Docusate Sodium Senna/Cascara

CASE STUDY 1:
GINGER FOR USE IN MOTION SICKNESS

A female patient in her mid-twenties has been examining the herbals section of the community pharmacy in which you serve as an intern. She approaches you with a bottle of ginger in her hands. She says that she is driving to San Francisco from Omaha and suffers from motion sickness. She has used dimenhydrinate (Dramamine) in the past to control her motion sickness, but it makes her drowsy, and since she is going to share the driving responsibilities with her roommate, she does not want to use it. She has read that ginger can be used to control the nausea and vomiting associated with motion sickness. She asks you if that is true, should she use ginger, and what are the side effects? What do you tell her?

Discussion

Zingiber officinale, commonly known as ginger, grows in warm climates such as India, Jamaica, and China. The part of the plant that is used for its therapeutic benefits is the rhizome. It is aromatic and a source of the dried powder spice. Ginger is used as a carminative, stimulant, diuretic, and for its antiemetic properties.[1-3,5]

The aroma of ginger is due to the volatile oil (1 to 3 percent bisabolene and zingiberene). The pharmacologically active compounds are contained within the oleoresin and include gingerol and shogaol. Both possess cardiotonic activity with positive inotropic effects on animal hearts. Shogaol is the more potent of the two compounds and has major antitussive properties compared to dihydrocodeine phosphate.[5] Shogaol is produced by the degradation of the gingerols and formed during drying and extraction. It decreases GI motility when given IV but increases GI motility when orally administered. Shogaols are twice as pungent as the gingerols, which explains why dried ginger is more potent than fresh. Both shogaol and gingerol are cardiotonic at high doses and cardiodepressant at lower doses. Gingerol is a potent inhibitor of prostaglandin synthesis.[6] The major components of ginger oil are sesquiterpine hydrocarbons, zingiberene, and bisabolene.

Not much is known about the pharmacology of ginger in humans. Ginger has been the subject of several clinical trials to assess efficacy in treating motion sickness, with positive results. A single double-blind study was conducted to compare the effects of 940 mg of powdered ginger root, 100 mg of dimenhydrinate (Dramamine), and a placebo for the prevention of motion sickness.[7] Thirty-six subjects were given preparations and placed blindfolded in a rotating chair. The results were as follows:

Compound	Average Time on Chair
Ginger	5.5 minutes
Dimenhydrinate	3.5 minutes
Placebo	1.5 minutes

Half of the subjects given ginger stayed on the chair for the full six minutes of the test. Nobody in the other two groups completed the test. In general, it took longer for the group given ginger to begin feeling sick, but once the vomiting center was activated, sensations of nausea and vomiting progressed at the same rate in all three groups. Other studies have shown that ginger is effective in relieving seasickness.[8] German authorities have subsequently concluded that 2 to 4 grams per day of ginger is effective for preventing motion sickness and useful as a digestive aid.[2]

In experimental rats, ethanol and acetone extracts of the dried rhizome inhibited gastric secretion and produced antiulcer effects.[9] Other reported effects of ginger are as a cardiotonic, antipyretic, analgesic, antitussive, and sedative.[2,3,10,11] Ginger is warming and stimulating, promoting gastric secretion and aiding absorption of food. It is excellent for easing indigestion, colic, and flatulence. Ginger reportedly alleviates the nausea and vomiting resulting from cancer chemotherapy.[10,11] Because it also produces stimulating effects on the heart and circulation it is a good choice for chronic cold hands and feet.

Unlike antihistamines which act on the CNS directly, the effects of ginger in decreasing motion sickness are said to be due to the compounds working directly on the GI tract. Adverse effects are not reported. Due to its multiple effects on platelet aggregation and possible prolongation of bleeding times, ginger should be used with caution in patients on oral anticoagulant therapy and its use avoided in pregnancy or during lactation.[1,4]

For this patient, the use of ginger to control her motion sickness seems appropriate.

CASE STUDY 2:
LICORICE AND DEGLYCYRRHIZINATED LICORICE

A 58-year-old male patient has been recently diagnosed with congestive heart failure and he has been placed on a digitalis preparation. In the course of taking a patient history, you note that he has been previously diagnosed with a peptic ulcer. You ask if he is taking any medications, OTC or herbal, for this. After some discussion, he reveals that he has been told by friends that licorice is useful in calming the stomach and for helping prevent ulcers, so he has been ingesting it regularly. What advice do you give this patient?

Discussion

Glycrrhiza glabra, or licorice, grows in subtropical climates with rich soil. The part cultivated for medicinal use is the roots and runners. The use of licorice dates back to the Roman empire when it was used as an expectorant and carminative. Today it is mostly used as a flavoring agent to mask bitter compounds like quinine, and it is also put in cough and cold remedies for its expectorant effects. Ninety percent of licorice today is used to flavor tobacco products. Anise oil is used to flavor licorice candy today because of the significant side effects that real licorice produces.[2,3,12]

Licorice contains a large variety of agents like ammonia and triterpenoids, but the main reason the root is cultivated is for the glycoside glycyrrhizin, which is 50 times sweeter than table sugar.[2] This glycoside is semisynthetically made into a succinic acid ester of the 18β-glycyrrhetic acid (carbenoxolone).[12] In the human body, the glycoside glycyrrhizin is hydrolyzed to glycyrrhetinic acid, which has a structure similar to the hormones of the adrenal cortex. The specific mechanism of action of carbenoxolone is unknown, but it does increase mucus secretions, increases the lifespan of gastric epithelial cells, inhibits back diffusion of hydrogen ions induced by bile, and possibly inhibits peptic activity.[12]

Glycyrrhetic Acid (Enoxolone)   Carbenoxolone

A controlled trial comparing carbenoxolone to cimetidine showed it to be less effective in treating gastric and duodenal diseases. The study showed that there was a 78 percent improvement of gastric symptoms with cimetidine and only a 52 percent improvement with carbenoxolone. A major disadvantage of carbenoxolone is the significant side effects that it causes such as edema, hypertension, and hypokalemia.[12] These are more pronounced in the elderly population and if a patient has renal and liver disease. Because carbenoxolone has direct effects on the renin-aldosterone-angiotensin axis, so it has an action like ACTH. There is an increased retention of sodium and water, which increases blood pressure and a ~~tion of potassium, which causes the hypokalemia.[13] Patien~~ high blood pressure, kidney disease, pregnancy, cirrhosis, disorders should be cautioned to avoid taking licorice.

Glycyrrhetinic acid has shown both anti-inflammatory activity in laboratory animals. This is probably explained PGE_2.[12] Mabey reports a case in which a woman with failur cortex was supported solely on a regular intake of licorice ~~cause of its cortisonelike effects.[14] It has recently been discovered that glycyrrhetinic acid inhibits 11-β-hydroxy steroid dehydrogenase in rats, and therefore potentiates the action of hydrocortisone in humans.[3] The flavonoids in licorice have recently been found to have strong antioxidant and antihepatotoxic activities.[9] Licorice also has a gentle laxative effect and it decreases stomach acid levels, so it can relieve heartburn. It heals stomach ulcers by spreading a protective gel over the stomach wall and also eases spasms of the large intestine. It can neutralize toxins such as diphtheria and tetanus, increases the flow of bile, and decreases blood cholesterol. Licorice also works like codeine in the throat to decrease irritations and has expectorant effects. Glycyrrhetinic acid has effects like aspirin and decreases fevers.[1-3,12]

It is well documented that 30 to 40 grams per day of licorice for nine months will cause lethargy, flaccid muscles, and dulled reflexes. Under these conditions, the patient will become hypokalemic and will experience myoglob-inuria. During World War II, a Dutch physician noted marked improvements in patients suffering from peptic ulcer disease when taking licorice, but the side effects, including swelling of the face and limbs, were enough to cause him to discontinue it. One man who had eaten two to three 36-gram licorice candy bars daily for six to seven years became so weak he could not get out of bed.

Thiazide diuretics will enhance potassium loss if taken concomitantly with glycyrrhizin; thus, so extreme hypokalemia, will be the end result. Also there is an increased sensitivity to digitalis glycosides when taken together with glycyrrhizin that can create digitalis intoxication. Spironolactone decreases the adverse side effects such as hypokalemia, but it also decreases the therapeutic benefits of the glycyrrhizin.[2]

Summary of Adverse Effects of Licorice
Hypertension
Edema
Hypokalemia
Muscle Weakness

Deglycyrrhizinated Licorice

The value of deglycyrrhizinated licorice, licorice from which all but 3 percent of the glycyrrhizin has been removed, is currently under study. Deglycyrrhizinated licorice exhibits a lower incidence of side effects, but most studies have not shown a clinical advantage over placebo. This may be due to a bioavailability problem, and recent studies are showing similar efficacy in the rate of gastric ulcer healing in patients treated with either deglycyrrhizinated licorice or cimetidine.[15] Several studies have been performed to evaluate the efficacy of deglycyrrhizinated licorice, but they are all inconclusive in showing a clinical response greater than placebo. Even though there have not been consistent results, neither do they show the serious side effects seen with carbenoxolone.[12]

A preparation combining deglycyrrhinized licorice with antacids is of proven value in the healing of gastric ulceration and is of equivalent efficacy compared to cimetidine and carbenoxolone.[16] One particular study showed that deglycyrrhinized licorice diminished acute gastric mucosal damage due to aspirin, prevented the potentiation of aspirin injury by bile acid, and did not greatly affect aspirin absorption. The failure of deglycyrrhinized licorice to reduce injury when given before aspirin suggests that the protective effect may only be temporary. Perhaps the effects are diminished because the deglycyrrhinized licorice may have left the stomach. Therefore combining aspirin with deglycyrrhinized licorice at the same time in one product may lessen gastric mucosal injury and decrease aspirin-induced ulcers.

In a trial involving 37 ambulant patients with chronic gastric ulcer, the efficacy of carbenoxolone and deglycyrrhizinated licorice were compared. The two groups were clinically and statistically similar. Each drug was given in the recommended dosage over a period of four weeks and the results were assessed by comparison of ulcer size shortly before and immediately after therapy. No significant statistical difference could be found between results obtained from either treatment.[17] For people who are suffering from both hypertension and gastric ulcers, deglycyrrhizinated licorice is preferred over licorice.

CASE STUDY 3:
PEPPERMINT AND INDIGESTION

A patient complaining of an upset stomach and gas comes to you for advice. He has read that peppermint is good for indigestion. He asks if this is true, and if so, what is the recommended treatment?

Discussion

Mentha piperita, also known as peppermint, is a hybrid of *Mentha spicata* (spearmint). It is a member of the mint family and has been used in Eastern and Western medicine for treatment of various conditions such as indigestion, nausea, sore throats, colds, and cramps. The most common use for it today is as a flavoring additive in many foods and drugs.[18]

Peppermint has a complex chemistry, consisting of 0.1 to 1 percent volatile oil composed mostly of menthol (29 to 48 percent), menthone (20 to 31 percent) and methyl acetate (3 to 10 percent). The rest of the oil is made up of trace amounts of more than 100 different compounds.[2,18]

Peppermint has a spasmolytic effect on smooth muscles and has been used in preparations for irritable bowel syndrome and abdominal pain. It is effective orally and the enteric coated capsule dosage form releases its contents in the large intestine in an unmetabolized state. It is best to take the enteric coated capsules between meals with no food. The volatile oils work directly on smooth muscle, resulting in decreased tone of the lower esophageal sphincter, and facilitate belching (carminative effect). The volatile oil of peppermint temporarily inhibits hunger pains in the stomach, but peristalsis resumes shortly with increased intensity, in essence stimulating the appetite. The spasmolytic activity is derived from the menthol, which is a calcium antagonist. The flavonoids found in the leaves of peppermint have bile-stimulating effects (choleretic) in dogs. In an experiment performed on guinea pigs given morphine prior to dosing to occlude the sphincter of Oddi, a single dose of IV essential oil of peppermint 1 mg/kg resulted in rapid opening of the sphincter. Interestingly, if the guinea pigs were given large doses (25 to 50 mg/kg) the sphincter constricted again.[18] The oil is recommended as an adjunct to colonoscopy, in which a diluted suspension of oil is sprayed on the endoscope to decrease colon spasm. Small quantities of azulene are found in the oil of peppermint and have been shown to have anti-inflammatory and antiulcerogenic effects in laboratory animals.[18]

Peppermint is regarded as generally safe for human consumption. The FDA recently declared the oil ineffective as a digestive aid and banned the use of it over the counter for that purpose. Menthol may cause allergic reactions such as contact dermatitis, flushing, and headache. Putting menthol ointment on the nostrils of babies has caused instant collapse and may cause choking sensations. Rats that have been fed high doses of peppermint oil (100 mg/kg) developed brain lesions.

Summary of Effects of Peppermint

Used extensively in food and drugs

Complex mix of more than 100 compounds

Menthol is the most abundant compound in the volatile oil
and is pharmacologically active in small doses

Documented success in treating digestive tract disorders

CASE STUDY 4: PSYLLIUM

A 50-year-old male patient visiting your pharmacy asks for advice about treating his constipation. He has heard that psyllium is a good laxative, and he wants to know just how effective it is and how he should use it. What is your advice?

Discussion

Plantago psyllium is native to the Mediterranean region, most often cultivated in Spain and southern France. The part of the plant that is used medicinally is the dried, ripe seed and the husk. These consist of up to 30 percent mucilage, mostly in the husk, and a mixture of monoterpene alkaloids, glycosides, and polysaccharides with D-xylose and L-arabinose as major residues.[9,19]

The main use of the psyllium seed is as a bulk laxative. When the seeds are soaked in water, they swell in size and their volume increases manyfold. The husk forms a gelatinous mass, thus keeping feces hydrated and soft. The resulting bulk promotes peristalsis and laxation. There are two different kinds of psyllium seed. Blond psyllium is a partly fermentable dietary fiber supplement that increases stool bulk and has mucosa-protecting effects. In one study, rats were fed 100 to 200 grams of blond psyllium seeds per kilogram in a fiber-free elemental diet for four weeks. Fecal fresh weight increased up to 100 percent, fecal dry weight increased up to 50 percent, and fecal water content increased up to 50 percent. The length and weight of the large intestine increased significantly. There were no reported changes in the small intestine.[9,19] Unsoaked seeds can cause GI problems. The other type is black psyllium, which is a gentler laxative.[14] It is important to note that the seeds should not be ground or chewed because they release a pigment that deposits in renal tubules.[9,19]

A recent European monograph indicates usage of psyllium for habitual constipation, anal fissures (where soft stool is desired), hemorrhoids, and postrectal surgery. It is also commonly indicated for irritable bowel syndrome, diverticulosis, and as an adjuvant therapy for diarrhea.[9] The most important factor in using psyllium is that it should be taken with a large quantity of water otherwise it is virtually ineffective.[4,19]

CASE STUDY 5: BILBERRY

MO, a 45-year-old female patient, comes to your pharmacy suffering from a mild case of diarrhea associated with a recent bout of a GI flu. She has heard that some herbal medicines are effective antidiarrheals, and one that she has heard about recently is bilberry. She asks if it is true and if it could be helpful for her, and if there are other medications, herbal or nonherbal, that she could use. What advice do you give her?

Discussion

Vaccinium myrtillus, more commonly known as bilberry, originates from Northern and Central Europe. They are black, coarsely wrinkled berries with many small, shiny brownish-red seeds that have a sweetly caustic taste. Bilberry is used in teas and topically for inflammation of mucus membranes of the mouth and throat. It was used during World War II to improve night vision and after the war it was confirmed through various studies that it could improve visual acuity.[20]

Bilberry consists of about 10 percent tannins, but most of the medicinally beneficial pharmacology comes from the 25 percent anthrocyanosides. The tannins are formed upon drying the fruit and once dried, they promote an antidiarrheal effect. Fresh fruit, therefore, will not have this effect. The drying process causes condensation of monomeric tannin precursors. The anthrocyanosides have vasoprotective and antiedema effects in experimental animals.[20] Oral doses of 25 to 100 mg/kg increased skin capillary permeability. Antiedema activity was found after IV or topical use.[20,21] Topically, it produced a mild anti-inflammatory effect on the mucus membranes of the mouth and throat. The IV dosage promoted and intensified arteriolar rhythmic diameter changes that aided in the redistribution of microvascular blood flow and interstitial fluid formation.[20]

A recent investigation using an anthrocyanidin pigment (IdB1027) found in bilberries showed it to have protective gastric effects without influencing acid secretion. Oral doses of 600 mg twice daily were administered to ten lab animals for ten days. The result was an increase in gastric mucosal release of prostaglandin E_2, which may explain its antiulcer and GI protective benefit.[20,22] Adverse effects associated with large doses are not found, and side effects or drug interactions have not been noted.

A summary of herbs used for GI disorders is given in Table 5.2.

Summary of Medicinal Effects of Bilberry Fruit
Vasoprotective

Antiedemic

Decreased vascular permeability

Gastroprotective

Intensifies arteriolar rhythmic diameter

TABLE 5.2. Herbal Medicines Commonly Used to Treat Gastrointestinal Disorders

Herbal medicine	Use	Reported active constituent	Precautions and interactions	Usual dosing
Aloes (*Aloe barbadensis*, *A. ferox*, *A. africana*, *A. spicata*)	Orally a strong cathartic and not usually recommended; atonic constipation	Anthraquinone glycoside constituents of leaf juice or latex	A drastic purgative, less toxic laxatives available. Contraindicated in patients with hemorrhoids, kidney disease, intestinal obstruction, abdominal pain, nausea, or vomiting. May color urine red.	Oral: 0.05-0.2 g of powdered aloe or dry extract.
Bilberry Fruit (*Vaccinium Myrtillus*)	Treatment of diarrhea, mild enteritis	Anthocyanosides	No known side effects or interactions.	Administered as a tea
Cascara (*Rhamnus purshiana*)	Stimulant laxative	Anthraquinone glycosides	Do not take if pregnant or lactating (passed into milk). Severe vomiting with fresh bark. Electrolyte imbalance, hypokalemia with misuse; potentiates toxicities of cardiac glycosides and thiazide diuretics.	Adult dose: 1g (½ tsp in 150 mL boiling water, strain). Effects seen in 6-8 hrs. Tea is bitter.

TABLE 5.2 (continued)

Herbal medicine	Use	Reported active constituent	Precautions and interactions	Usual dosing
Chamomile (*Matricaria recutita*)	Antispasmodic, anti-inflammatory; treatment of peptic ulcers, spasms of GI tract, inflammation of mouth and gums	Azulene components; sesquiterpene bisabolol compounds; various flavonoids	May cause allergic reactions (rare)	Adult dose: 3 g dried flower heads (1 heaping Tbsp) in 250 mL hot water, steep 10-15 min, strain. Taken TID-QID between meals.
Ginger (*Zingiber officinale*)	Treatment of motion sickness and nausea	"Pungent principles"; shogaol; gingerols; zingerone	May cause prolonged bleeding times; caution in patients on oral anticoagulant therapy. Reported to be an abortifacient, so avoid use in pregnancy or lactation.	Adult dose: 1 g 30 min prior to travel, then 0.5-1 g every 4 hrs (maximum daily dose 2-4 g). Dose prior to cancer chemotherapy is 1 g.
Licorice (*Glycyrrhiza glabra*; *G. uralensis*)	Treatment of peptic ulcer; expectorant	Glycyrrhizin (glycyrrhizic acid)	Considered unsafe. High doses (> 50 g/d) can cause pseudoaldosteronism leading to increased blood pressure, potassium loss, water retention. Contraindicated in pregnancy, and in patients on cardiac glycosides or thiazide diuretics.	Deglycyrrhizinated licorice may allow ulcer healing without side effects, but results inconclusive. Do not use longer than 4-6 weeks.

Peppermint (*Mentha piperita*)	Decreases muscle spasms of GI tract. Treatment of abdominal pain. Enteric coated capsules used to treat irritable bowel syndrome.	Essential oils (menthol and menthol esters)	Do not use in infants or small children; tea from leaves can cause laryngeal and bronchial spasms. Overuse can lead to heartburn and relaxation of lower esophageal sphincter.	Tea: 1-1.5 g (1 Tbsp) leaves in 160 mL of boiling water, steep for up to 10 min TID-QID. Dose of peppermint spirit (10% oil and 1% leaf extract) is 1 mL (20 drops) taken with water.
Psyllium (*Plantago arenaria, P. psyllium, P. indica, P. ovata*)	Bulk-forming laxative for constipation, irritable bowel syndrome.	Swelling of mucilaginous seed coat on contact with intestinal fluids	Allergic reactions (anaphylaxis —rare); interference with absorption of other drugs. Bezoars (GI blockage) may result if inadequate liquid intake. Wait 30-60 min between dosing.	7.5-10 g plus at least 150 mL water for each 5 g drug. Take 30-60 minutes after a meal.
Senna (*Cassia acutifolia; C. angustfolia, Senna. alexandrina*)	Cathartic, used to treat constipation.	Dianthrone glycosides; anthraquinone derivatives	Chronic use can result in electrolyte imbalance and potassium loss. May increase toxicity of cardiac glycosides and thiazide diuretics.	Tea made from 0.5-2 g (½-1 tsp) soaked in water 10-12 hrs or hot for 10 min. Effects seen in 10-12 hrs after ingestion. Do not take for more than 1 to 2 weeks.

REFERENCES

1. Tyler VE. *Herbs of Choice: The Therapeutic Use of Phytomedicinals,* The Haworth Press, Binghamton, NY, 1994.

2. Tyler VE. *The Honest Herbal: A Sensible Guide to the Use of Herbs and Related Remedies,* The Haworth Press, Binghamton, NY, 1993.

3. Newall CA, Anderson LA, Phillipson JD. *Herbal Medicines: A Guide for Health-Care Professionals,* Pharmaceutical Press, London, 1996.

4. Covington TR (Ed.). *The Handbook of Non Prescription Drugs,* American Pharmaceutical Association, Washington, DC, 1996.

5. DerMarderosian A (Ed.). "Ginger." In *The Lawrence Review of Natural Products,* Facts and Comparisons, St. Louis, MO, 1986.

6. Kiuchi F, Shibuya M, Sankawa U. Inhibitors of prostaglandin biosynthesis from ginger. *Chem Pharm Bull 30:* 754-757 (1982).

7. Mowrey DB, Clayton DE. Motion sickness, ginger and psychophysics. *Lancet i:* 655-657 (1982).

8. Grontved A, Brask T, Kambskard J, Hentzer E. Ginger root against seasickness. A controlled trial on the open sea. *Acta Otolaryngol 105:* 45-49 (1988).

9. Leung AY, Foster S. *Encyclopedia of Common Natural Ingredients Used in Foods, Drugs, and Cosmetics* (Second Edition), John Wiley & Sons, New York, 1996.

10. Barnett RA. Ginkgo, ginger, garlic, ginseng. *Remedy September/October:* 33-36, 38-39 (1996).

11. Tyler VE. What pharmacists should know about herbal remedies. *JAPhA NS36:* 29-37 (1996).

12. DerMarderosian A (Ed.)."Licorice." In *The Lawrence Review of Natural Products,* Facts and Comparisons, St. Louis, MO, 1989.

13. Stewart PM, Wallace AM, Valentino R, Burt D, Shackleton CH, Edwards CR. Mineralocorticoid activity of liquorice: 11-beta-hydroxysteroid dehydrogenase deficiency comes of age. *Lancet ii:* 821-824 (1987).

14. Mabey R. *The New Age Herbalist,* Simon and Schuster, New York, 1988.

15. Chandler RF. Herbal remedies in modern pharmacy: Licorice, more than just a flavor. *Can Pharm J 118:*422-423 (1985).

16. Morgan RJ, Nelson LM, Russell RI, Docherty C. The protective effect of deglycyrrhinized liquorice against aspirin and aspirin plus bile acid-induced gastric mucosal damage, and its influence on aspirin absorption in rats. *J Pharm Pharmacol 35:* 605-607 (1983).

17. Wilson JA. A comparison of carbenoxolone sodium and deglycyrrhizinated liquorice in the treatment of gastric ulcer in the ambulant patient. *Brit J Clin Prac 26:* 563-566 (1972).

18. DerMarderosian A (Ed.)."Peppermint." In *The Lawrence Review of Natural Products,* Facts and Comparisons, St. Louis, MO, 1990.

19. Robbers JE, Speedie MK, Tyler VE. *Pharmacognosy and Pharmacobiotechnology,* Williams and Wilkins, Baltimore, MD, 1996.

20. DerMarderosian A (Ed.). "Bilberry Fruit" In *The Lawrence Review of Natural Products,* Facts and Comparisons, St. Louis, MO, 1996.

21. Lietti A, Cristoni A, Picci M. Studies on *Vaccinium myrtillus* anthocyanosides. 1. Vasoprotective and antiinflammatory activity. *Arzniemittel-Forschung 26:*829 (1976).

22. Mertz-Nielsen A, Munck LK, Bukhave K, Rask-Madsen J. A natural flavonoid, IdB1027, increases gastric luminal release of prostaglandin E2 in health subjects. *Ital J Gastroenterol 22:*288 (1990).

Chapter 6

Herbal Medications and Nutraceuticals Used to Treat Rheumatoid or Osteoarthritis

Jan V. Beckwith, PharmD

INTRODUCTION

"Arthritis" has become a catchall term used by the general public to refer to almost any symptom of joint disease. In fact, osteoarthritis (OA) and rheumatoid arthritis (RA) are just two of at least 100 diseases generally classified as rheumatic diseases. In addition, joint involvement can be a symptom of a number of other systemic diseases. Rheumatoid arthritis is an inflammatory process of the connective tissue that occurs two to three times more commonly in women than in men.[1] Osteoarthritis, by far the most common of the joint diseases, is a noninflammatory degeneration primarily of the cartilage and bone that occurs equally in both men and women. Osteoarthritis generally appears as part of the aging process.[1]

The degeneration that occurs in osteoarthritis is attributed to wear and tear on weight-bearing joints. Joint cartilage is composed of an extracellular matrix that holds chondrocytes, proteoglycans, and water, but contains no blood vessels, nerves, or lymph structures. The pumping action of joint motion transports molecules into and out of cartilage, and enhances blood circulation to synovial tissues that line the joints. Therefore both inactivity and excess activity adversely affect the circulation of nutrients and wastes that may result in unhealthy joints.[2] Normally, a balance exists between formation and degradation of both cartilage and the bone beneath the cartilage (subchondral bone). When this balance is disrupted, the result is increased cartilage destruction and increased bone synthesis around joint surfaces. By the time symptoms appear, damage may have been occurring for some time.[1,3]

The disease process seen with rheumatoid arthritis involves an inflammatory process that results in an increase in the number of inflammatory and connective-tissue destructive mediators within the synovial lining of the joints. The concentration of these mediators varies, depending upon the cause of the inflammation. This variation may partially explain the differences in symptoms, as well as in results seen in research and drug development related to rheumatoid arthritis. Mediators include prostanoids (prostaglandins), enzymes (proteinases, collagenases, stromelysins, etc.), leukotrienes, and cytokines.[4,5] Cytokines are proteins with potential proinflammatory actions, which include the interleukins (IL) and tumor necrosis factors (TNF).[5,6] Cytokines not only promote destruction of matrix, but also inhibit matrix synthesis.[7,8]

Production of these mediators involves release of arachidonic acid, which is then acted on either by cyclooxygenases or by lipoxygenases to form the pro-inflammatory mediators.[6] Development of drugs that will block the arachidonic acid cascade, either by preventing release of arachidonic acid itself, or by blocking cyclooxygenases or lipoxygenases, is a major area of research in rheumatoid arthritis.[4] Aspirin (acetylsalicylic acid), for example, inhibits cyclooxygenases, resulting in decreased formation of prostaglandins and therefore decreased inflammation.[9] Salicylic acid, on the other hand, does not inhibit cyclooxygenase but still has anti-inflammatory activity,[6] suggesting that other mechanisms play a role in the effectiveness of anti-inflammatory drugs.

Although the early course of rheumatoid arthritis can include temporary remissions, the disease often progresses to disabling damage and deformity. Initial therapy includes rest, physical therapy, and aspirin or another non-steroidal anti-inflammatory drug (NSAID).[10] NSAIDs block the formation of arachidonic acid, but they do not seem to prevent damage to bone and cartilage. They may take up to two weeks to reduce inflammation, and they may cause severe adverse effects such as GI bleeding. Glucocorticoids may be of therapeutic benefit, but they also have serious side effects, such as steroid psychosis, exacerbation of preexisting diabetes, and aseptic necrosis. [1,10,11]

Beginning disease-modifying antirheumatic drugs (DMARDs) within three months of diagnosis is frequently recommended for any patient who is not in remission. These drugs include hydroxychloroquine (HCQ), sulfasalazine (SSZ), methotrexate (MTX), injectable or oral gold salts, azathioprine (AZA), and D-penicillamine (DP). All of these have side effects, ranging from rash and diarrhea to thrombocytopenia and myelosuppression, which may limit or restrict their use. Although not curative, surgery is an option in extreme cases.[10]

Proper diagnosis of rheumatoid arthritis and osteoarthritis is essential. Other diseases or problems, such as Lyme disease and even stress fractures, can present similar symptoms but require different therapy. Osteoarthritis is noninflammatory and usually presents with bony swelling and mild or no tenderness. In contrast, the swelling of rheumatoid arthritis accompanied by inflammation is usually symmetrical, soft, and tender. Synovial fluid in inflammatory joint disease, or rheumatoid arthritis, is translucent with low viscosity and contains 2,000 to 100,000 white blood cells/µL. In contrast, synovial fluid in noninflammatory joint disease, or osteoarthritis, is transparent with normal (high) viscosity and fewer than 2,000 white blood cells/µL.[1,2] With both types of arthritis, joints are stiff in the mornings, or after periods of disuse. Stiffness lasts for thirty minutes or more with rheumatoid arthritis, but disappears within fifteen to thirty minutes with osteoarthritis. Laboratory and X-ray studies may help differentiate between the various rheumatic diseases and other disorders.[1]

When pain is present in conjunction with osteoarthritis, allopathic drug therapy often begins with aspirin or another NSAID. However, the potential for adverse reactions to NSAIDs makes the use of acetaminophen a safer first choice.[12] Intra-articular glucocorticoids can provide relief for severe pain when there are signs of inflammation.[1,12] The main therapy for osteoarthritis is therapeutic exercise and rehabilitation, including weight reduction, muscle conditioning, use of canes or walkers to relieve pressure, braces, and short-term splinting.[12] Surgery is a last resort.[1]

Many nutraceutical and herbal products have been used traditionally to treat both rheumatoid arthritis and osteoarthritis. Scientific and clinical studies show that some of these products may have beneficial effects. Many studies have tested the effects of herbs on induced inflammation in rats and other mammals. Most of these studies involve inducing edema by injection of carrageenan or another irritant into the rat's paw. Paw size is then compared between animals receiving either injectable or oral test preparations. This is an accepted method, used in numerous studies, for testing the comparative anti-inflammatory properties of various drugs and herbs.

We must recognize the limitations of relying purely on controlled laboratory studies to predict the efficacy of herbal and traditional therapies that may be supported within the experience of traditional healing. Patients are sometimes "cured" by methods that have not been validated through any testing that has as yet been devised. Furthermore, some therapies may not be validated until new tools and approaches are added to our research and development methods.

CASE STUDY 1: ARTICULIN-F

TC is a 55-year-old slightly obese male diagnosed four years ago with osteoarthritis. Radiological changes show increased density of the subchondral bone in both knees, and he has some joint deformity. He was a professional hockey player at one time. He has knee stiffness in the morning that disappears about 20 minutes after he begins moving, and has distal interphalangeal involvement in the hand. Three months ago, after becoming discouraged by lack of improvement in his condition, TC visited an Ayurvedic practitioner and was given a preparation called Articulin-F which he takes as two capsules every eight hours after food. His pain has almost disappeared. His morning stiffness only lasts about 15 minutes now, and he sleeps much better. He has recently begun to complain of abdominal pain.

Discussion

TC exhibits several risk factors associated with osteoarthritis, including increasing age, obesity, and a profession that results in joint trauma.[2] He should be counseled on weight loss as a means to reduce his symptoms, since the stress of weight on damaged joints has been shown to accelerate damage.[12,13]

Articulin-F contains *Withania somnifera* root 450 mg, *Boswellia serrata* oleo-gum resin 100 mg, *Curcuma longa* rhizome 50 mg, and 50 mg of zinc.[14] This combination has been reported to be effective in reducing the clinical symptoms of both rheumatoid and osteoarthritis.[14] Forty-two patients seen at a clinic in India with symptoms of osteoarthritis were given either placebo or Articulin-F three times per day after meals for three months.[14] After a two-week wash-out period, the patients were switched to the other arm of the study for another three months. Although all measurement scores decreased at least slightly in both groups, severity of pain and disability scores were decreased significantly in the active treatment group compared with the placebo group. Erythrocyte sedimentation rate and radiological assessment did not show a significant decrease in either group.[14]

Withania somnifera, also known as Ashwagandha, is a member of the Solanaceae family.[15,16] The active ingredients are believed to be steroidal lactones (withanolides). Extracts have been shown to have anti-inflammatory activity in rats when 1 g/kg is injected into paws after inflammation is initiated by formalin.[17] Results are comparable to 10 mg/kg hydrocortisone and 50 mg/kg of phenylbutazone,[17] although the mechanism is not known.[15] Oral administration has caused CNS depression and sedation in rats. TC should be cautioned about potentiation of other CNS depressants, especially barbiturates and ethanol. *Withania* has also been shown to increase the lethal effects of amphetamine.[15]

Boswellia serrata, from the family Burseraceae, also known as salai guggul or salai gugal, has been shown in animal models and in vitro to inhibit the activation of complement, an inflammatory mediator.[18] It does not affect the cyclooxygenase pathway, but is a specific inhibitor of 5-lipoxygenase, resulting in a decrease in leukotriene production.[9] The clinical result is a prevention of inflammatory degradation of connective tissue.[18,19] Salai guggul oral doses of 50 to 200 mg/kg significantly reduced swelling as measured by both carrageenan and formaldehyde-induced rat paw edema.[20] Short-term safety of salai guggul has been shown in animal models at doses up to 100 mg/kg IV or 500 mg/kg intradural.[20]

Anecdotal reports from veterinary medicine indicate that *B. serrata* does not reverse or cure arthritis. Symptoms reoccur when the herb is stopped.[21] Although the gum resin of *Boswellia serrata* has sedative and analgesic effects, no side effects have been reported.[22,23] The recommended dose for treatment of osteoarthritis is 400 mg three times per day.[22] The dose given to TC is only 200 mg three times per day.

Curcuma longa is the yellow-orange dye from the commonly known kitchen spice, turmeric, a member of the Zingiberaceae family. Curry powder contains 28 percent turmeric.[16] Turmeric is said to inhibit the arachidonic acid cascade and leukotriene biosynthesis which gives it anti-inflammatory activity.[9,24] However, curcuma is not absorbed well orally and high doses must be given to achieve anti-inflammatory effects.[16,25] Studies have determined that doses of 400 to 600 mg three times per day are necessary.[22] TC's dose is much lower, only 300 mg/day. However, the literature mentions improvement in morning stiffness, walking time, and joint swelling for 18 patients with rheumatoid arthritis who were given an oral dose of 120 mg/day for two weeks.[25]

Although some sources report no side effects, others recommend using with caution during pregnancy, and the German Commission E monograph states that *Curcuma* is contraindicated in patients with obstruction of the biliary tract, and should be used with caution in patients with gallstones.[24] Long-term use frequently results in gastrointestinal disturbances and may cause gastric ulcers.[16,24] Therefore, TC's abdominal complaints should be evaluated to rule out these potentially serious conditions. The reason for inclusion of zinc (Jasad Bhasma) in the formulation of this medication is not explained.

Each of the herbal products in this formula has exhibited anti-inflammatory effects individually, although generally at higher doses than what is found in Articulin-F, indicating that a synergistic effect is possible in this combination. Articulin-F, although not arresting or reversing the course of TC's osteoarthritis, appears to have decreased his symptoms. He should maintain regular follow-up for gastrointestinal symptoms and if gastric ulceration is suspected should discontinue the *Curcuma longa* portion of the medication immediately and begin appropriate ulcer therapy. No studies have investigated the effectiveness of preventive measures against gastrointestinal damage while taking this herb. However, appropriate ulcer prevention prophylaxis should be considered.

CASE STUDY 2: CAPSAICIN

WP is a 60-year-old housewife who has noticed symptoms of osteoarthritis for the past two years. Although she has gained ten pounds over the past six months, she is not overweight. She has played tennis regularly for many years, but now has moderate morning stiffness. Increased pain in her hip and elbow when she exercises has prevented her from maintaining her previous level of activity. A history of peptic ulcer disease indicates that WP is not a candidate for NSAIDs. She has heard that topical capsaicin may relieve her pain. How should WP be counseled about use of capsaicin?

Discussion

Capsaicin is derived from *Capsicum frutescens, Capsicum annuum,* or any of several other hot chili peppers of the Solanaceae family. It is available commercially as a 0.025 percent and 0.075 percent cream, to be applied topically four times per day. Pain relief may not appear for two or three days, and patients should continue regular application for at least four weeks in order to gain maximum effect.[2,16,22,26] Some patients experience local burning and may stop therapy, although this side effect is transient and usually ceases to be a problem within ten days of initiating therapy.[2] Patients should be cautioned to use plastic gloves during application, or to wash their hands with soap or vinegar, since capsaicin is only slightly soluble even in hot water, and if accidentally transmitted to mucous membranes or eyes can cause extreme irritation and discomfort.[2,27]

Topical capsaicin has been used effectively to treat, among other conditions, the pain of rheumatoid arthritis, osteoarthritis, shingles, diabetic neuropathy, and phantom limb pain.[26] Studies in patients with RA or OA show mixed results. A study of 21 patients (14 with OA and 7 with RA) showed a decrease in pain severity only in the OA group compared to the RA group.[22,28] On the other hand, another study of 101 patients (70 with OA and 31 with RA) showed slightly more pain relief for RA patients than for either the OA group or a placebo group.[28] Studies cannot be truly blinded because of the burning sensation caused by capsaicin application, and this situation may contribute to inconclusive study results.

Capsaicin depletes substance P from peripheral nerve endings. Substance P is active in the transmission of pain impulses from the periphery to the spinal cord. Therefore, even though the source of the pain remains unchanged, the patient does not feel it.[22,26] This situation may be detrimental to a patient such as WP who plans to resume repetitive or stressful activities. Lack of pain perception may result in overuse of the affected joint, which may promote joint degeneration. However, since muscle conditioning has been shown to improve pain and motion parameters in osteoarthritis,[12] WP can be advised to use capsaicin for pain relief in conjunction with a physical therapy and retraining program in an attempt to maintain an acceptable level of physical activity.

CASE STUDY 3: CHINESE HERBS

JC, a 40-year-old female, presents with symptoms of weakness, tingling in her fingers, and nausea. Hypotension and bradycardia are seen upon examination. Her medical history includes a diagnosis of rheumatoid arthritis, for which she has recently started taking a Chinese herbal product labeled Kuei-chih-chia-ling-chu-fu-tang. Is there any ingredient in this product that could be causing her symptoms?

Discussion

The contents of this product were identified as cinnamon, ginger, atractylodes (red), peony, jujube, hoelen, licorice, and aconite.[29] The ingredient of most concern is aconite, which is usually derived from *Aconitum napellus* or *Aconitum columbianum* of the family Ranunculaceae. Although there are over 170 species of *Aconitum*, most of them contain the toxic alkyloid aconitine.[30] Common names for this plant include monkshood, friar's cap, helmet flower, soldier's cap, and wolfsbane.[15] Although aconite is seldom used in the United States because of its toxicity, Chinese herbal formulas prescribed for chronic rheumatoid arthritis frequently contain aconite.[15,29] Proper processing can detoxify aconite, although there are numerous reports in the literature of aconite poisoning from herbal products.[15,31] Symptoms include burning of the oral membranes and numbness of the throat with difficulty in speaking, vomiting and diarrhea, paresthesia, sweating, visual disturbances, hypotension, and cardiac arrhythmias that do not respond to usual emergency measures. Aconite has a low margin of safety, meaning that differences in processing or errors in administration are potentially fatal. Death is usually a result of cardiac arrhythmias or respiratory depression. There are no antidotes to aconite poisoning. Therapy consists of respiratory and cardiac support and electrolyte replacement in cases of diarrhea and fluid loss. Weakness and sensory disturbances may persist after recovery.[24]

Another ingredient in this formula that has been shown in clinical trials to contribute to relief of rheumatoid arthritis symptoms is ginger.[22,32,33] Ginger oil significantly reduced artificially induced inflammation in rat paw and knee joints compared to placebo.[33] Other reports advocate the food intake of 50 grams of raw ginger daily, but the effectiveness of this dose is illustrated by only one case.[32] Although ginger is considered nontoxic, it has been noted to inhibit thromboxane synthetase (a platelet aggregation inducer), and to be a prostacyclin (inhibitor of platelet aggregation) agonist.[16,34] Platelet aggregation inhibition has been reported after excessive dietary intake of ginger and after 5 g of dry ginger taken in combination with a fatty meal.[32,34] However, although the potential for prolonged bleeding time and interaction with anticoagulant drugs should be considered, the therapeutic use of ginger is generally considered safe.[34,35] Large amounts of ginger should be avoided during pregnancy and during times in chemotherapy or after surgery when bleeding is a concern.[35]

Of the other ingredients in this formula, cinnamon is usually used to treat gastrointestinal disorders and diarrhea.[24] Licorice is also used for gastrointestinal disorders, including peptic ulcers. Animal studies have shown some anti-inflammatory activity from licorice.[15] Mineralocorticoid toxicity, especially hypertension and hypokalemia, limits licorice to short term use (no more than six weeks).[16,24] Some authors caution that preparations containing the whole root are safe and that it is only the licorice extract that is responsible for reported toxicity.[36]

Peony flowers were used in folk medicine to treat rheumatism, but their efficacy for any therapeutic use has not been proven.[24] There is little or no evidence in the English language literature for use of atractylodes, jujube, or hoelen to treat arthritis. Without clinical studies to prove or disprove efficacy, synergistic effects cannot be ruled out.

CASE STUDY 4: DEVIL'S CLAW AND FEVERFEW

LV is a 37-seven-year-old female with rheumatoid arthritis of six months' duration. She has been taking aspirin 325 mg, three tablets four times per day for the past three months. She has had no side effects from the drug, but her arthritis symptoms (morning stiffness, inflammation, and tenderness) seem to be getting worse. She has been reading the literature and is apprehensive about trying any of the second-line, or disease-modifying antirheumatic drugs (DMARDs). She has read about herbal products, namely devil's claw and feverfew, that might alter her disease with few side effects and she would like to try them first. Should she try them?

Discussion

The popular herbal literature enthusiastically supports the use of both devil's claw and feverfew for treatment of arthritis. However, actual studies do not support the effectiveness of either one of these herbal products. Devil's claw is the common name for an herbal plant native to Africa whose botanical name is *Harpagophytum procumbens*.[15,24] It is of the family Pedaliaceae, and its active ingredients are iridoid glycosides.[15] The most active glycoside, harpagoside, is found in the roots and a trace is found in the leaves, but none is found in the flowers, stems, or ripe fruits.[15] However, the specific compound in devil's claw responsible for its anti-inflammatory activity has not been demonstrated,[35] and this uncertainty may contribute to conflicting study results. The commercial product Arko-caps contains devil's claw.[22]

Studies in rats and humans have shown mixed results using devil's claw for treatment of inflammation and arthritis.[22,37,38,39] Contradictory reports may result from a lack of consistency between preparations, but most likely from the fact that devil's claw is not active orally.[15,40] It has also been shown not to affect arachidonic acid, cyclooxygenase, or lipoxygenase pathways.[37,38] Some effectiveness has been shown when extracts are injected subcutaneously, beside the knee joint, as supportive therapy.[24] Because one patient reported side effects including frontal headache, tinnitus, anorexia, and gastrointestinal discomfort during oral use it would not be safe for LV to add this herb to her present regimen.[22,35,41] The German Commission E monograph also contraindicates its use in patients with gastric and duodenal ulcers.[24]

Feverfew is the plant *Tanacetum parthenium*, family Asteraceae. Most studies show little or no anti-inflammatory effectiveness when given orally.[42,43] Although its mechanism of action is complicated and not totally understood, it appears that it does not inhibit cyclooxygenation of arachidonic acid, but rather may block the synthesis of thromboxane.[35,42] The mechanism is probably different than that of salicylate's prostaglandin inhibition.[15] One placebo-controlled, parallel study in 40 patients with inadequately controlled rheumatoid arthritis investigated dried, powdered feverfew leaf, equivalent to two medium-sized leaves, given daily for six weeks.[43] No benefit was shown. Although some literature says that NSAIDs or steroids may interfere with the effectiveness of feverfew, the patients in this study were allowed to continue with their existing anti-inflammatory treatments. It should be noted that even with concomitant NSAID administration, there were no reports of adverse effects in the patients taking feverfew, other than minor tongue ulceration noted in one patient.[43]

Feverfew's main use is for the treatment of migraine headaches.[16] However, the quality of commercial products varies widely, which may be the reason for its demonstrated lack of efficacy in some studies. Assays for the active ingredient, parthenolide, in products available in the United States showed that two out of three contained no parthenolide at all.[16,22]

Because of the potential for decreased platelet aggregation,[15,42] if LV decides to try feverfew, she should be monitored for increased bleeding tendency.

CASE STUDY 5:
GLUCOSAMINE AND CHONDROITIN SULFATE

Although physical therapy has improved her range of motion, WP, the 60-year-old housewife described in Case Study 2, desperately wants to resume the active lifestyle that she feels has kept her healthy for 60 years. She has discovered advertisements for glucosamine sulfate that claim it will "bind to the connective tissue matrix of the joints," and advertisements for glucosamine plus chondroitin sulfate. Should she take one or both of these, and will binding to matrix restore the cartilage that has been destroyed by her osteoarthritis and allow her to play tennis again?

Discussion

Glucosamine, the 2-amino derivative of glucose, chemically known as 2-amino-2-deoxyglucose, is found in the matrix of cartilage.[15,44] It is a substrate of proteoglycan and also stimulates the synthesis of proteoglycans.[44,45] Animal studies have shown that it is incorporated into articular cartilage after both parenteral and oral administration.[45] The effectiveness of glucosamine is not related to inhibition of the cyclooxygenases or to an effect on the arachidonic acid cascade, and therefore its mechanism of action is different from NSAIDs.[46] Early studies show that it may rebuild damaged cartilage and prevent further degeneration.[47] Glucosamine is obtained either by extraction from cartilage or by chemical synthesis.[48]

Clinical trials on small numbers of patients indicate that patients have significant reduction in pain and joint tenderness when given glucosamine in doses of 500 mg tid. A six-to-eight-week trial by Pujalte and colleagues, in which 12 patients were given glucosamine and 12 patients were given placebo resulted in an 80 percent reduction in pain and joint tenderness compared to a 20 percent reduction in the placebo group.[47] Two patients failed to report in each group and were not accounted for. Another placebo-controlled study using 80 patients (40 in each group) measured pain, joint tenderness, and restriction of active and passive movement, and showed a clinically significant decrease in all symptoms in the glucosamine group over the placebo group.[3] In addition, after 30 days of therapy, ten of the 40 patients on glucosamine reported being pain free, and nine of those 40 patients completely regained their mobility. Electron microscopy of cartilage samples in this study indicated that the cartilage from patients taking glucosamine had been repaired. However, samples were only taken from two patients, and there were no before and after comparisons.

A frequently quoted article comparing ibuprofen with glucosamine reports pain scores for 18 patients given glucosamine and 20 patients given ibuprofen.[49] The dose of ibuprofen is only 400 mg tid. Two patients dropped out of the glucosamine group, which originally numbered 20, and were not accounted for. As would be expected, the ibuprofen reduced pain scores more quickly than the glucosamine. However, after four weeks, patients taking glucosamine reported slightly less pain than patients taking ibuprofen. No patients became pain free within the time of the study and no effects on movement were measured.

In a short-term study by Crolle and D'Este, 30 patients with concomitant diseases sufficiently serious to cause hospitalization were treated with glucosamine.[50] Patients were allowed to continue current medications, including unspecified antibiotics, antidepressants, and medications for diabetes, circulatory, liver, and lung disorders. No interactions were reported during the three weeks of the study. One half of the patients were given a daily IM injection of glucosamine 400 mg daily for seven days. They were then switched to an oral dose of 500 mg tid. The other half (15 patients) were given a daily IM injection of a reference drug, a piperazine/chlorbutanol combination, for seven days, followed by 14 days of oral placebo. The overall symptom score, including pain and function restrictions, decreased significantly clinically for the glucosamine group as compared to the placebo group but did not reach statistical significance.

The time to walk 20 meters was measured and this time also decreased for the glucosamine group.

Administration of high doses of glucosamine (2700 mg/kg and 2149 mg/kg respectively) to rats and dogs for periods of six to 12 months did not cause any lesions in the GI tract or in other organs.[44] Other studies measured blood glucose before and after administration of glucosamine and did not show any significant changes.[3,50] However, in vitro studies show that glucosamine desensitizes beta cells to stimulation.[51,52] Therefore, the potential exists for disturbances of glucose regulation in patients who take glucosamine and who have preexisting conditions of altered glucose utilization or diabetes. These patients should monitor their blood sugar regularly. Based on efficacy data, glucosamine appears to be a logical nutraceutical medication for WB to try, keeping in mind that long-term safety studies are not complete.

Chondroitin sulfate is a glycosaminoglycan. In cartilage, chondroitin combines with proteoglycans, which bind with another glycosaminoglycan, hyaluronic acid. This combination forms aggregates that are an integral part of the cartilage matrix.[8,53] Chondroitin stimulates both synthesis of proteoglycans and hyaluronan formation.[54] Hyaluronan, in addition to being a backbone of cartilage matrix, acts as a joint lubricant and shock absorber and has been proposed to have a protective role in inflammatory cartilage damage.[55] However, results of studies on the use of hyaluronan in arthritis have been mixed and its role in therapy is still being investigated. Hyaluronan must be given by intra-articular injection since its high molecular weight may limit its oral absorption and hence its bioavailability.[55,56] In addition, its activity varies with its molecular weight and commercial formulas cannot be considered therapeutically equivalent, a factor that complicates both research and therapy.[55] Studies are currently being done to investigate the effects of coadministration of hyaluronan with chondroitin sulfate, glucosamine, and proteolysis inhibitors for treatment of arthritis, but sufficient evidence is not available to recommend their use.[12]

CASE STUDY 6: TRIPTERYGIUM WILFORDII

CS, a 37-year-old Asian female, comes into the clinic visibly upset. She fears she may be pregnant. She has missed her last two menstrual periods and her stomach feels uncomfortable, although she has not vomited. Her medical history includes rheumatoid arthritis, which has been only partially controlled by NSAIDs and occasional steroids. She states that she has taken NSAIDs infrequently and has discontinued steroids since she began taking 15 ml per day of an unknown herbal liquid given to her by a Chinese physician about six months ago. She was told to take an antacid with the herb but has since discontinued the antacid. Upon examination some swelling was noted in the knuckles of her thumbs and in her great toes. A pregnancy test was negative and her laboratory screening was within normal limits. She states that her menstrual cycle has always been regular and that she does not exercise excessively. The Chinese physician was contacted and the herb identified as *Tripterygium wilfordii*. He expressed surprise at the patient's amenorrhea, since he had been monitoring for blood, liver, and kidney function, and she had tolerated the herb well, denying any menstrual irregularities. How has the herb affected CS?

Discussion

Tripterygium wilfordii, or yellow vine, is known to cause amenorrhea, and in at least one reported male patient has caused decreased numbers of spermatozoa.[57] Hypermenorrhea and oligomenorrhea have also been reported.[58] Two reports from China evaluate a total of 192 cases of rheumatoid arthritis, juvenile rheumatoid arthritis, or ankylosing spondylitis for which *Tripterygium wilfordii* was administered.[57,58] These studies conclude that *Tripterygium wilfordii* is more effective than conventional NSAIDs, although neither study used controls and measurements were subjective. A blinded, placebo-controlled study conducted in a strain of mice genetically modeled to represent human rheumatoid arthritis resulted in significantly decreased arthritis scores and mortality in the *Tripterygium wilfordii*-treated group compared to the placebo group.[59] The herb has been shown to decrease prostaglandin E_2 synthesis and inhibit interleukin-2 production by T cells.[59]

In addition to menstrual disturbances, *Tripterygium wilfordii* has exhibited toxic effects such as perioral blisters and mouth ulcers, conjunctivitis, mild hair loss, petechiae, pigmentation of the face, anorexia, and stomach discomfort (probably accounting for CS's symptoms). Patients have experienced an increase in infections such as lymphadenitis and cellulitis, which may indicate that the herb has immunosuppressive activity.[58] These adverse reactions are attributed to a component of the whole herb rather than to the isolated total glycosides.[57] Therefore, *Tripterygium wilfordii* is a classic example of how important it is that herbs be used only by experienced healers or physicians who have knowledge of proper preparation techniques.

Table 6.1 presents a summary of information about herbs and nutraceuticals used to treat arthritis.

TABLE 6.1. Herbs and Nutraceuticals Used to Treat Arthritis

Herbs	Notes and comments
*Aconite (monkshood)[15] Aconitum napellus A. columbianum	Must be processed correctly to avoid toxicity. Found in many Chinese herbal remedies for RA.
Alfalfa[15,60] Medicago sativa	Anti-inflammatory activity not documented. Must be prepared properly since some parts are toxic. Contaminants have caused one death—reputable sources are critical.
Arnica[15,16,24] Arnica montana	Toxicity can result in death when used orally. Used topically as a counterirritant.
Ash tree[61,62] Fraxinus excelsior	Combined with P. tremula and S. virgaurea as Phytodolor N. Interferes with arachidonic acid cascade. Studies on effectiveness for arthritis ongoing.
Birch[63] Betula verrucosa, B. pubescens	Not an effective anti-inflammatory.
Bromelain (Pineapple)[15,28,64] Ananas comosus	Proteolytic enzyme used to treat edema and soft tissue inflammation. Affects prostaglandin synthesis, but studies ongoing to prove usefulness for arthritis.
Black Cohosh[15] Cimicifuga racemosa	Used mostly for estrogenic effects. Traditionally used for rheumatic disorders but little evidence of efficacy.
Bogbean[24] Menyanthidis folium	Usually used to stimulate gastric juice and saliva. Little documentation for use in arthritis.
Bupleurum root (various species)[65,66] Bei Chai Hu, Saiko	Most commonly used as an antipyretic. Blocks histamine-induced capillary permeability. One report of adult respiratory distress syndrome (ARDS).
*Capsaicin[2,12,28] Capsicum frutescens	Effective topical analgesic for OA and RA. Caution not to overuse joint when pain decreases.
Celery[15,24] Apium graveolens	Used traditionally to treat arthritis, but effectiveness not documented. May cause allergy and photo-dermatitis. Contraindicated in kidney inflammation.
Comfrey[15,16,24] Symphytum officinale	Used topically as an anti-inflammatory. Hepatotoxic and carcinogenic when taken orally.
*Devil's Claw[37,38,39,40,41,67] Harpagophytum procumbens	Studies show lack of efficacy for treating arthritis. May be inactivated by stomach acid.
*Feverfew[15,42,43,68] Tanacetum parthenium T. microphyllum	Mixed reports of effectiveness in RA. Amount of active components varies in products. NSAIDs may reduce efficacy. Chewing leaves can cause mouth ulceration.

*Ginger Zingiber officinale	Case reports indicate effectiveness for arthritis, not a traditional use. May prolong bleeding time.
Goldenrod[24,61,62] Solidago virgaurea	Combined with *P. tremula* and *F. excelsior* as Phytodolor N. Spasmolytic, antihypertensive, and diuretic effects. May not be effective orally as anti-inflammatory.
Meadowsweet[24] Filipendula ulmaria	Used primarily for colds, chills, etc. Arthritis use not documented.
Mussel extract[43]	Not proven effective in RA.
Mustard[15,24] Brassica nigra, B. alba	Used topically as counterirritant. Undiluted, is one of the most toxic essential oils. Can cause ulceration if applied too long.
Nettle[15,24] Urtica dioica	Herb used as tea for rheumatism. Fruit used topically as dressing. Either use not adequately documented.
Oats[15,24] Avena sativa	Tea used to lower uric acid levels, not documented. Oat straw traditionally used as soothing bath.
*Salai guggul[9,18,19,23] Boswellia serrata	Suppresses arthritis symptoms. No side effects reported.
Sarsaparilla[16,69] Smilax aristolochiaefolia and others	Only use is as a flavoring agent (not a source of testosterone). Often adulterated.
Skullcap[15,66] Scutellaria lateriflora	Animal studies of *S. baicalensis* show anti-inflammatory effect.
*Turmeric[9,24,25,67,70] Curcuma longa	Effective anti-inflammatory. Not absorbed well orally. Long-term use may cause gastric ulcers.
White poplar[61,62] Populus tremula	Combined with *F. excelsior* and *S. virgaurea* as Phytodolor N. Less effective than *F. excelsior* and *S. virgaurea*. Salicin content may account for activity.
Willow bark[15,16,24] Salix purpurea Salix fragilis and others	Used as an analgesic. Salicin is converted to salicylic acid, but may be subtherapeutic. Not shown to affect platelet function.
*Withania (Ashwagandha)[14,15,16, 67] Withania somnifera	Anti-inflammatory activity documented by animal studies and folk medicine. Has CNS effects and may interact with CNS depressants and amphetamines.
*Yellow vine[57,58,59,66] Tripterygium wilfordii	Reduces symptoms of joint inflammation. May affect menstrual cycle and sperm count. Toxic if not prepared properly.
Yucca (Joshua tree)[15] Yucca spp.	Efficacy for treating arthritis not adequately documented.

* Reviewed in chapter.

REFERENCES

1. Berkow R (ed.). *Merck Manual of Diagnosis and Therapy*, Sixteenth Edition. Rahway, NJ: Merck Research Laboratories, 1996.
2. Kraus VB. Pathogenesis and treatment of osteoarthritis. *Med Clin North Am.* 1997; 81(1):85-112, January.
3. Drovanti A, Bignamini AA, Rovati AL. Therapeutic activity of oral glucosamine sulfate in osteoarthrosis: A placebo-controlled double-blind investigation. *Clin Ther* 1980; 3(4):260-272.
4. Ahern MJ, Smith MD. Rheumatoid arthritis. *Med J Aust.* 1997; 166(3): 156-161, February 3.
5. Ali H., Haribabu B, Richardson RM, Snyderman R. Mechanisms of inflammation and leukocyte activation. *Med Clin North Am.* 1997; 81(1):1-28, January.
6. Winyard PG, Blake DR. Antioxidants, Redox-regulated transcription factors, and inflammation. *Adv Pharmacol.* 1997; 38:403-421.
7. Månsson B, Carey D, Alini M, Ionescu M, Rosenberg LC, Poole AR, Heinegård D, Saxne T. Cartilage and bone metabolism in rheumatoid arthritis. *J Clin Invest.* 1995; 95(3):1071-1077, March.
8. Poole AR, Ionescu M, Swan A, Dieppe PA. Changes in cartilage metabolism in arthritis are reflected by altered serum and synovial fluid levels of the cartilage proteoglycan aggrecan. *J Clin Invest.* 1994; 94(1):25-33, July.
9. Ammon HPT, Safayhi H, Mack T, Sabieraj J. Mechanism of antiinflammatory actions of curcumine and boswellic acids. *J Ethnopharmacol.* 1993; 38(2-3): 113-119, March.
10. American College of Rheumatology Ad Hoc Committee on Clinical Guidelines. Guidelines for the management of rheumatoid arthritis. *Arthritis Rheum.* 1996; 39(5):713-722, May.
11. Spencer-Green G. Drug treatment of arthritis: update on conventional and less conventional methods. *Postgrad Med.* 1993; 93(2):129-138, 140, May 15.
12. Block JA, Schnitzer TJ. Therapeutic approaches to osteoarthritis. *Hosp Pract Off Ed.* 1997; 32(2):159-164, February 15.
13. Sharif M, George E, Shepstone L, Knudson W, Thonar EJA, Cushnaghan J, Dieppe P. Serum hyaluronic acid level as a predictor of disease progression in osteoarthritis of the knee. *Arthritis Rheum.* 1995; 38(6):760-767, June.
14. Kulkarni RR, Patki PS, Jog VP, Gandage SG, Patwardhan B. Treatment of osteoarthritis with a herbomineral formulation: A double-blind, placebo-controlled, cross-over study. *J Ethnopharmacol.* 1991; 33(1-2):91-95, May-June.
15. Hagemann RC (Ed.). *The Lawrence Review of Natural Products.* St. Louis, MO: Facts and Comparisons, 1996.
16. Tyler VE. *Herbs of Choice: The Therapeutic Use of Phytomedicinals.* Binghamton, NY: The Haworth Press, 1994.
17. Sudhir S, Budhiraja RD, Miglani GP, Arora B, Gupta LC, Garg KN. Pharmacological studies on leaves of *Withania somnifera. Planta Med.* 1986; (1):61-63, February.

18. Kapil A, Moza N. Anticomplementary activity of boswellic acids—an inhibitor of C3-convertase of the classical complement pathway. *Int J Immunopharmacol.* 1992; 14(7):1139-1143, October.

19. Reddy GK, Chandrakasan G, Dhar SC. Studies on the metabolism of glycosaminoglycans under the influence of new herbal anti-inflammatory agents. *Biochem Pharmacol.* 1989; 38(20):3527-3534, October 15.

20. Singh GB, Atal CK. Pharmacology of an extract of salai guggal ex-*Boswellia serrata*, a new non-steroidal anti-inflammatory agent. *Agents Actions.* 1986; 18(3/4): 407-412, June.

21. Puotinen CJ. *Herbs to Relieve Arthritis.* New Canaan, CT: Keats Publishing, 1996

22. Werbach MR, Murray MT. *Botanical Influences on Illness.* Tarzanna, CA: Third Line Press, 1994.

23. Kar A, Menon MK. Analgesic effect of the gum resin of *Boswellia serrata* Roxb. *Life Sci.* 1969; 8(19):1023-1028, October 1.

24. Bisset NG (ed.). *Herbal Drugs and Phytopharmaceuticals.* Boca Raton, FL: CRC Press, 1994.

25. Ammon HP, Wahl MA. Pharmacology of *Curcuma longa.* *Planta Med.* 1991; 57(1):1-7, February.

26. Robbers JE, Speedie MK, Tyler VE. *Pharmacognosy and Pharmacobiotechnology.* Baltimore, MD: Williams & Wilkins, 1996.

27. Tyler VE. *The Honest Herbal,* Third Edition. Binghamton, NY: The Haworth Press, 1993.

28. Watson CPN. Topical capsaicin as an adjuvant analgesic. *J Pain Symptom Manage.* 1994; 9(7):425-433, October.

29. Tsung P-K, Hsu H-Y. *Arthritis and Chinese Herbal Medicine.* Long Beach, CA: Oriental Healing Arts Institute, 1987.

30. Rumack BH, Hess AJ, Gelman CR. (Eds.). *POISINDEX® system.* Englewood, CO: MICROMEDEX, Inc., (Edition expires 5/31/97).

31. Thorat S, Dahanukar S. Can we dispense with Ayurvedic samskaras? *J Postgrad Med.* 1991; 37(3):157-159, July.

32. Srivastava KC, Mustafa T. Ginger *(Zingiber officinale)* in rheumatism and musculoskeletal disorders. *Med Hypotheses.* 1992; 39:342-348, December.

33. Sharma JN, Srivastava KC, Gan EK. Suppressive effects of eugenol and ginger oil on arthritic rats. *Pharmacology* 1994; 49(5):314-318, November.

34. De Smet PAGM, Keller K, Hänsel R, Chandler RF. (Eds.). *Adverse Effects of Herbal Drugs,* Third Edition. Berlin: Springer-Verlag, 1997.

35. Newall CA, Anderson LA, Phillipson JD. *Herbal Medicines: A Guide for Health-Care Professionals.* London: Pharmaceutical Press, 1996.

36. Mowrey DB. *The Scientific Validation of Herbal Medicine.* New Canaan, CT: Keats Publishing, 1986.

37. Moussard C, Alber D, Toubin M-M, Thevenon N, Henry J-C. A drug used in traditional medicine, *Harpagophytum procumbens:* No evidence for NSAID-like effect on whole blood eicosanoid production in human. *Prostaglandins Leukot Essent Fatty Acids.* 1992; 46(4):283-286, August.

38. Whitehouse LW, Znamirowska M, Paul CJ. Devil's claw *(Harpagophytum procumbens):* No evidence for anti-inflammatory activity in the treatment of arthritic disease. *Can Med Assoc J.* 1983; 129(3):249-251, August 1.

39. McLeod DW, Revell P, Robinson BV. Investigations of *Harpagophytum procumbens* (Devil's Claw) in the treatment of experimental inflammation and arthritis in the rat. *Br J Pharmacol.* 1979; 66(1):140P-141P, May.

40. Lanhers MC, Fleurentin J, Mortier F, Vinche A, Younos C. Anti-inflammatory and analgesic effects of an aqueous extract of *Harpagophytum procumbens. Planta Med.* 1992; 58(2):117-123, April.

41. Grahame R, Robinson BV. Devil's claw *(Harpagophytum procumbens):* Pharmacological and clinical studies (letter). *Ann Rheum Dis.* 1981; 40(6):632, December.

42. Makheja AN, Bailey JM. The active principle in feverfew (letter). *Lancet.* 1981; 2(8254):1054, November 7.

43. Pattrick M, Heptinstall S, Doherty M. Feverfew in rheumatoid arthritis: A double blind, placebo controlled study. *Ann Rheum Dis.* 1989; 48(7):547-549, July.

44. Setnikar I, Pacini MA, Revel L. Antiarthritic effects of glucosamine sulfate studied in animal models. *Arzneimittelforschung.* 1991; 41(5):542-545, May.

45. Reichelt A, Förster KK, Fischer M, Rovati LC, Setnikar I. Efficacy and safety of intramuscular glucosamine sulfate in osteoarthritis of the knee. *Arzneimittelforschung.* 1994; 44(1):75-80, January.

46. Setnikar I, Cereda R, Pacini MA, Revel L. Antireactive properties of glucosamine sulfate. *Arzneimittelforschung.* 1991; 41(2):157-161, February.

47. Pujalte JM, Llavore EP, Ylescupidez FR. Double-blind clinical evaluation of oral glucosamine sulphate in the basic treatment of osteoarthrosis. *Curr Med Res Opin.* 1980; 7(2):110-114.

48. Setnikar I, Palumbo R, Canali S, Zanolo G. Pharmacokinetics of glucosamine in man. *Arzneimittelforschung.* 1993; 43(10):1109-1113, October.

49. Vaz AL. Double-blind clinical evaluation of the relative efficacy of ibuprofen and glucosamine sulphate in the management of osteoarthrosis of the knee in out-patients. *Curr Med Res Opin.* 1982; 8(3):145-149.

50. Crolle G, D'Este E. Glucosamine sulphate for the management of arthrosis: A controlled clinical investigation. *Curr Med Res Opin.* 1980; 7(2):104-109.

51. Zawalich WS, Zawalich KC. Glucosamine-induced desensitization of β-cell responses: Possible involvement of impaired information flow in the phosphoinositide cycle. *Endocrinology.* 1992; 130(6):3135-3142, June.

52. Crook ED, Zhou J, Daniels M, Neidigh JL, McClain DA. Regulation of glycogen synthase by glucose, glucosamine, and glutamine: Fructose-6-phosphate amidotransferase. *Diabetes.* 1995; 44(3):314-320, March.

53. Shinmei M, Miyauchi S, Machida A, Miyazaki K. Quantitation of chondroitin 4-sulfate and chondroitin 6-sulfate in pathologic joint fluid. *Arthritis Rheum.* 1992; 35(11):1304-1308, November.

54. Conte A, Volpi N, Palmieri L, Bahous I, Ronca G. Biochemical and pharmacokinetic aspects of oral treatment with chondroitin sulfate. *Arzneimittelforschung.* 1995; 45(8):918-925, August.

55. Goa KL, Benfield P. Hyaluronic acid: A review of its pharmacology and use as a surgical aid in ophthalmology, and its therapeutic potential in joint disease and wound healing. *Drugs.* 1994; 47(3): 536-566, March.

56. Laurent TC, Fraser JRE. Hyaluronan. *FASEB J.* 1992; 6:2397-2404, April.

57. Gao ZG, Zang AC, Bai RX. Radix *Tripterygium wilfordii* hook F in rheumatoid arthritis, ankylosing spondylitis and juvenile rheumatoid arthritis. *Chin Med J.* 1986; 99(4):317-320, April.

58. Juling G, Shixiang Y, Xichun W, Shixi X, Deda L. *Tripterygium wilfordii* hook f in rheumatoid arthritis and ankylosing spondylitis. *Chin Med J.* 1981; 94(7):405-412, July.

59. Gu WZ, Banerjee S, Rauch J, Brandwein SR. Suppression of renal disease and arthritis, and prolongation of survival in MRL-*lpr* mice treated with an extract of *Tripterygium wilfordii* Hook F. *Arthritis Rheum.* 1992; 35(11):1381-1386, November.

60. De Smet PAGM (Ed.). *Adverse Effects of Herbal Drugs* 1. New York: Springer-Verlag, 1992.

61. von Kruedener S, Schneider W, Elstner EF. A combination of *Populus tremula, Solidago virgaurea* and *Fraxinus excelsior* as an anti-inflammatory and antirheumatic drug: A short review. *Arzneimittelforschung.* 1995; 45(2):169-171.

62. el-Ghazaly M, Khayyal MT, Okpanyi SN, Arens-Corell M. Study of the anti-inflammatory activity of *Populus tremula, Solidago virgaurea* and *Fraxinus excelsior. Arzneimittelforschung.* 1992; 42(3):333-336.

63. Klinger W, Hirschelmann R, Süss J. Birch sap and birch leaves extract: Screening for antimicrobial, phagocytosis-influencing, antiphlogistic and antipyretic activity. *Pharmazie.* 1989; 44(8):558-560, August.

64. Cooreman WM, Scharpé S, Demeester J, Lauwers A. Bromelain, biochemical and pharmacological properties. *Pharm Acta Helv.* 1976; 51(4):73-97.

65. McNamara S. *Traditional Chinese Medicine.* New York: Basic Books, 1996.

66. Huang KC. *The Pharmacology of Chinese Herbs.* Boca Raton, FL: CRC Press, 1993.

67. Iwu MM. *Handbook of African Medicinal Plants.* Boca Raton, FL: CRC Press, 1993.

68. Abad MJ, Bermejo P, Valverde S, Villar A. Anti-inflammatory activity of hydroxyachillin, a sesquiterpene lactone from *Tanacetum microphyllum. Planta Med.* 1994; 60(3):228-231, June.

69. Osborne F, Chandler F. Sarsaparilla. *CPJ-Can Pharm J.* 1996; 129:48-51, June.

70. Huang HC, Jan TR, Yeh SF. Inhibitory effect of curcumin, an anti-inflammatory agent, on vascular smooth muscle cell proliferation. *Eur J Pharmacol.* 1992; 221(2-3):381-384, October 20.

Chapter 7

Herbal Medications, Nutraceuticals, and Diabetes

Lucinda G. Miller, PharmD, BCPS

INTRODUCTION

Diabetes mellitus is a syndrome characterized by impaired glucose tolerance and/or a deficiency or an absolute lack of insulin, which is needed to regulate blood glucose (sugar). Insufficient insulin results in hyperglycemia (high blood glucose levels). High fasting (≥ 140 mg/dl) or random (≥ 200 mg/dl) venous plasma glucose concentrations are highly suggestive of diabetes mellitus. Typically, patients present with polyuria (increased urination), polydipsia (increased thirst), polyphagia (increased appetite and food intake), and fatigue. Left untreated, retinopathy, nephropathy, and neuropathy (eye, kidney, and nerve damage, respectively) may result. Fourteen million Americans have diabetes classified as either Type I (insulin-dependent diabetes mellitus) or Type II (non-insulin-dependent diabetes mellitus). Type I diabetics will require exogenous insulin to adequately control blood sugar levels. Type II diabetics, which comprise approximately 90 percent of the diabetic population, may be able to control their blood sugar with diet, exercise, and oral medications. Oral medications include acetohexamide (Dymelor), chlorpropamide (Diabinese), tolazamide (Tolinase), tolbutamide (Orinase), glimepiride (Amaryl), glipizide (Glucotrol), glyburide (Diabeta, Micronase), metformin (Glucophage), and acarbose (Precose). Strict blood sugar control with monitoring of levels at least four times a day was associated with a 76 percent decrease in retinopathy, 39 percent decrease in microalbuminuria, and a 60 percent decrease in clinical neuropathy.[1] However, a two- to threefold increase in severe hypoglycemia was also noted.[1] Obviously, diabetes mellitus requires close control of the blood sugar in order to minimize or avoid adverse outcomes. Any substance that affects blood sugar may adversely affect the patient's blood sugar control. Herbal products are no exception.

CASE STUDY 1: MOMORDICA CHARANTIA

AL is a 28-year-old Asian male diagnosed with Type I diabetes as a child. His blood glucose is controlled with an average level of 118 mg/dl and a hemoglobin A_1C of 8 percent. He monitors his blood sugar four times a day with adjustment of insulin as required. However, for the last week, 30 percent of his readings have indicated blood sugars of less than 40 mg/dl. When asked if he is taking any other medications, he denies use of over-the-counter medications but mentions he has recently seen an herbalist who recommended *Momordica charantia* (karela) for his diabetes mellitus. How do you integrate this information with his clinical presentation?

Discussion

Momordica charantia, also known as karela, has been referred to as both a vegetable and a fruit. It is indigenous to Asia and South America and has been advocated for the oral treatment of diabetes mellitus.[2] It can be found in combination with *Allium sativum* (garlic), another less-potent product thought to lower blood glucose, in curry.[3] When taken in conjunction with an oral sulfonylurea, chlorpropamide, the dose of the latter needed to be reduced, although this report specified neither the starting nor adjusted final dose.[3] Juice extracted from fresh karela was found to be more potent than when slices of karela were fried in vegetable oil.[4] Hence if a patient is alternating between juice extract and frying the sliced vegetable, blood glucose levels will vary accordingly, with greater decreases in blood sugar following juice ingestion. Karela has been shown to improve glucose tolerance without inducing hyperinsulinemia or reducing intestinal absorption.[4,5] The mechanism of *Momordica charantia*'s ability to lower blood glucose is unknown, but in studies in diabetic rabbits it has been proposed to possess a direct mechanism similar to insulin.[6] The drug does not seem to act indirectly by stimulating insulin release as alloxan causes permanent destruction of beta cells, and karela was found effective in lowering blood glucose in alloxan-treated rabbits.[7] The increased frequency of AL's hypoglycemia could be related to karela ingestion. AL should be advised that hepatic damage (hepatic portal inflammation) and testicular lesions in dogs have been reported with excessive consumption of cerasee (a component of the wild variety of *M. charantia*).[8] He should be advised to discontinue karela use.

CASE STUDY 2: CHROMIUM PICOLINATE

BC is a 42-year-old Type II diabetic patient who is trying to lose weight. He is presently well-controlled on metformin 750 mg/day and glipizide 20 mg/day. He is advised by a friend that chromium picolinate will not only help him lose weight but will also assist in controlling his diabetes. Do you concur with the friend?

Discussion

The data regarding the efficacy of chromium in diabetes is conflicting. Anderson suggests that chromium increases insulin activity and reduces the amount of insulin required to control blood sugar.[9] The underlying premise of chromium's efficacy is believed to be related to glucose tolerance factor (GTF). Chromium, when combined with two molecules of nicotinic acid, forms a biologically active complex called GTF, which enhances insulin activity.[10] The National Research Council of the National Academy of Sciences recommends a chromium intake of 50 to 200 mcg/day, yet the typical North American diet contains less than 50 mcg/day attributable in part to chromium removal in our cereal refinement process.[11-13] Plasma chromium concentrations are lower in diabetic patients than in nondiabetic control patients and depressed plasma chromium levels are related to elevated glucose concentrations.[14-16] However, bear in mind that plasma chromium levels are extremely variable and may not reflect body stores; relatively high levels may be found in blood or urine in patients whose blood stores are nearly exhausted.[17] Yet, 13 diabetic patients supplemented with $CrCl_3$ 2 mg daily for three months showed improvement in diabetic control with significantly lower blood glucose (from 259 mg/dl to 119 mg/dl), compared to 13 controls whose fasting blood glucose did not change significantly.[18] During a six-week administration of 200 mcg/day of chromium picolinate, fasting blood glucose decreased on average 32 mg/dl (18 percent) and hemoglobin A_1C decreased 1.2 mg/dl (10 percent, n = 11).[19] Following one to two months of supplementation with high-chromium yeast, insulin requirements decreased 20 to 45 U/day (baseline 60-130 U/day) in five diabetic patients.[20] These reports, however, suffer from small sample size.

Well-designed placebo-controlled studies, however, have not been able to replicate these beneficial effects of chromium. In a prospective, double-blind, placebo-controlled, crossover study of 28 patients receiving chromium picolinate 200 mcg/day or placebo for two months, no statistically significant difference was noted in glucose control.[10] Twenty-six elderly subjects (aged 65 to 74 years) with persistent impaired glucose tolerance were randomized to receive either chromium-rich yeast (160 mcg/Cr/day) or placebo for six months. No significant change in oral glucose tolerance tests (glucose dose 75 g; 0, 1, and 2 hour blood glucose respectively) was noted.[21] In a larger study evaluating urinary excretion of chromium in 185 diabetics and 185 control patients, urinary excretion of chromium was not significantly different from controls.[22] Supporters explain these findings, however, by postulating that chromium functions only as a nutrient and not as a therapeutic agent; if one is consuming sufficient amounts of a nutrient, additional intake should not lead to improvements; hence, the patients in these studies may have had sufficient chromium levels at baseline.[9] Others contend that a relative lack of nicotinic acid may block a beneficial effect of chromium supplementation.[23] Additionally, concurrent use of diuretics may deplete chromium stores.[24]

The potential carcinogenic effects of chromium have been explored. The epidemiologic evidence of chromium carcinogenicity is from occupationally exposed individuals mainly among workers in the bichromate-producing industry and in chromate-pigment manufacturing.[25] However, in these populations, the workers are exposed not only to different chromium compounds but to other toxic metals such as lead and nickel. Accordingly, the general view is that the evidence for chromium carcinogenicity is limited to lung cancer but no epidemiologic studies have documented increased cancer risk in individuals exposed to chromium alone.[26] Zinc chromate as well as calcium chromate has been identified as a potent carcinogen.[27] Evidence also suggests that water-soluble chromates may be more potent carcinogens than those with low solubility.[27] It is unlikely, however, that humans exposed to chromium at doses of 200 mcg/day will incur an increased risk for cancer.

Given the conflicting data, the following statements and recommendations can be made:

1. Brittle diabetics may note changes in insulin requirements based on chromium intake
2. Brewer's yeast is a known chromium source and should be asked about when taking a drug history
3. Diuretics may lower chromium, hence worsening the diabetic state
4. Chromium is an area worthy of more study; holds promise

Since BC's blood glucose is well controlled, it is unlikely that any further benefit will be derived from chromium supplementation. In fact, to add chromium now may lower blood glucose beyond a desirable range. However, BC should be advised that future studies may outline a place for chromium in the treatment of diabetes mellitus.

CASE STUDY 3: GINSENG

EF is a 62-year-old patient with Type II diabetes who is well-controlled with acarbose (Precose) 50 mg three times daily with meals. It has been recommended to her to begin taking ginseng tablets to further lower her blood glucose. Is this a good recommendation in light of her current therapy and response? What side effects can she expect from ginseng?

Discussion

Ginseng is one of the most touted herbs, with purported efficacy for diabetes as well as anemia, atherosclerosis, depression, edema, hypertension, and ulcers.[28] Ginseng has also been promoted as an aphrodisiac but this effect is unsubstantiated.[29] It has also been characterized as an adaptogen, which is a substance that improves the ability of an organism to adapt to differing external or internal disturbances.[30] Immunostimulatory effects have also been ascribed to ginseng with enhancement of RNA and protein biosyntheses resulting from ginseng administration.[31-35] Ginseng's activity has been attributed to 2 to 3 percent ginsenosides (triterpene saponins), of which ginsenosides Rg_2, Rc, Rd, Rb_1, Rb_2, and Rb_0 are considered quantitatively the most important.[29] Specifically, five glycans with strong hypoglycemic activity have been isolated from the root.[36,37] These glycans are panaxans Q, R, S, T, and U, which markedly reduce blood glucose in normal and alloxan-induced hyperglycemic mice.[38,39] It was found that the hypoglycemic effects of the panaxans from Japanese ginseng were weaker than those from Korean and Chinese ginseng and within the Japanese ginseng, the composition varied remarkably from lot to lot, although all isolated polysaccharides exhibited some hypoglycemic activity.[38] The variation in the polysaccharide composition of the Japanese ginseng was attributed to differences in strain and/or place of production. In the rat model, ginseng's hypoglycemic effect is due to a significant rise in liver glucokinase activity.[40] Rats treated with ginsenoside-Rb2 showed a significant decrease of 30 percent in blood glucose levels by the sixth day, compared to a control group corresponding with a 31 percent decrease in the gluconeogenic enzyme activity in the liver.[40]

Few reports of severe side effects secondary to ginseng exist despite the fact that nearly six million people ingest ginseng regularly in the United States.[41] The most commonly reported side effects are nervousness and excitation but these will diminish with continued use or with dosage reduction.[41] An estrogenlike effect has been noted in women as mammary nodularity and vaginal bleeding.[42-44] An inability to concentrate was reported following long-term use.[45] (See Table 7.1.)

TABLE 7.1. Adverse Effects Attributed to Ginseng

diarrhea
gynecomastia
hypertension
inability to concentrate
insomnia
mammary nodularity
nervousness
neonatal androgenization (weak association)
skin eruptions
vaginal bleeding

A much-publicized report of stimulation, well-being, increased motor and cognitive efficiency, diarrhea, skin eruptions, nervousness, sleeplessness, and hypertension was noted in a study of 133 patients ingesting relatively large doses of the root (more than 3 g/day) for up to two years.[46] Referred to as the "ginseng abuse syndrome," this report has been disputed on the basis that it was an open study and concomitant drugs such as caffeine were allowed during the study period. Additionally, some patients were taking up to 15 g/day.[47] Maternal use of Siberian ginseng tablets during pregnancy has been associated with a case of neonatal androgenization.[48] This association, however, has not been replicated and has been attributed to an undetermined peculiarity of the subject.[49] Dr. Awang, upon evaluating the product in question, found it in fact did not contain any ginseng but rather *Periploca sepium;* hence the association is highly questionable.[47]

Ginseng composition and potency varies according to the location where grown, the season when harvested, method of curing, and age of the root.[50] Additional problems of adulteration and purity beset ginseng products. Some preparations have been adulterated with phenylbutazone, aminopyrine, or mandrake root.[51,52] Hence if a patient presents with gastrointestinal distress and agranulocytosis, an adulterant such as phenylbutazone should be suspected. Purity has also been issue. When studied, 60 percent of ginseng samples contained substandard quality ginseng and 25 percent did not contain any ginseng.[52] Total panaxoside ginseng concentrations for 24 products varied from 0.26 to 6.85 mg per 250 mg sample.[53] This degree of variance is unacceptable.

Given the spectrum of potential side effects secondary to ginseng, the relative lack of standardization and the expense, EF should continue with acarbose and defer use of ginseng at this time.

CASE STUDY 4: EPHEDRA

JR is a 48-year-old patient with Type II diabetes stabilized on regular insulin 20 units before meals and 10 U NPH/Reg at bedtime. During the afternoon for the last week, his blood sugars have been elevated. He denies use of any over-the-counter medications such as decongestants but upon further questioning states he is using Formula One to increase his energy level after lunch. Formula One contains ma huang and *Cola nitida*. What is causing the increases in his blood glucose?

Discussion

The active ingredient of ma huang is ephedra, whose active constituent is ephedrine. Known to increase both systolic and diastolic blood pressure, it is also known to elevate blood glucose.[54] Although its ability to increase blood glucose is less than that observed following epinephrine administration, it is enough to disturb glucose control in a brittle diabetic patient. The blood glucose response to ephedrine is variable. Although pronounced increases of plasma glucose have been noted following administration of 20 mg of ephedrine when combined with 200 mg caffeine, ephedrine when administered alone at 40 mg/day demonstrated no significant changes in blood glucose.[55,56] JR would be well advised to avoid use of ephedrine-containing products, especially when combined with caffeine.

The Texas Department of Health attempted to ban Formula One. The FDA alleged that the product was a health hazard and unsafe following the death of a woman in her early forties while playing tennis in Austin, Texas, in May 1994. Formula One, which contains both ephedra (ma huang) and caffeine *(Cola nitida)*, is thought to be particularly dangerous and should be avoided by diabetics.[57]

JR should avoid any product, whether herbal or over-the-counter, that will disturb blood glucose control. This includes ephedrine, which is contained in ma huang and Formula One.

CASE STUDY 5: FENUGREEK

AM is a 52-year-old white male with non-insulin-dependent diabetes (NIDDM) who has been stabilized for the past five years on glyburide 20 mg/day with average blood glucoses ranging from 90 to 120 mg/dl and average hemoglobin A_1C of 5 to 7. Yesterday he developed polyuria, polydipsia, and weight loss of two pounds. As the day progressed, he developed malaise and by evening was experiencing diffuse abdominal tenderness, nausea, and vomiting. By morning, he was barely arousable and had shortness of breath with deep respirations with a fruity odor. His wife brought him to the emergency room.

Upon examination, AM's face is flushed and his lips and tongue are parched. There are rapid respirations early and deep Kussmaul respiration later. His breath has a fruity odor. His pulse is rapid (115 beats/minute), brisk, and regular. His blood pressure is 105/60. He is very drowsy and his reflexes are diminished. His intake laboratory data demonstrated a pH = 7.25, serum bicarbonate of 13 mEq/L, serum potassium of 5.4 mEq/L, blood sugar of 425 mg/dl, and WBCs of 15,000/mm^3. Urinalysis revealed moderate ketones and 2 percent glucose and emitted a maple syrup odor. Upon questioning, his wife reports AM had discontinued his therapy due to nausea, epigastric fullness, and heartburn experienced while taking glyburide. He decided to discontinue glyburide one week ago and began an herbal remedy called fenugreek. An EKG is started, hydration is begun, and the patient is treated for diabetic ketoacidosis (DKA). How do you advise this patient regarding future herb use?

Discussion

The most common side effects of glyburide are gastrointestinal, including nausea, epigastric fullness, and heartburn. These side effects are usually dose-related and most likely would have subsided with a dose reduction (the usual maintenance dose for glyburide is 1.25 to 20 mg/day). The return of nausea accompanied by vomiting is directly related to deteriorating blood glucose and ensuing DKA.

Fenugreek *(Trigonella foenum-graecum)* has a rich history as a folk remedy for various ailments including diabetes as well as hyperlipidemia, cellulitis, boils, tuberculosis, baldness, ulcers, and fungal infections.[40,58] It is listed as the principal ingredient of Lydia Pinkham's Vegetable Compound, an old panacea with a high alcohol content. The seeds contain several alkaloids including trigonelline, carparine, and gentianine.[40] When the seed is roasted, trigonelline is degraded to nicotinic acid.

When used for diabetes mellitus, the fenugreek seeds exerted a modest and transient hypoglycemic effect in healthy and mildly diabetic animals, but was ineffective in severely diabetic animals.[59-64] Trigonelline and perhaps its by-product, nicotinic acid, have been identified as the active constituents.[61,62] In healthy dogs, the fenugreek seeds reduced glucagon and somatostatin concentrations but there was no indication of altered insulin secretion.[50,63,65] Fifty to 60 percent of the seeds is fiber and may constitute another potential mechanism of fenugreek's beneficial effect in diabetic patients.[65]

The maple syrup smell of AM's urine is due to fenugreek consumption. Preparation of fenugreek tea by boiling seed in water is a common Ethiopian folk remedy for diarrhea and vomiting. A nine-day-old boy had been given this tea by a parent for his gastroenteritis and when admitted to the hospital was found to have urine with a maple syrup odor indistinguishable from the smell of the tea itself.[66] For these patients, it is important to rule out the presence of "maple syrup urine" disease (an inborn metabolism error).

Hence, while fenugreek has a folk remedy history and some animal evidence to indicate a hypoglycemic effect, it should never be relied on totally for diabetes mellitus management. As was the case with AM, a diabetic patient can quickly enter a life-threatening situation if the blood glucose is not adequately controlled. This case exemplifies the need for open communication between the patient and the health care provider. Simple alteration of AM's glyburide dose may have been all that was needed.

CASE STUDY 6: GS$_4$

BB is a 53-year-old male with diabetes mellitus. He has been adequately treated with glyburide 10 mg/day and insulin (14 units NPH/7 units Regular before breakfast and 8 units NPH/4 units Regular before dinner). BB also uses his Accu-Check blood glucose monitoring system three to four times a day. His average blood glucoses are 115 mg/dl. On office visits, hemoglobin A$_1$C averages 7 to 8 percent. Two months ago, he began GS$_4$ therapy 400 mg/day. At today's office visit he reports he has discontinued glyburide and has decreased his insulin requirements to 10 units NPH/5 units Regular before breakfast and 6 units UNPH/3 units Regular before dinner. Today his office blood glucose is 135 mg/dl and his hemoglobin A$_1$C is 10 percent. How do you interpret this patient's office visit?

Discussion

GS$_4$ is an herbal product of *Gymnema sylvestre* leaf extract in use for diabetes mellitus for at least 65 years.[67] At doses of 400 mg/day in a study of 26 patients with insulin-dependent diabetes mellitus, insulin requirements decreased by half with a corresponding improvement in fasting blood glucose (average reduction: 232 to 152 mg/dl) and glycosylated hemoglobin A$_1$C ($p < 0.001$).[68] In this study a patient treated with concomitant Lente insulin with Euglucon (glibenclamide, glyburide) was able to discontinue glyburide after six months of GS$_4$ therapy. Another patient experienced a variable response with frequent hypoglycemic episodes. Found to have brittle diabetes, the patient was advised not to continue GS$_4$ use. In this report, the authors speculate that GS$_4$ enhances endogenous insulin activity perhaps by regeneration and revitalization of residual beta cells in insulin-dependent diabetes mellitus based on their C-peptide assay before and after GS$_4$ therapy.[68] Hence residual pancreatic function would be necessary for *Gymnema sylvestre* leaf extract to have any effect.

In another report of 22 patients with Type 2 diabetes mellitus treated with GS$_4$ 400 mg/day, five patients were able to discontinue their conventional drug (i.e., glyburide) while maintaining blood glucose homeostasis with GS$_4$ alone.[69] They speculated without laboratory evidence that GS$_4$'s mechanism of action may involve inhibition of liver metabolism of insulin. A reliable preparation of *Gymnema sylvestre* with a standardized content is needed before its use can be advocated. Certainly brittle diabetics should avoid its use.

GENERAL COMMENTS

Other entities used for their blood glucose-lowering effects and beneficial effects for diabetes mellitus are listed in Tables 7.2 and 7.3. Controlled scientific studies evaluating these products for use in patients with diabetes are lacking. Not included in these tables is *Vaccinium myrtillus*. It has been claimed to reduce insulin requirements but animal data suggest an association with renal carcinogenicity (increased occurrence of renal adenoma and epithelial hyperplasia of the renal papilla) and hepatocarcinogenicity (hepatocellular adenoma).[70-72] Given these data, it is inadvisable to recommend use of these herbs for diabetes at this time.

A patient diagnosed with diabetes mellitus should be questioned regarding the use of the above herbal products. This is especially important for a patient suffering spurious blood glucose readings despite stable drug administration, diet, and physical activity. Because patients may be reluctant to admit to such use, the clinician must impress on the patient that for effective control to be achieved, open communication is a must.

Clearly, any patient striving to achieve consistent and optimal blood glucose control must have a reliable and consistent hypoglycemic agent. This can be achieved with conventional medications such as insulin, sulfonylureas, acarbose, and metformin. However, herbal products may vary from lot to lot and may introduce unacceptable variability in the patient's blood glucose levels. Diabetic patients should closely adhere to their medical practitioner's advice and avoid additional products that will introduce unacceptable variability into their blood glucose control.

A summary of agents reviewed in this chapter is presented in Table 7.4.

TABLE 7.2. Herbs and Nutraceuticals Affecting Blood Glucose

Agents Advocated for Their Antidiabetic Effects	
Agaricus bisporus	*Galega officinalis*
Agrimonia eupatoria	*Ganoderma lucidim*
alfalfa	garlic (*Allium* sp.)
Aloe vera	ginger
Amanta phalloides	ginseng
Amorphophallus konjoe	goat's rue
Anemarrhena asphodeloides	goldenseal
Atractylodes japonica	*Gymnema sylvestre*
Blighia sapida	*Hammada salicornia*
bramble leaf	
(*Rubus fruticosus folium*)	
(Nervosana Mixtur)	
buchu leaves	Jerusalem artichoke
burdock	(*Helianthus tuberosa*)
	Job's tears
	(*Coix lacryma-jobi*)
Cassia alata	*Juniperus communis*
celery	
chromium	*Lavandula stoechas*
Coccinia indica	*Lithospermum officinale*
corn silk	*Lythrum salicaria*
Coprinus comatus	
Coriandrum sativum	
cumin	manganese
Cuminum nigram	marshmallow
	Melia azardirachta
	myrrh
damiana	
	neem (*Azadrachta indica*)
elecampane	nettle
Emericella quadrilineata	
eucalyptus extract	
	onion (*Allium cepa*)
	Opuntia streptacantha
false unicorn root	*Oryza sativa*
fenugreek	
Ficus bengalensis	
fringe tree bark	*Phaseolus vulgaris*
(old man's beard,	prickly pear cactus
snow drop tree, phyllyrin)	(*Opuntia ficus indica*)

TABLE 7.2 *(continued)*

Agents Advocated for Their Antidiabetic Effects	
Quercus infectoria	tansy *Tecoma stans* *Teucrium olverianum*
Rubus fruticosus	*Tinospora crispa* *Trigonella foenun-graecum* (fenugreek)
Saccharum officinarum sage *Salvadora persica* *Salvia lavandulifolia* selenium synthalin *Syzygium jambolana*	uva ursi vanadium wild yam (*Dioscorea dumetorum* tuber)

Hyperglycemics	
devil's claw	hydrocotyle
elecampane	licorice
figwort	ma huang *(Ephedra)*
ginseng, panax	

TABLE 7.3. Herbs Affecting Blood Glucose and Associated Adverse Effects

Herbs Affecting Blood Glucose	Associated Adverse Effects
Aconitum carmichaelie	subject to poison control in some Australian states
Arctium lappa (burdock root)	Commission E states root is not permitted for therapeutic use; usefulness not documented adequately; no risks are known however
Artemisia abbysinica	essential oil should not be used; listed as unsafe by FDA (1975)
Catharanthus roseus	subject to poison control in some Australian states
Echinacea spp. (coneflower)	contraindicated in progressive systemic diseases (e.g, tuberculosis, MS) according to Commission E; associated with metabolic worsening in some diabetic patients; should not be used more than three weeks
Eleutherococcus senticosus	should not be given to patients whose blood pressures exceed 180/90 mmHg; palpitations, pressure headaches, and arrhythmias have been reported in the Russian literature
Lupinus termis	*Lupinus* extracts cause "crooked calf disease," a congenital abnormality in bovine stock
Momordica charantia (karela, bitter melon)	hepatic necrosis has been associated with excessive intake; testicular lesions have occurred in dogs
Taraxacum officinalis (dandelion root)	contraindicated in biliary obstruction empyema of gallbladder and ileus; can produce poisoning especially in children (nausea, vomiting, diarrhea, arrhythmias)
Vaccinium myrtillus (huckleberry)	doses > 1g may result in nausea, vomiting, diarrhea, fibrillations, dyspnea, cyanosis, delirium and collapse; hemolytic anemia, cachexia, hepatic steatosis, and hair depigmentation have been reported; fatal doses range from 2 to 12 g

TABLE 7.4. Summary

Karela may sufficiently lower blood glucose to merit a decrease in insulin, sulfonylureas, or other oral medications in order to avoid or minimize the incidence of hypoglycemia.
Karela juice will exact a greater decrease in blood glucose than when slices of karela are fried.
Korean or Chinese ginseng may exert a greater hypoglycemic effect than Japanese ginseng.
Brewer's yeast as a source of chromium may cause a decrease in blood glucose and introduce unfavorable variability in blood glucose control if the clinician is unaware of concomitant use.
Diuretics (e.g., hydrochlorothiazide) may increase excretion of chromium, thereby reducing chromium's effectiveness in decreasing blood glucose.
Herbal products containing ephedra (e.g., ma huang, Formula One) may increase blood glucose necessitating an increase in insulin or oral hypoglycemic requirements.
Gymnema sylvestre (GS_4) may decrease requirements for insulin and glyburide but it should not be relied on for blood glucose control, especially in brittle diabetics.
Fenugreek exerts a modest and transitory effect on blood glucose in part due to the fibrous content of seeds; urine may emit maple syrup odor.
Comparative efficacy of chromium picolinate versus other salts is lacking; however, the possibility exists of variable blood glucose effects with each preparation.

MEDICINAL AND PHARMACEUTICAL
CHEMISTRY ASPECTS

Chromium when bound to picolinate forms an organic water-soluble complex with improved bioavailability compared to inorganic chromium salts.[10] Chromium also forms complexes with other organic acids such as ascorbic acid (vitamin C) and citric acid, exerting similar solubility and biopharmaceutical properties. Although unstudied, it is feasible that if coadministered with ascorbic acid, chromium may have a more pronounced effect on blood glucose. Hence products bound to certain salts (e.g., picolinate) may have a greater effect on blood glucose than that observed when chromium is bound to other salts (e.g., chloride). If a patient is using two different chromium products of differing salts, this may account for variability in blood glucose.

Zinc may adversely affect chromium absorption. Chromium absorption is increased in animals fed a zinc-deficient diet.[73] Conversely, it was shown that if chromium is administered concomitantly with zinc, chromium absorption was markedly decreased. Hence, these products should not be taken together.

In order to exert its hypoglycemic effects, chromium is complexed with endogenous stores of niacin (nicotinic acid, vitamin B_5) to form GTF as previously described. In this endogenous capacity, niacin does not exert its hyperglycemic effects. In fact, for chromium to fully exert its hypoglycemic effects, niacin must be present. For patients refractory to chromium's beneficial hypoglycemic effects, niacin deficiency should be considered. Niacin supplementation may be necessary. Although not adequately defined, it is unlikely that large doses will be required; hence it is unlikely that the patient will encounter the adverse effects associated with therapeutic doses of niacin such as flushing, gastrointestinal upset, and hepatotoxicity.

Editor's note: The possibility of chromium-induced nephrotoxicity has recently been addressed in the literature following a case report on renal failure developing in a patient taking chromium picolinate (600 mcg/daily), terazosin, hydrochlorothiazide, and verapamil.[74] Previously unreported secondary to trivalent chromium, hexavalent chromium has been reported to cause acute tubular necrosis in industrial poisoning.[75] The Environmental Protection Agency states that daily ingestion of as much as 70,000 mcg of trivalent chromium is safe.[75] Whether chromium picolinate in doses commonly ingested can cause nephrotoxicity is currently being debated in the literature.[76] Until fully resolved, it would be prudent for the clinician to intermittently monitor serum creatinine and blood urea nitrogen (BUN) in patients known to be ingesting chromium picolinate.

REFERENCES

1. Diabetes Control and Complications Trial Research Group. The effect of intensive treatment of diabetes on the development and progression of long-term complications in insulin-dependent diabetes mellitus. *N Engl J Med* 1993;329:977-986.

2. Pons JA, Stevenson DS. The effect of *Momordica charantia* in diabetes mellitus. *Puerto Rico Journal of Public Health and Tropical Medicine* 1943;19:196-215.

3. Aslam M, Stockley IH. Interaction between curry ingredient (karela) and drug (chlorpropamide). *Lancet* 1979;i:607.

4. Leatherdale BA, Panesar RK, Singh G, Atkins TW, Bailey CJ, Bignell AHC. Improvement in glucose tolerance due to *Momordica charantia* (karela). *Br Med J* 1981;282:1823-1824.

5. Gupta SS, Seth CB. Effect of *Momordica charantia* linn (karela) on glucose tolerance in albino rats. *J Indian Med Assoc* 1962;39:581-584.

6. Akhtar MS, Athar MA, Yaqub M. Effect of *Momordica charantia* on blood glucose level of normal and alloxan diabetic rabbits. *Planta Med* 1981;42:205-212.

7. Larner J, Haynes C. Insulin and hypoglycemia drugs, glycogen. In: Gilman GG, Goodman LS, Rall TW, Murad F, eds., *The Pharmacological Basis of Therapeutics*, Fifth Edition, New York, Macmillan Publishing, 1975:1507-1528.

8. Anderson RA. Chromium, glucose tolerance and diabetes. *Bio Trace Elem Res* 1992;32:19-24.

9. Lee NA, Reasner CA. Beneficial effect of chromium supplementation on serum triglyceride levels in NIDDM. *Diabetes Care* 1994;17:1449-1452.

10. Anderson RA, Kozlovsky A. Chromium intake, absorption and excretion of subjects consuming self-selected diets. *Am J Clin Nutr* 1985;41:1177-1183.

11. Committee on Dietary Allowances, Food and Nutrition Board, National Research Council. *Recommended Dietary Allowances*, Ninth Edition, Washington, DC, National Academy of Sciences, 1980.

12. Mossop RT. Trivalent chromium in atherosclerosis and diabetes. *Cent Afr J Med* 1991;37:369-373.

13. Morris BW, Kemp GJ, Hardisty CA. Plasma chromium and chromium excretion in diabetes. *Clin Chem* 1985;31:334-335.

14. Morris BW, Griffiths H, Kemp GJ. Effect of glucose loading on concentrations of chromium in plasma and urine of healthy adults. *Clin Chem* 1988;34:1114-1116.

15. Morris BW, Griffiths H, Kemp GJ. Correlations between abnormalities in chromium and glucose metabolism in a group of diabetics. *Clin Chem* 1988;34:1525-1526.

16. Liu V. Detection of chromium deficiency. In: Shapcott D, Hubert J, eds., *Chromium in Nutrition and Metabolism*, New York, Elsevier/North Holland Biomedical Press 1979:113-127.

17. Mossop RT. Effects of cril on fasting glucose, cholesterol and HDL in diabetics. *Cent Afr J Med* 1983;29:80-82.

18. Doisy RJ, Streeten DHP, Souma ML, Kalafer ME, Rekant SL, Dalakos TG. In: Mertz W, Cornatzer, eds., *Newer Trace Elements in Nutrition*, New York, Marcel Dekker, 1971:155-168.

19. Evans GW. Improved blood glucose trial with chromium picolinate in a six-week trial. *Int J Biosco Med Res* 1989;11:163.

20. Uusitupa MIJ, Mykkanen L, Sitonen O et. al., Chromium supplementation in impaired glucose tolerance of elderly: Effects on blood glucose, plasma insulin, C-peptide and lipid levels. *Br J Nutrition* 1992;68:209-216.

21. El-Yazigi A, Hanna N, Raines DA. Urinary excretion of chromium copper, and manganese in diabetes mellitus and associated disorders. *Diabetes Res* 1991;18:129-134.

22. Carter JP, Kattar A. Urinary excretion of chromium in diabetes patients. *Am J Clin Nutr* 1968;21:195.

23. Mossop RT. The diabetogenic effect of thiazides and the relation to chromium. *Cent Afr J Med* 1985;31:129-131.

24. DeFlora S, Serra D, Basso C, Zanacchi P. Mechanistic aspects of chromium carcinogenicity. *Arch Toxicol* 1989;13 (Suppl):28-39.

25. Langard S. Chromium carcinogenicity: A review of experimental animal data. *Sci Total Environ* 1988;71:341-350.

26. Langard S. One hundred years of chromium and cancer: A review of epidemiological evidence and selected case reports. *Am J Ind Med* 1990;17:189-215.

27. Tyler VE. Ginseng and related herbs. In: *The Honest Herbal,* Binghamton, NY: The Haworth Press, 1993: 153-158.

28. Bisset NG, ed. *Herbal Drugs and Phytopharmaceuticals: A Handbook for Practice on a Scientific Basis.* Boca Raton, FL, CRC Press, 1994.

29. Merson FZ. *Adaptation, Stress and Prophylaxis.* Berlin-Heidelberg-New York/Tokyo, Springer, 1984.

30. Jie YH, Cammisuli S, Baaiolini M. *Agents Action* 1984;15:386.

31. Singh VK, George CX, Singh N, Agarwal SS, Gupta BM. Combined treatment of mice with *Panax ginseng* extract and interferon inducer: Amplification of host resistance to Semliki Forest virus. *Planta Med* 1983;47:234.

32. Singh VK, Agarwal SS, Gupta BM. Immunomodulatory activity of *Panax ginseng* extract. *Planta Med* 1984;50:462.

33. Lu ZQ, Dice JF. Ginseng extract inhibits protein degradation and stimulates protein synthesis in human fibroblasts. *Biochem Biophy Res Comm* 1985;126:636-640.

34. Iijima M, Higasha T. Effect of ginseng saponins on nuclear ribonucleic acid (RNA) metabolism. II. RNA polymerase activities in rats treated with ginsenoside. *Chem Pharm Bull* 1979;27:2130.

35. Konno C. Isolation and hypoglycemic activity of panaxans A, B, C, D and E glycans of *Panax ginseng* roots. *Planta Medica* 1984;50:434

36. Tomoda M, Shimada K, Konna C, Sugiyama K, Hikino H. Partial structure of Panaxan A, a hypoglycemic glycan of *Panax ginseng* roots. *Planta Medica* 1984;50:436-438.

37. Konno C, Murakami M, Oshima Y, Hikino H. Isolation and hypoglycemic activity of panaxans Q, R, S, T and U, glycans of *Panax ginseng* roots. *J Ethnopharmacol* 1985;14:69-74.

38. Oshima Y, Konno C, Hikino H. Isolation and hypoglycemic activity of panaxans I, J, K, and L, glycans of *Panax ginseng* roots. *J Ethnopharmacol* 1985;14:255-259.

39. Yokozawa T, Kobayashi T, Oura H, Kawashima Y. Studies on the mechanism of the hypoglycemic activity of ginsenoside-Rb_2 in streptozotocin-diabetic rats. *Chem Pharm Bull* 1985;33:869-872.

40. Hebel SK, ed. *Lawrence Review of Natural Products.* St. Louis, Facts and Comparisons, 1996.

41. Punnonen R, Lukola A. Oestrogen-like effect of ginseng. *Br Med J* 1980;281:1110.

42. Palmer BV, Montgomery ACV, Monteiro JCMP. Ginseng and mastalgia. *Br Med J* 1978;1:1284.

43. Greenspan EM. Ginseng and vaginal bleeding. *JAMA* 1983;249:2018.

44. Hammond TG, Whitworth JA. Adverse reactions to ginseng. *Med J Aust* 1981;1:492.

45. Siegel RK. Ginseng abuse syndrome: Problems with the panacea. *JAMA* 1979;241:1614-1615.

46. Castleman M. Ginseng: Revered and reviled. *The Herb Quarterly* 1990;48: 17-24.

47. Awang DVC. Maternal use of ginseng and neonatal androgenization. *JAMA* 1991;266:363.

48. Waller DP, Martin AM, Farnsworth NR, Awang DV. Lack of androgenicity of Siberian ginseng. *JAMA* 1992;267:2329.

49. Tyler VE. Performance and immune deficiencies. In: *Herbs of Choice,* Binghamton, NY: The Haworth Press, 1994: 171-186.

50. Reis CA, Sahud MA. Agranulocytosis caused by Chinese herbal medicine: Dangers of medications containing aminopyrine and phenylbutazone. *JAMA* 1975; 231:352.

51. Abramowicz M. Adulterated herbal products. *The Medical Letter* 1979;21:29.

52. Liberti LE, DerMarderosian A. Evaluation of commercial ginseng products. *J Pharmaceutical Sci* 1978;67:1487-1489.

53. Ziglar W. Ginseng products may not contain ginseng. *Whole Foods* 1979; 2(4):48-53

54. Weiner N. Norepinephrine, epinephrine and the sympathomimetic amines. In: Gilman AG, Goodman LS, Rall TW, Murad F, eds. *The Pharmacological Basis of Therapeutics*, New York, Macmillan Publishing Company, 1985:145-180.

55. Astrup A, Toubro S. Thermogenic, metabolic and cardiovascular responses to ephedrine and caffeine in man. *Int J Obes Relat Metabol Disord* 1993;17 suppl 1:S41-43.

56. Paquot N, Schneiter P, Jequier E, Tappy L. Effects of glucocorticoids and sympathomimetic agents on basal and insulin-stimulated glucose metabolism. *Clin Physiol* 1995;15:231-240.

57. Blumenthal M, King P. Ma huang: Ancient herb, modern medicine, regulatory dilemma: A review of the botany, chemistry, medicinal uses, safety concerns, and legal status of ephedra and its alkaloids. *HerbalGram* 1995;34:22-26,43,56-57.

58. Tyler VE. Fenugreek. In: *The Honest Herbal,* Binghamton, NY: The Haworth Press 1993: 131-132.

59. Ajgaonkar SS. Herbal drugs in the treatment of diabetes: A review. *IDF Bull* 1979;24:10-17.

60. Swanston-Flatt SK, Day C, Flatt PR. Traditional plant treatments for diabetes: Studies in normal and streptozotocin diabetic mice. *Diabetologia* 1990;33:462-464.

61. Shani J, Goldschmied A, Joseph B, Aharonseon Z, Sulman FG. Hypoglycemic effect of *Trigonella foenum-graecum* and *Lupinus termis* (leguminosae) seeds and their major alkaloids in alloxan-diabetic and normal rats. *Arch Int Pharmacodyn Ther* 1974;210:27-37.

62. Mishinsky J, Joseph B, Sulman FG, Golschmied A. Hypoglycaemic effect of trigonelline. *Lancet* 1967:2:1311-1312.

63. Ribes G, Sauvarie Y, Baccou JC, Valette G, Chenon D, Trimble ER, Loubatieres-Mariani MM. Effects of fenugreek seeds on endocrine pancreatic secretions in dogs. *Ann Nutr Metab* 1984;28:37-43.

64. Ajabnoor MA, Tilmisany AK. Effect of *Trigonella foenum-graecum* on blood glucose levels in normal and alloxan-diabetic mice. *J Ethnopharmacol* 1988;22: 45-49.

65. Madar Z, Abel R, Samish S, Arad J. Glucose-lowering effect of fenugreek in non-insulin dependent diabetics. *Eur J Clin Nutr* 1988;42:51-54.

66. Bartley GB, Hymd H, Andreson BD, Clairmont AC, Maschke SP. "Maple syrup" urine odor due to fenugreek ingestion. *N Engl J Med* 1981;305:467.

67. Mhaskar SK, Caius JF. A study of Indian medicinal plants. II: *Gymnema sylvestre R. Br. Indian Medical Research Memoirs* 1930:16:2-75.

68. Shanmugasundaram ERB, Rajeswara G, Baskaran K, Kumar BRJ, Shanmugasundaram KR, Arhmath BK. Use of *Gymnema sylvestre* leaf extract in the control of blood glucose in insulin-dependent diabetes mellitus. *J Ethnopharmacol* 1990;30:281-294.

69. Baskaran K, Ahamath BK, Shanmugasundaram KR, Shanmugasundaram ERB. *J Ethnopharmacol* 1990;30:295-305.

70. Bailey CJ, Day C. Traditional plant medicines as treatments for diabetes. *Diabetes Care* 1989;12:553-565.

71. Devillers J, Boule P, Vasseur P et. al., Environmental and health risks of hydroquinone. *Ecotoxicol Environ Safety* 1990;19:327-354.

72. Shibata MA, Hirose M, Tanaka H, Asakawa E, Shirai T, Ito N. Induction of renal cell tumors in rats and mice, and enhancement of hepatocellular tumor development in mice after long-term hydroquinone treatment. *Jpn J Cancer Res* 1991;82:1211-1219.

73. Hahn CJ, Evans GW. Absorption of trace metals in the zinc-deficient rat. *Am J Physiol* 1975;228:1020-1023.

74. Wasser WG, Feldman NS, D'Agati VD. Chronic renal failure after ingestion of over-the-counter chromium picolinate. *Ann Intern Med* 1997;126;410.

75. Mertz W. Risk assessmant of essential trace elements: New approaches to setting recommended dietary allowances and safety limits. *Nutr Rev* 1995;53: 179-185.

76. Michenfelder HJ, Shepherd M. Over-the-counter chromium and renal failure. *Ann Intern Med* 1997;127:655.

Chapter 8

Herbal Medications, Nutraceuticals, and Hypertension

Lucinda G. Miller, PharmD, BCPS
Louis A. Kazal Jr., MD

INTRODUCTION

Hypertension is one of the most frequently encountered chronic conditions, estimated to affect 50 million Americans.[1] A normal blood pressure of adults aged eighteen years and older is defined as a systolic less than 130 mmHg and a diastolic pressure less than 85 mmHg.[1] Stage 1 (mild) hypertension, based on an average of at least two readings at separate visits after initial screening, is defined as a systolic pressure of 140 to 154 mmHg and a diastolic pressure of 90 to 99 mmHg.[1] In 1972, only 51 percent of hypertensive patients were cognizant of their elevated blood pressure but by 1988, due to educational efforts, this percentage has risen to 65 percent.[2] Yet, only 21 percent of individuals have obtained optimal blood pressure control.[1] Untreated hypertension is a significant risk factor for the development of cardiovascular morbidity and mortality including, but not limited to, myocardial infarction, congestive heart failure, renal failure, stroke, blindness, left ventricular hypertrophy, and sudden death.

Patients fortunate enough to have their hypertension diagnosed should seek adequate treatment. Diuretics (e.g., hydrochlorothiazide) are considered the drugs of choice for elderly or black patients who do not have contraindications for their use.[3-6] In addition to thiazide diuretics, beta-blockers (e.g., propranolol, metoprolol) have been shown to decrease morbidity and mortality secondary to hypertension. Angiotensin-converting enzyme (ACE) inhibitors (e.g., captopril, enalapril, lisinopril) are especially usefully in hypertensive patients with concomitant congestive heart failure or diabetes mellitus.[7,8]

LK wishes to thank Anthony F. Valdini, MD, for his collegial support and Ms. Eva Grabarek for her tireless secretarial efforts.

Losartan is the first of a new class of antihypertensives referred to as angiotensin II antagonists. Calcium channel blockers (e.g., nifedipine, verapamil, diltiazem) are potent vasodilators used to treat ischemic heart disease and have also found use in reducing blood pressure.[9] Other agents considered appropriate as antihypertensive monotherapy are peripheral $alpha_1$-antagonists (e.g., prazosin, doxazosin, terazosin) and central $alpha_2$-agonists (e.g., clonidine, guanabenz, guanfacine, and methyldopa). Third- and fourth-line agents include adrenergic antagonists (e.g., reserpine, guanethidine) and direct vasodilators (e.g., hydralazine). With appropriate therapy the risk of stroke can be decreased by 42 percent, whereas coronary artery disease mortality is reduced by only 15 percent.[10]

All of these agents have side effects. Diuretics are associated with hypokalemia and increases in cholesterol.[11] In a study of 514 individuals, it was found that patients receiving non-potassium-sparing diuretics had an increased risk of sudden cardiac death (relative risk = 1.8; 95 percent CI, 1.0 to 3.1) when compared to a reference group treated with other potassium-sparing diuretics.[12] Lethargy, sedation, fatigue, and impaired exercise tolerance are noted in some patients receiving beta-blockers.[13,14] ACE inhibitors have caused cough, dysgeusia, neutropenia, and hyperkalemia.[15] Calcium channel blockers have been associated with headache, dizziness, peripheral edema, and flushing.[16] More serious in nature, reports of increased mortality (risk ratio = 1.16; 95 percent CI, 1.01 to 1.33) in patients with coronary heart disease and a 60 percent increase in the adjusted risk rates for myocardial infarctions (risk ratio = 1.57; 95 percent CI, 1.21 to 2.04; p < 0.001) following calcium channel blocker use have dampened enthusiasm for their use, especially nifedipine.[17,18] These are but a few of the side effects encountered, which have led many to raise quality-of-life issues with antihypertensive therapies.[19,20]

Studies undertaken to address these issues have found antihypertensives vary in quality-of-life issues generally as a correlate of their side effect profile. In a study of 626 men, it was found that patients taking captopril, compared to patients taking methyldopa, scored significantly higher (p < 0.05 to < 0.01) on measures of well-being and life satisfaction and had fewer side effects.[21] When compared to propranolol, patients taking captopril had fewer side effects and less sexual dysfunction with greater improvement in general well-being (p < 0.05 to 0.01). More such studies are needed to address quality-of-life issues. Until then, patients are asked to balance improved blood pressure control and its associated benefits (e.g., decreased incidence of stoke) with adverse effects of drugs. Many patients have elected to augment or substitute their allopathic therapies with herbal remedies. Is this advantageous or deleterious? That issue will be addressed in this chapter.

CASE STUDY 1: LICORICE

KJ is a 30-year-old white male who presents to the family medicine clinic with a blood pressure of 145/105 mmHg. He has no family history of hypertension. He is a nonsmoker and only occasionally consumes alcohol. His lipid profile is cholesterol = 190 mg/dl, HDL cholesterol 70 mg/dl, and triglycerides = 122 mg/dl, his blood glucose is 100 mg/dl, and he weighs 180 pounds. His potassium is 3.2 mEq/l. He has no concomitant conditions. On two subsequent visits, his blood pressures are 155/110 mmHg and 148/115 mmHg. He is diagnosed with moderate hypertension. He is begun on propranolol 40 mg bid. Two weeks later, his blood pressure is 130/98 mmHg. His propranolol dose is gradually increased over the next month to 120 mg SR once daily. At his next office visit (two weeks later), his blood pressure is mildly improved (130/100 mmHg) but he complains of muscle weakness. His potassium level today is 3.0 mEq/l. Upon further questioning, it is found that he chews tobacco.

Discussion

Licorice is a chewy black confection extracted from the plant root *Glycyrrhiza glabra*.[22] The hemisuccinate derivative of glycyrrhetinic acid is carbenoxolone, widely used in the treatment of duodenal and gastric ulcers.[23] Licorice is 50 times sweeter than sugar and hence has found widespread use as a sweetener, especially in candies.[24] However, most licorice candies contain little or no licorice but rather are flavored with anise oil.[24] Approximately 90 percent of licorice is used in chewing tobacco, cigars, pipe tobaccos, and cigarettes, with some use in authentic licorice candy primarily in Europe.[24] Authentic licorice, however, can also be obtained as an herbal product advocated for use as an expectorant, antimicrobial, for Addison's disease, acne, pimples, frostbite, irritability, and as an antispasmodic for treatment of stomach ulcers and in prophylaxis.[25,26]

Pseudohyperaldosteronism presenting as hypertension, hypokalemia, renal potassium wasting, metabolic alkalosis, sodium retention, and depressed renin is associated with licorice use. In one report, 20 percent of patients receiving licorice for the treatment of peptic ulcers developed hypertension and edema.[27] An 85-year-old man presented with a blood pressure of 160/110 mmHg, profound muscle weakness most prominent in limb girdles, and hypokalemia, following a 50-year history of chewing eight to twelve three-ounce (85 g) bags of chewing tobacco daily and swallowing the associated saliva.[28] This chewing tobacco contained 8.3 percent (w/w) licorice paste with a corresponding glycyrrhizinic acid content of 0.15 percent. This translated into daily consumption of 680 to 1020 g of product and 0.88 to 1.33 g of glycyrrhizinic acid, which is sufficient to cause hypertension. Unlike many tobacco chewers, this patient swallowed the saliva, expectorating only the well-chewed tobacco leaf, hence enhancing the probability of resulting toxicity. Within ten days of discontinuing chewing tobacco use and with potassium replenishment, this 85-year-old man resumed normal blood pressure and muscle strength. KJ should be questioned regarding the manner of his chewing tobacco use. Given his clinical profile, he may be swallowing his chewing tobacco saliva as well.

Licorice-induced hypertension mimics apparent mineralocorticoid excess. Licorice produces an acquired 11-beta-hydroxylase deficiency.[29] In such a deficiency, the patient cannot convert 11-deoxycortisol or deoxycorticosterone into the active glucocorticoids, cortisol and corticosterone, respectively. The resulting increase in the mineralocorticoid deoxycorticosterone promotes sodium retention, hypertension, and hypokalemia.[29] It has been further observed that the hypertensinogenic effect may be centrally mediated. An infusion of glycyrrhizic acid into a lateral ventricle of rat brain at doses less than that associated with hypertension when infused subcutaneously cause hypertension without affecting sodium.[30]

Severe hypokalemia has been observed in patients as a result with associated myopathy.[31,32] In one of the reports, protypical for this condition, a 35-year-old man developed acute myopathy, hypokalemia (K = 2.1 mEq/l), hypertension (170/110 mmHg), metabolic alkalosis ($pCO_2 = 55$) and depressed plasma renin (0.46 ng/ml/h; normal: 5 to 39 ng/ml/h) and serum aldosterone (12 ng/ml; normal: 16 to 80 ng/ml).[33] This patient's acute myopathy was characterized by complete paralysis of proximal muscles of the arms and shoulder girdles, weakness of muscles of the forearms and hands, weakness of proximal leg muscles (he could barely raise his legs from the bed) and moderate weakness of posterior and anterior neck muscles, areflexia, and a complaint of distal tingling without objective sensory loss.

For the previous two years, this man had ingested one or two bags of tablets of pure licorice daily, equating to 20 to 40 grams daily. He began this practice after he stopped smoking. After licorice discontinuation and potassium replacement, this patient's paralysis resolved by the third hospital day. After 1300 mEq of potassium, his potassium levels were restored to normal by day 10. His blood pressure remained high for two weeks (160/105 mmHg) but decreased to 140/90 mmHg by day 20. The persistence of hypokalemia and hypertension after licorice withdrawal has been attributed to glycyrrhizinic acid's effect on renal tubular excretion, which persists for days despite discontinuation.[32]

Treatment for hypertension associated with licorice usually can be accomplished with product discontinuation. Upon discontinuation, the blood pressure should return to baseline within ten days to three weeks.[28,34,35] For those cases where the blood pressure necessitates treatment, spironolactone should be initiated.[36]

Licorice root is contraindicated in patients with cholestatic liver disease, liver cirrhosis, hypertension, hypokalemia, severe renal insufficiency, and pregnancy, according to German Commission E monographs.[37] Furthermore, French authorities advise against concurrent use with corticosteroids principally because of probable electrolyte imbalances.[38] The clinician should be observant for this potential interaction as corticosteroids may be associated with gastrointestinal upset, which may prompt a patient to self-medicate with licorice, known for its gastrointestinal soothing effects. The intact adrenals are required for licorice ingestion to cause hypertension; hence, in the setting of inadequate adrenal function, licorice may not elicit a hypertensive response but when corticosteroid supplementation is supplied, adrenal function may be restored sufficiently to elicit the hypertensive effect of licorice.[39,40] Documented clinical experience for this potential interaction is lacking.

Other potential interactions include oral contraceptives and thiazide diuretics. According to Italian investigators, elevation of plasma renin activity by oral contraceptives may predispose patients to the ill effects of licorice.[41] In their study of 24 healthy subjects, fluid retention secondary to licorice ingestion occurred more frequently in the premenstrual period or when patients were taking oral contraceptives. Of interest is the finding that a woman in this study taking estrogen and progestin did not undergo side effects such as renal sodium retention.[41] There are no reports of angiotensin converting inhibitors (e.g., captopril, enalapril, lisinopril) or angiotensin II receptor blockers (e.g., losartan, valsartan) interacting with licorice but surveillance is advised. Thiazide diuretics are known to promote potassium depletion and may predispose the patient to licorice toxicity.[42] Concurrent administration is ill-advised.

CASE STUDY 2: YOHIMBINE

RV is a 58-year-old white male with hypertension (BP = 145/98 mmHg; HR 70 beats/minute) and mild anxiety. He is treated successfully with clonidine 0.2 mg bid with an attendant blood pressure of 122/88 mmHg. At his next office visit, he reports being less anxious but is also experiencing xerostomia, sedation, and impotence. His physician recommends he begin yohimbine to address the impotence. He obtains yohimbine and ingests 20 mg daily. Two weeks later, his impotence has diminished but his blood pressure is 150/100 mmHg. The patient states he has been compliant with clonidine, which concurs with pharmacy refill records. He also complains of a return of the anxiety and pruritic scaly skin and desquamation of the palms. Antinuclear antibody, anti-Sjogren syndrome-A/Ro antigen, anti-SS-B/La antigen, antinuclear ribonucleoprotein (nRNP), C_3, and C_4 values were all negative or within normal limits. His erythrocyte sedimentation rate (ESR) was 75 mm/h (normal: 15 mm/h). To what do you ascribe RV's loss of blood pressure control and new constellation of side effects?

Discussion

Clonidine is a central alpha-adrenergic stimulant that inhibits sympathetic cardioaccelerator and vasoconstrictor centers, reduces sympathetic outflow from the CNS, and decreases peripheral resistance, heart rate, and blood pressure.[43] It also causes sedation, dry mouth, drowsiness, and impotence (16 percent). Yohimbine has been advocated for male impotence due to its ability to block presynaptic alpha$_2$-adrenergic receptors, thereby decreasing blood outflow from the corporeal bodies of the penis.[44-47] It has been associated with a 43 to 80 percent effectiveness rate.[45-47] A two- to three-week latency between onset of yohimbine therapy and improvement in erectile function is encountered at a dosage of 18 mg daily (6 mg thrice daily).[45] In contrast, no latency is observed with the following side effects in this study, which are also attributed to alpha$_2$ adrenoreceptor blockade:

- increased anxiety
- accelerated heart rate
- increased circulating levels of catecholamines
- elevated blood pressure

It is particularly troublesome that yohimbine is associated with increased blood pressure because it will often be used for impotence associated with antihypertensives (e.g., clonidine, beta-blockers). In a study of 25 white adult patients with uncomplicated essential hypertension, yohimbine (21.6 mg) was associated with maximal increases in systolic blood pressure of 10 ± 2 mmHg (range: 4 to 26 mmHg) and in diastolic blood pressure of 5 ± 1 mmHg (range 2 to 17 mmHg) with a corresponding significant increase in plasma norepinephrine (NE) and 3,4-dihydroxyphenylglycol (DHPG) levels.[48] This observation has been confirmed in other studies in which statistically significant increases in diastolic blood pressure occur secondary to yohimbine therapy.[49,50] In another study of 17 white men aged 23 to 37 years, dose-dependent increases in postdrug steady-state values of arterialized plasma NE were observed ($p < 0.005$).[51] It has been proposed that yohimbine augments release of NE from sympathetic nerves, increasing reuptake and intraneuronal metabolism of the transmitter.[48] Others have proposed that yohimbine increases NE release into the bloodstream by the following mechanisms:[52]

1. Blockade of inhibitory alpha$_2$-adrenergic receptors on vascular smooth muscles with vasodilation causing reflexive increases in sympathetic outflow
2. Direct stimulation of sympathetic outflow from the brain
3. Blockade of inhibitory alpha$_2$-adrenergic receptors on sympathetic nerve endings, enhancing NE release for a given amount of sympathetic traffic

Yohimbine, however, has not been observed to alter NE clearance.[51-52] Of interest is the observation that 40 percent of patients with essential hypertension ($n = 19$) exhibited pressor hyperresponsiveness during yohimbine administration as compared to normotensive control subjects ($n = 19$).[52] A bolus yohimbine challenge test results in a 13 ± 2 percent increase in mean arterial pressure in normotensive patients and 17 ± 2 percent in hypertensive patients.[52] Hence hypertensive patients may be more vulnerable to the hypertensive effects of yohimbine. The increase in RV's blood pressure was probably based on this evidence.

Yohimbine has been associated with side effects related to and independent of its ability to block alpha$_2$ receptors (see Table 8.1). Increased blood pressure, heart rate, and anxiety as well as piloerection could all be expected as a correlate of increased NE. Cold sweaty hands and an urge to void also relate to the vasoconstrictor properties of NE. Manic-like symptoms have occurred, especially in patients with preexisting bipolar diathesis.[53]

In one patient, 10 mg of yohimbine elicited tremulousness and generalized restlessness within one hour.[53] A 20-year-old woman with postpartum depression experienced talkativeness, lacrimation, rhinorrhea tremor, and a tingling sensation in her feet within one hour of receiving 20 mg of yohimbine.[53] This observation is felt to be consistent with reports of increased noradrenergic activity as measured by 3-methoxy-4-hydroxy-phenylglycol (MHPG) in the cerebrospinal fluid of manic patients.[54] In a study of ten normal male volunteers, the most commonly reported side effect was restlessness.[55] Uneasiness, irritability, and easy fatigability have also been reported but completely resolved within 36 hours of yohimbine discontinuation.[55] Cutaneous drug eruptions, progressive renal failure, and a lupuslike syndrome have also been reported secondary to yohimbine.[56]

TABLE 8.1. Side Effects Associated with Yohimbine

piloerection	lupus-like syndrome
bronchospasm	increased blood pressure
rhinorrhea	accelerated heart rate
lacrimation	increased anxiety
fine rest tremor	cutaneous drug eruption
unusual taste and smell	restlessness
cold, sweaty hands	irritability
urge to void	precipitation of manic symptoms
fatigue	panic attacks
tingling sensation in feet	

A 42-year-old black man developed pruritic, scaly skin, fever, chills, malaise, periorbital edema, desquamation of the palms, eosinophilia (eosinophils: 19 percent) and an elevated erythrocyte sedimentation rate (87 mm/h) one day after ingesting three 5.4 mg doses of yohimbine.[56]

Broncho-spasm has also been reported with yohimbine.[57] A 60-year-old man with a history of transplant for idiopathic cardiomyopathy presented to the emergency room with a ten-day history of cough productive of copious amounts of clear white sputum and progressive shortness of breath immediately following initiation of yohimbine 5.4 mg three times a day for impotence. Upon examination, he was afebrile, had expiratory sneezes, and rhonchi bilaterally. His chest X-ray findings were normal as were his blood studies except for a white blood cell count of 12,400 cells/mm³. Yohimbine was discontinued, and he was treated with sulfamethoxazole/ trimethoprim followed by albuterol inhaler and theophylline for three weeks. This adverse effect was attributed to an increase in cholinergic activity secondary to yohimbine.[57] Despite these side effects, yohimbine is relatively safe. Even in a massive overdose (100 2-mg tablets), the only side effects were tachycardia, hypertension, and anxiety of brief duration (19 hours).[58] The return of anxiety symptoms and cutaneous drug reaction is consistent with other reported side effects of yohimbine.

Yohimbine has the ability to interact with other drugs, most notably those with adrenergic effects. Tricyclic antidepressants and other drugs known to interfere with neuronal uptake or metabolism of NE may exacerbate NE's effect when coadministered with yohimbine.[48] It has been shown that yohimbine when given concomitantly with desipramine decreases the density of brain beta adrenergic receptors more rapidly than when either agent is given alone.[59-60] This speaks to the synergistic effect of these two agents and the reflex downregulation that may occur when given together. However, yohimbine has been used successfully with clomipramine to combat orthostatic hypotension induced by the latter.[61] In this study of 12 patients with depression and clomipramine-induced orthostatic hypotension, yohimbine 4 mg tid induced a significant increase in blood pressure.[61] This effect was observed after the first dose and persisted for 17 to 24 hours. Since this effect extended beyond five half-lives ($t_{1/2} = 36$ minutes), it is most likely that the interaction is pharmacodynamic and not pharmacokinetic.[58] Another potential interaction involves clonidine, which possesses both alpha$_1$ and alpha$_2$ agonist activity; when coadministered with yohimbine, the alpha$_1$ activity is unopposed, resulting in hypertension.[58] RV's hypertension could be explained in this context in addition to yohimbine's hypertensive effect independent of coadministration with clonidine.

Before attributing any side effect or potential drug-drug interaction to yohimbine, it would be prudent to determine first if the product in question actually contains yohimbine. Products claiming to contain 500 mg of yohimbe bark extract in each tablet, upon assay, contained caffeine and no yohimbine.[62] Once again, this exemplifies that standardization and regulation by an independent agency is needed for the herbal industry.

CASE STUDY 3: GARLIC

VZ is a 48-year-old black female diagnosed with uncomplicated essential hypertension. Her blood pressure has been adequately controlled with losartan 25 mg bid. On today's visit her blood pressure is low at 110/60 mmHg, and she smells strongly of garlic. How do you interpret her blood pressure in terms of garlic consumption?

Discussion

Garlic enjoys a long history of reputed efficacy in the treatment of hypertension, hyperlipidemia, and diabetes mellitus.[63] In one study of 26 patients, 85 percent of patients receiving garlic experienced antihypertensive effects with an average decrease in systolic blood pressure of 12.3 mmHg and 6.5 mmHg diastolic blood pressure.[64] Twenty-five percent of these patients experienced a decrease in systolic blood pressure of 20 mmHg or more. Allimin, containing 4.75 grains of garlic concentrate equivalent to 0.31 g of desiccated garlic and 2.375 grains of desiccated parsley (to offset garlic's malodorous presentation), was administered to these patients as two tablets three times a day.[64] The findings of this study were confirmed by two additional studies. Piotrowski found 40 percent of patients (n = 100) experienced a 20 mmHg or greater decline in systolic blood pressure (following 0.6 to 1.2 g daily of dialyzed, alcoholic garlic extract).[65] This occurred within one week of initiating garlic therapy. Pektov found a moderate hypotensive effect in 67 hypertensive patients with a decrease in systolic blood pressure of 20 to 30 mmHg and of 10 to 20 mmHg for diastolic blood pressure.[66]

In a 12-week, blinded, randomized, placebo-controlled study of 47 ambulatory patients administered 200 mg thrice daily of garlic powder, diastolic blood pressure decrease 11.5 percent (102 mmHg to 89 mmHg; $p < 0.01$).[67] In a meta-analysis of eight trials evaluating the antihypertensive effect of garlic including 415 subjects all using the same dried garlic powder (Kwai), it was concluded that while three studies showed a significant decrease in systolic blood pressure and four in diastolic blood pressure, garlic use should be reserved for patients with mild hypertension only.[68] These authors felt there was still insufficient evidence to recommend garlic use as routine. Additionally, it has been noted that garlic composition may differ according to region and seasonal conditions, which could result in a varying dose.[69] Also, at least seven cloves of garlic each day are required to exert beneficial effects, which many patients will find unacceptable due to its odoriferous nature.[69]

Garlic is not without side effects (see Table 8.2). Allergic contact dermatitis has been reported.[70] Such garlic-sensitive patients are believed to be reacting to diallyl disulfide, allyl propyl disulfide, allyl mercaptan, and/or allicin.[71] Other reported side effects include nausea, diaphoresis, light-headedness, and burning sensations of the upper GI tract of 15 minutes duration.[72] Anorexia, nausea, severe vomiting, diarrhea, marked weight loss, metorrhagia, and menorrhagia have been reported following 0.25 mg three times daily of garlic essential oil.[73] However, in another study patients receiving up to 60 g of crude garlic daily for three months experienced no side effects.[74] Caution, however, should be exercised when used in excessive amounts. Spontaneous spinal epidural hematoma occurred in an 87-year-old man who ingested 2000 mg of garlic daily to prevent heart disease.[75] He denied use of nonsteroidal anti-inflammatory drugs, aspirin, or other medications known to precipitate bleeding disorders. He developed complete bilateral sensory and motor paralysis in the lower extremities and loss of sensation at about the T6 level. Prothrombin time (PT) and partial thromboplastin time (PTT) were 12.7 and 22.3 seconds, respectively. Platelet

TABLE 8.2. Side Effects of Garlic

allergic contact dermatitis	vomiting
nausea	diarrhea
diaphoresis	metorrhagia
light-headedness	menorrhagia
burning sensation in GI tract	spinal epidural hematoma

count was 178,000, although the bleeding time was prolonged to 11.5 minutes (normal: 3 minutes). A computed tomographic scan demonstrated a posterior extradural mass at the T9-T10 level with dural sac displacement. A bilateral thoracic laminectomy from T8 to T10 resulted in return of motor function and sensation in the lower extremities. This patient's condition was attributed to garlic's ability to inhibit normal platelet function.[75] This is validated in a study where essential oil of garlic in a daily dose of 120 mg for 20 days resulted in a significant (p < 0.001) decrease in platelet aggregation from 30.37 percent to 21.21 percent (n = 34).[76] Other toxicities have been observed as well. When 50 mg daily of garlic powder was administered to rats, degenerative changes were observed after 45 days and severe testicular lesions were seen after 70 days.[77] It is difficult, however, to extrapolate animal data to humans.

No drug-drug interactions have been reported to date but neither has there been active surveillance for such interactions. Garlic extracts can inhibit serum and liver enzymes; hence, if drug-metabolizing enzymes are affected, drugs excreted via hepatic metabolism (e.g., diazepam, see Table 8.3) will be affected.[78] Also, other drugs that inhibit hepatic metabolism (e.g., cimetidine, see Table 8.4) may at least additively and perhaps synergistically interact with garlic. Given the ability of garlic to adversely affect platelet function as noted by Rose et al.,[75] it would be prudent to avoid concomitant use of drugs known to also affect platelet function such as NSAIDs (e.g., indomethacin), aspirin, and dipyridamole. Because anticoagulants (e.g., warfarin) have also been associated with epidural hematomas, concomitant use with garlic is not advisable.[79,80] More study is needed to determine if statistical and/or clinical significance is obtained.

TABLE 8.3. Drugs That Are Extensively Metabolized by the Liver

alprazolam (Xanax)	cortocosteroids (e.g., prednisone; Deltasone)	propranolol (Inderal)
amitriptyline (Elavil, Endep)	cyclosporine (Sandimmune, Neoral)	terfenadine (Seldane)
astemizole (Hismanal)	desipramine (Norpramin)	theophylline (Theodur)
carbamazepine (Tegretol)	diazepam (Valium)	triazolam (Halcion)
cisapride (Propulsid)	imipramine (Tofranil)	warfarin (Coumadin)
clozapine (Clozaril)	phenytoin (Dilantin)	

TABLE 8.4. Drugs That Inhibit Liver Metabolism

cimetidine (Tagamet)	erythromycin (E-Mycin, EES)	nefazodone (Serzone)
ciprofloxacin (Cipro)	fluoxetine (Prozac)	paroxetine (Paxil)
clarithromycin (Biaxin)	fluvoxamine (Luvox)	ritonavir (Norvir)
diltiazem (Cardizem)	itraconazole (Sporanox)	
enoxacin (Penetrex)	ketoconazole (Nizoral)	

CASE STUDY 4: HERBAL DIURETICS

EH is a 48-year-old black male with primary essential hypertension. His blood pressure has been adequately controlled with hydrochlorothiazide (HCTZ) 25 mg/day. At his most recent physician office visit, his potassium was 3.3 mEq/L so he was begun on potassium chloride supplementation. Since the latter caused gastrointestinal distress EH elected to try an herbal diuretic, dandelion *(Taraxacum officinale)*, and discontinued HCTZ without notifying his physician. EH contracted an upper respiratory infection and consulted with his physician. At that time his blood pressure had risen to 140/96 mmHg. Why did the herbal diuretic not control his hypertension and in fact, cause an increase in his blood pressure?

Discussion

Diuretics such as HCTZ increase the rate of urine flow and increase the excretion of sodium (natriuresis) and an accompanying anion, usually chloride.[81] Because NaCl is the body's major determinant of extracellular fluid volume, diuretics are especially useful. Thus, diuretics are recommended for hypertension because they reduce extracellular fluid volume by decreasing total body NaCl content, thereby decreasing vascular resistance and blood pressure. In contrast, herbal diuretics are not diuretics but, more accurately, aquaretics.[82] Herbal aquaretics increase blood flow to the kidneys with a subsequent increase in urine, but neither sodium nor chloride resorption is decreased. Hence these electrolytes are retained. As a consequence, osmotic pressure will increase as extracellular fluid is drawn into the vessel to equilibrate with the remaining NaCl. This increased intravascular fluid volume will translate into increased vascular resistance with a corresponding increase blood pressure. Hence, not only is the blood pressure not controlled, but with herbal diuretics, the patient's hypertension may in fact be worse than at baseline. See Table 8.5 for a listing of herbal aquaretics.

TABLE 8.5. Herbal Aquaretics

adonis	heartsease
agrimony	hydrangea
bearberry	lady's mantle
buchu	larch
dandelion	sassafras

CASE STUDY 5: GRAPEFRUIT AND GINSENG

VL is a 65-year-old white male diagnosed with hypertension after obtaining three readings averaging 145/110 mmHg. He is begun on nifedipine and titrated to a maintenance dose of 60 mg SR once daily. He monitors his blood pressure at home with DynaPulse, a computerized monitoring system, logging the following blood pressure readings over the next two weeks: 138/98, 130/95, 120/85, 110/78, 100/60, 135/95, 138/100 mmHg. The patient notes beginning to take nifedipine with grapefruit juice based on his neighbor's report of being better able to control his blood pressure in this nutritionally-based manner. At this time his blood pressure recorded as the 110/60 mmHg reading. However, VL began to feel lethargic, dizzy, and tired and began taking ginseng. After several days of ginseng ingestion, his blood pressure readings were 135/95 and 138/100 mmHg. The patient also complains of enlargement of his breasts. VL was compliant with his nifedipine regimen during this time as verified with pharmacy records, and VL has no other concomitant conditions. How do you explain VL's labile blood pressure and gynecomastia?

Discussion

Grapefruit juice contains flavonoids (naringenin, quercetin, and kaempferol), which inhibit the metabolism of dihydropyridine calcium channel blockers (nifedipine, felodipine, nitrendipine, and nisoldipine).[83] This interaction is not noted with orange juice, which does not contain all three of these flavonoids. Other sources of these flavonoids include tea, onions, and apples.[83] Quercetin may be the main inhibitor of cytochrome P-450IIIA4. Clinically, this has been demonstrated in a 63-year-old white man diagnosed with hypertension with a blood pressure of 205/105 mmHg.[83] When treated with isosorbide, hydralazine, terazosin, and felodipine, his blood pressure was 190/95 mmHg. He discontinued hydralazine and began drinking six ounces of grapefruit juice with his felodipine and terazosin, resulting in a blood pressure of 155/81 mmHg, further decreasing to 141/74 mmHg six months later. To determine if his blood pressure decrease was related to grapefruit juice ingestion, he discontinued grapefruit juice for ten days, which resulted in an increase of blood pressure to 175/97 mmHg. With resumption of grapefruit ingestion and maintenance of felodipine (10 mg/day) and terazosin (20 mg/day), his blood pressure remained controlled at 144/82 mmHg. Subsequent studies have shown grapefruit juice increases felodipine maximal concentrations by 170 to 270 percent and the area under the curve (AUC) 192 to 299 percent.[84-88] Additionally, grapefruit juice increases the AUC of nifedipine by 134 percent and the AUC of nitrendipine by 140 percent (maximal concentrations unchanged).[89,90] Hence, even if the patient is taking the same amount of grapefruit juice with consistent flavonoid potency every day, this will still introduce considerable variability in blood levels of the concomitant calcium channel blocker.

In addition, ginseng has been noted to affect blood pressure with both increases and sometimes decreases, meaning that this also introduces another determinant of blood pressure variability for VL.[25,91-93] Furthermore, ginseng content varies widely. When studied, 60 percent of ginseng samples contained substandard quality ginseng and 25 percent did not contain any ginseng.[94] Total panaxoside ginseng concentrations for twenty-four products varied from 0.26 to 6.85 mg per 250 mg sample. Therefore, differences in blood pressure could be related to variances in ginseng purity.

Gynecomastia has been reported for both calcium channel blockers (specifically nifedipine, verapamil, and diltiazem) and ginseng.[16,95] When the two are taken concomitantly, the patient is at increased risk for the development of gynecomastia. VL should be counseled to discontinue both grapefruit juice and ginseng intake to reduce the lability of his blood pressure and to reduce or eliminate gynecomastia.

CASE STUDY 6: CHINESE HERBS

HMT is a 48-year-old Asian woman of Chinese descent who presents to the family medicine clinic with a blood pressure of 138/112 mmHg. She has had three previous readings taken by her pharmacist averaging 142/115 mmHg. She has self-medicated with a Chinese herbal tea advocated for hypertension containing Dai-saiko-to and Saiko-ka-rhykotsu-boreito but was urged by her pharmacist to seek physician care given her continued high readings. How do you advise her regarding her use of this herbal tea and treatment of her hypertension?

Discussion

Chinese herbal remedies are steeped in a several-thousand-year history of use. Most, however, have not been rigorously studied by Western methods. Limited studies for those that have been studied indicate that some of these remedies have not proven as efficacious as Western remedies. Such remedies are Dai-saiko-to and Saiko-ka-rhykotsu-boreito. Dai-saiko-to contains in the following ratios: *Bupleuri radix*-6, *Pinelliae tuber*-4, *Zingiberis rhizoma*-1,

Scutellariae radix-3, *Zizyphi fructus*-3, *Paeoniae radix*-3, *Aurantii fructus immaturus*-2, and *Rhei phizoma*-1. The Saiko-ka-ryukotsu-boreito mixture ratios are *Bupleuri radix*-5, *Pinelliae tuber*-4, *Zingiberis rhizoma*-1, *Scutellariae radix*-2.5, *Zizyphi fructus*-2.5, *Cinnamomi cortex*-3, *Hoelen*-3, *Ginseng radix*-2.5, *Ostreae testa*-2.5 and *Fossila ossis mastodi*-2.5. In an open randomized trial of thirty outpatients with mild to moderate essential hypertension, patients received either Dai-saiko-to or Saiko-ka-ryukotsu-boreito three times daily after each meal for three months (7.5 g/day, each).[96] After three months of therapy, the blood pressures remained unchanged but high-density lipoprotein-cholesterol increased significantly ($p < 0.05$).[96] Of interest is the ginseng component of Saiko-ka-ryukotsu-boreito, which has a predominantly hypertensive effect. Hence it is not surprising that blood pressure did not decrease given this component. Also of note is the presence of *Radix scutellariae* in both remedies. *Radix scutellariae* is the root of *Scutellaria baicalensis,* commonly known as Huangqin in China and Ogon or Wogon in Japan.[97] The major flavonoid is baicalin, which has been associated with hepatotoxic reactions.[98,99] Hepatitis and jaundice have been reported following three days to two months of use.[98] It would be prudent to obtain liver function tests (LFTs) in HMT. HMT would be better treated with a first-line Western medication such as a diuretic, a beta-blocker, or an ACE inhibitor.

Black and colleagues conducted a randomized study in 45 patients comparing Western medicine (thiazide diuretic and propranolol) with Chinese medicine (a mixture of 12 herbs).[100] The 12-herb mixture contained:

- *Rhizoma gastrodiae* (gastrodia tuber)
- *Ramulus uncariae* cum *uncis* (uncaria stem with hooks)
- *Concha holiotidis* (sea-ear shell)
- *Cortex eucommia* (eucommia bark)
- *Radix achyranthis* (*Bidentatae achyranthes* roots)
- *Os draconis ustum* (ignited dragon's bone)
- *Rhizoma aliamatis* (water plantain tuber)
- *Radix scutellarie*
- *Rhizoma rehmannia praeporata*
- *Salvia paeoniac alba* (white peony root)
- *Helianthus annuus* L.
- *Salvia miltiorrhiza*

After 23 days of therapy, Western medicine resulted in a decrease from 173/107 to 141/90 mmHg, whereas there was no change in blood pressure for those patients taking the Chinese mixture (169/108 to 166/106 mmHg).[100] However, other Chinese herbal medicinals do hold considerable promise.

Tetrandrine, the alkaloid extracted from the Chinese medicinal herb *Radix stephania tetrandrae,* and daurisoline, the alkaloid extracted from *Menispermum dauricum* have calcium channel blocking abilities, which may explain their usefulness in hypertension.[101-103]

Clearly more study is needed with Chinese herbal medicinals to identify those that are as, if not more, efficacious than our Western medicines. Given their many thousand years of usefulness, it is very likely that more compounds like tetrandrine and daurisoline will be identified.

CASE STUDY 7: FISH OIL

DS is a 53-year-old white male with a fifteen-year history of hypertension currently controlled with 50 mg of atenolol. His blood pressure usually averages 130/80 mm/Hg, but during the last two visits blood pressures were 126/78 mmHg and 124/76 mmHg, respectively. He reported making no changes in his medication but had started himself on four grams of fish oil per day that he purchased from a health food store after he read about the benefits of fish oil supplementation in a nutrition magazine. DS had been using the supplement for six months without any side effects. He had no fishy aftertaste as some of his friends had complained. How do you advise him regarding continued use?

Discussion

There is no evidence that fish oil supplements (*n*-3 fatty acids) lower blood pressure in normotensive people.[104,105] However, in hypertensive subjects, evidence suggests that supplementation of the diet with fish oil does have a beneficial effect on blood pressure.[105-108] A meta-analysis of studies evaluating the efficacy of fish oil in untreated hypertensive patients concluded that greater than three grams of fish oil per day significantly reduced blood pressure, both clinically and statistically.[105] The average decline in systolic and diastolic blood pressures was 5.5 and 3.5 mmHg, respectively. Another meta-analysis of placebo-controlled trials found a dose-related blood pressure lowering response to fish oil supplements in patients with untreated hypertension.[108] The year that these meta-analyses were published, a randomized crossover trial reported no hypotensive effect by fish oil supplements in 18 subjects with untreated mild hypertension.[109] However, a later study of 78 persons with untreated mild hypertension found a decrease in blood pressure similar to the above-mentioned meta-analysis (Appel et al.) in individuals receiving four grams of fish oil daily.[106] Despite the overall encouraging findings, generalization of the results of these studies must be done with caution. For example, most patients in the studies subjected to meta-analysis by Appel and colleagues were middle-aged white males.

The concomitant use of fish oil supplements by hypertensive patients already on antihypertensive medication has received limited attention. The addition of 3.4 g (85 percent *n*-3 preparation) fish oil in the diet of hypertensive patients using beta-blockers ($n = 29$), diuretics ($n = 3$), or both ($n = 11$) further lowered blood pressure (3.1/1.8 mmHg) with statistical significance.[110] The authors recognized the decline as small from a clinical perspective but noted that the accompanying 21 percent reduction in plasma triglycerides they found could be an important benefit in patients with hypertension taking these types of antihypertensive medication. An earlier study demonstrated that fish oil supplements reduced blood pressure comparably to propranolol or fish oil alone.[111] In 18 previously untreated hypertensive males with hyperlipidemia, the hypotensive effect of fish oil supplements in addition to nifedipine was no different than nifedipine alone.[112] However, fish oil lowered trigylceride/VLDL-cholesterol levels by 24 percent, and the same effect was maintained when nifedipine was given in addition to fish oil, but there was also a significant reduction (12 percent) in total cholesterol. Another study of hypertensive patients was not able to demonstrate that the combination of dietary fish oil supplementation and sodium restriction augmented the antihypertensive effect of angiotension converting enzyme (ACE) inhibitors more than sodium restriction alone, but there was a 27 percent decline in plasma triglycerides in the group that received fish oil.[113]

There are a variety of potential biochemical mechanisms by which *n*-3 fatty acids may lower blood pressure, but it is unclear which one or combination is at work, or if there are unknown processes. It appears that the incorporation of *n*-3 fatty acids into cell membranes may reduce vascular resistance by tipping the balance between vasodilating and vasoconstricting prostaglandins. They inhibit the production of thromboxane A_2 (vasoconstrictor), increase the production of thromboxane A_3 (less vasoconstrictive), and stimulate the formation of prostaglandin I_3 (vasodilator).[105,106,109,114] Also, *n*-3 fatty acids reduce blood viscosity by increasing red blood cell deformability[105,109,114] and may affect the arterial baroreceptor mechanism.[105,106]

The long-term benefits and effects of the use of fish oil supplements for the treatment of hypertension are unknown. Thus far, fish oil supplements seem to be well tolerated and safe. In one study, no patient (n = 55) during a two-year trial stopped fish oil treatment (12 g/day) due to side effects or complications.[115] This appears to be consistent with other studies in which subjects were given fish oil daily for weeks to years; few subjects dropped out because of adverse effects. The most common side effects were unpleasant taste, halitosis, eructation, heartburn, flatulence, and diarrhea. Since *n*-3 fatty acid supplements have been shown to prolong bleeding time, inhibit platelet aggregation, and decrease thromboxane A_2, some have raised concern about an increased risk of bleeding. However, bleeding has not been reported as a complication in studies evaluating the efficacy of fish oil supplementation in the treatment of hypertension and other diseases. In fact, fish oil was not found to increase bleeding problems in a study of patients on aspirin or warfarin[116] or in surgical patients.[117] This does not mean that fish oil can be recommended irrespective of underlying medical problems or the use of an antiplatelet medication or anticoagulants. Clinical judgment and caution should be exercised in each individual's case.

MEDICINAL AND PHARMACEUTICAL CHEMISTRY ASPECTS

The form in which glycyrrhizin is administered will have therapeutic impact. It has been shown that the bioavailability of glycyrrhizin and glycyrrhetic acid is lower if administered as licorice extract rather than as glycyrrhizin itself.[41] Hence the hypertensive effect may be more profound if glycyrrhizin itself is administered.

Patients considering use of garlic would be well advised to closely examine the nature of their garlic preparation. Dried garlic preparations contain alliin, the nonodorous precursor to ajoene, the anticlotting agent, and allicin, the antibacterial component.[102] Allinase is required to convert alliin to allicin and ajoene but when dried garlic is consumed, stomach acids destroy the enzyme. Hence, if dried garlic preparations are employed, they must be enteric coated.

Table 8.6 is a list of herbs that may have an effect on blood pressure. Table 8.7 summarizes information about herbs reviewed in this chapter.

TABLE 8.6. Herbs with Purported Effects on Blood Pressure

HYPOTENSIVES	
agrimony	mistletoe
asafoetida	nettle
avens	*Os draconis ustum* (ignited dragon's bone)
calamus	parsley
celery	pokeroot
chotachand	prickly ash, northern
cohosh, black	prickly ash, southern
Concha holiotidis (sea-ear shell)	*Radix achyranthis* (*Bidentatae achyranthes* roots)
Cortex eucommia (eucommia bark)	*Radix scutellariae*
corn silk	*Radix stephania tetrandrae* (tetrandrine)
Dai-saiko-to	*Ramulus uncariae cum uncis* (uncaria stem with hooks)
devil's claw	*Rhizoma aliamatis* (water plantain tuber)
elecampane	*Rhizoma gastrodiae* (gastrodia tuber)
English hawthorne	*Rhizoma rehmannia praeporata*
fenugreek	sage
Fucus (*Laminaria* species, kelp, seaweed)	Saiko-ka-rhykotsu-boreito
fumitory	*Salvia paeoniac alba* (white peony root)
garlic	shepherd's purse
ginger	squill
ginseng, *panax*	St. John's wort
goldenseal	vervain
Helianthus annuus L.	wild carrot
hellebore	yarrow
horseradish	*Salvia miltiorrhiza*
Laminaria japonica (ne-kombu; seaweed)	

HYPERTENSIVES	
bayberry	ginger
broom	ginseng
capsicum	licorice
cohosh, blue	khat
cola	ma huang (ephedra)
coltsfoot	mate
Eleutherococcus species	vervain
gentian	aquaretics (e.g., dandelion; see Table 8.5)

TABLE 8.7. Summary

Yohimbine may be used to treat impotence secondary to antihypertensive use but may increase blood pressure.
Yohimbine should not be coadministered with tricyclic antidepressants or clonidine.
Garlic may be useful for mild hypertension but its routine use is not recommended.
Avoid concomitant use of garlic with NSAIDs, anticoagulants and drugs that inhibit liver metabolism (e.g., cimetidine) and drugs that may be affected by liver inhibition (e.g., propranolol, diazepam).
Herbal diuretics (e.g., goldenrod) are actually aquaretics and may worsen hypertension.
Licorice may induce hypertension accompanied by hypokalemia mimicking syndromes of apparent mineralocorticoid excess.
Patients taking oral contraceptives or thiazide diuretics may be predisposed to licorice toxicity if taken concomitantly.
Grapefruit juice if administered concomitantly with nifedipine may result in a clinically significant decrease in blood pressure.
Most Chinese herbal medicinals have not been studied by Western means. Tetrandrine *(Radix stephania tetrandrae)* and daurisoline *(Menispermum dauricum)* may possess calcium channel blocking activity.

REFERENCES

1. The Joint National Committee on Detection, Evaluation and Treatment of High Blood Pressure. The fifth report of the national committee on detection, evaluation and treatment of high blood pressure (JNC V). *Arch Intern Med* 1993; 153:154-183.

2. National High Blood Pressure Education Program. National high blood pressure education program working group report on hypertension in diabetes. *Hypertension* 1994;23:145-158.

3. Arradondo J. Tailoring antihypertensive drug therapy for black patients. *J Nat Med Assoc* 1987;79:149-154.

4. Veterans Administration Cooperative Study Group on Antihypertensive Agents. Comparison of propranolol and hydrochlorothiazide for the initial treatment of hypertension: I. Results of short-term titration with emphasis on racial differences in response. *JAMA* 1982;248:1996-2003.

5. Lopez LM. Hypertension in the elderly: Conventional wisdom revisited. *Pharmacotherapy* 1991;11:225-236.

6. Epstein M. Hypertension in the elderly. Part 11. *Geriatric Med Today* 1990;9:28-45.

7. Packer M, Lee WH, Yushak M, Medina N. Comparison of captopril and enalapril in patients with severe chronic heart failure. *N Engl J Med* 1986; 315:847-853.

8. D'Angelo A, Sartori L, Gambaro G, Giannini S, Malvasi L, et al., Captopril in the treatment of hypertension in type I and type II diabetic patients. *Postgrad Med J* 1986;62 (Suppl 1):69-72.

9. Robinson BF. Calcium-entry blocking agents in the treatment of systemic hypertension. *Am J Cardiol* 1985;55:102B-106B.

10. Kaplan NM. Cardiovascular risk reduction: The role of antihypertensive treatment. *Am J Med* 1991;90 (Suppl 2A):19S-20S.

11. Kasiske BL, Ma JA, Kalil SN, Louis TA. Effects of antihypertensive therapy on serum lipids. *Ann Intern Med* 1995;122:133-141.

12. Hoes AW, Grobbee De, Lubsen J, Mall in't Veld AJ, van der Does E, Hofman A. Diuretics, beta-blockers and the risk for sudden cardiac death in hypertensive patients. *Ann Intern Med* 1995;123:481-487.

13. Lim PO, MacFadyen RJ, Blarkson PBM, MacDonald TM. Impaired exercise tolerance in hypertensive patients. *Ann Intern Med* 1996;124 (1 pt 1):41-55.

14. Gengo FM, Gabos C. Central nervous system considerations in the use of beta-blockers, angiotensin-converting enzyme inhibitors, and thiazide diuretics in managing essential hypertension. *Am Heart J* 1988;116:305-310.

15. DiBianco R. Adverse reactions with angiotensive converting enzyme (ACE) inhibitors. *Medical Toxicol* 1986;1:122-141.

16. Olin BR., Ed. *Facts and Comparisons,* St. Louis, MO: Facts and Comparisons, 1996.

17. Furberg CD, Psaty BM, Meyer JV. Nifedipine: Dose-related increase in mortality in patients with coronary heart disease. *Circulation* 1995;92:1326-1331.

18. Psaty BM, Heckbert SR, Koepsell TD et al., The risk of myocardial infarction associated with antihypertensive drug therapies. *JAMA* 1995;274:620-625.

19. McCorvey E, Wright JT, Culbert JP, McKenney JM, Proctor JD, Annett MP. Effects of hydrochlorothiazide, enalapril and propranolol on quality of life and cognitive and motor function in hypertensive patients. *Clin Pharm* 1993;12:300-305.

20. Rakel RE. Antihypertensive therapy and quality of life. *Am Fam Physician* 1987;35:221-226.

21. Croog SH, Levine S, Testa MA et al., The effects of antihypertensive therapy on the quality of life. *N Engl J Med* 1986;314:1657-1664.

22. Walker BR, Edwards CRW. Licorice-induced hypertension and syndromes of apparent mineralocorticoid excess. *Endocrin Metab Clin N Amer* 1994;23:359-377.

23. Reynolds JEF, Ed. *Martindale The Extra Pharmacopoeia,* Twenty-ninth Edition, London: The Pharmaceutical Press, 1989.

24. Tyler V. Licorice. In: *The Honest Herbal.* The Haworth Press, Binghamton, NY, 1993:197-199.

25. Bisset NG, Ed. *Herbal Drugs and Phytopharmaceuticals: A Handbook for Practice on a Scientific Basis.* CRC Press: Boca Raton, FL, 1994.

26. Davis EA, Morris DJ. Medicinal uses of licorice through the millennia: The good and plenty of it. *Molecul Cell Endocrinol* 1991:78;1-6.

27. Revers FE. Heeft succus liquirtae een genezende werking op de maagzweer? *Nederl T Geneesk* 1947:90:135-137.

28. Blachley JD, Knochel JP. Tobacco chewer's hypokalemia: Licorice revisited. *N Engl J Med* 1980;302:784-785.

29. Gomez-Sanchez CE, Gomez-Sanchez EP, Yamakita N. Endocrine causes of hypertension. *Sem Nephrol* 1995;15:6-15.

30. Gomez-Sanchez EP, Gomez-Sanchez CE. Central hypertensinogenic effects of glycyrrhizic acid and carbenoxolone. *Am J Physiol* 1992;236:E1125-E1130.

31. Santeusanio E, Nunzi E, Natali P, et al. Hypokalemic myopathy in arterial hypertension. *Min Med* 1982;73:2279-2286.

32. Epstein MT, Espiner EA, Donald RA, Hughes H. Liquorice toxicity and the renin-angiotensin-aldosterone axis in man. *Br Med J* 1977;1:209-210.

33. Corsi FM, Galgani S, Giacanelli M, Piazza G. Acute hypokalemic myopathy due to chronic licorice ingestion: Report of a case. *Ital J Neurol Sci* 1983;4:493-497.

34. Beretta-Piccoli C, Salvade G, Crivelli PL, Weidmann P. Body sodium and blood volume in a patient with licorice-induced hypertension. *J Hypertension* 1985;3:19-23.

35. Wash LK, Bernard JD. Licorice-induced pseudoaldosteronism. *Am J Hosp Pharm* 1975;32:73-74.

36. Salassa RM, Mattox VR, Rosevear JW. Inhibition of mineralocorticoid activity of licorice by spironolactone. *J Clin Endocrinol* 1962;22:1156.

37. Anonymous. Bekanntmachung uber die Zulassung und Registrierung von Arzneimeitteln. Bundesanzeiger (herausgegeben von Bundesminister der Justiz) (German Commission E Monograph series) 1992.

38. Anonymous. Avis aux fabricants concernant les demandes d'autorisation de mise sur le marche des medicaments a base de plantes. *Fasiccule special no. 90/22 bis.* Paris: Direction de la Pharmacies et du Medicament, Ministere des Affaires Sociales et de la Solidarite, 1990.

39. Stewart PM, Wallace AM, Valentino R, Burt D, Shackleton CHL, Edwards CRW. Licorice and hypertension. *Lancet* 1987;ii:821-823.

40. Edwards CRW. Lessons from licorice. *N Engl J Med* 1991;325:1242-1243.

41. Bernardi M, D'Intino PE, Trevisani F et al., Effects of prolonged ingestion of graded doses of licorice by healthy volunteers. *Life Sci* 1994;55:863-872.

42. Hollifield JW. Licorice intoxication. *J Tenn Med Assoc* 1974;67:584-585.

43. Hoffmann BB, Lefkowitz RJ. Catecholamines, sympathomimetic drugs, and adrenergic receptor antagonists. In Hardman JG, Limbird LE, Molinoff PG, Ruddon RW, Eds., *Goodman & Gilman's The Pharmacological Basis of Therapeutics.* McGraw-Hill Health Professions Division, New York, 1996:100-248.

44. Baum N. Treatment of impotence. *Postgrad Med* 1987;81:133.

45. Morales A, Condra M, Owen JA, Surridge DH, Fenemore J, Harris C. Is yohimbine effective in the treatment of organic impotence? Results of a controlled trial. *J Urol* 1987;137:1168-1172.

46. Morales A, Surridge DHC, Marshall PG, Fenemore J. Nonhormonal pharmacological treatment of organic impotence. *J Urol* 1982;128:45.

47. Margolis R, Preito P, Stein L, Chinn S. Statistical summary of 10,000 male cases using afrodex in treatment of impotence. *Curr Ther Res* 1971;13:616.

48. Grossman E, Rosentahl T, Peleg E, Holmes C, Goldstein DS. Oral yohimbine increases blood pressure and sympathetic nervous outflow in hypertensive patients. *J Cardiovasc Pharmacol* 1993;22:22-26.

49. Musso NR, Vergassola C, Pende A, Lotti G. Yohimbine effects on blood pressure and plasma catecholamines in human hypertension. *Am J Hypertens* 1995;8:565-571.

50. Damase-Michel C, Tran MA, Llau ME et al., The effect of yohimbine on sympathetic responsiveness in essential hypertension. *Eur J Clin Pharmacol* 1993;44:199-201.

51. Murburg MM, Villacres EC, Ko GN, Veith RC. Effects of yohimbine on human sympathetic nervous system function. *J Clin Endocrinol Metab* 1991; 73:861-865.

52. Goldstein DS, Grossman E, Listwak S, Folio CJ. Sympathetic reactivity during a yohimbine challenge test in essential hypertension. *Hypertension* 1991; 18 (Suppl 3):40-48.

53. Price LH, Charney DS, Heninger GR. Three cases of manic symptoms following yohimbine administration. *Am J Psychiatry* 1984;141:1267-1268.

54. Swann AC, Secunda S, Davis J, et al., CFS monoamine metabolites in mania. *Am J Psychiatry* 1983;140:396-400.

55. Goldberg MR, Hollister AS, Robertson D. Influence of yohimbine on blood pressure, autonomic reflexes and plasma catecholamine in humans. *Hypertension* 1983;5:772-778.

56. Sandler B, Aronson P. Yohimbine-induced cutaneous drug eruption, progressive renal failure and lupus-like syndrome. *Urology* 1993;41:343-345.

57. Landis E, Shore E. Yohimbine-induced bronchospasm. *Chest* 1989;96:1424.

58. Friesen K, Palatnick W, Tenebein M. Benign course after massive ingestion of yohimbine. *J Emerg Med* 1993;11:287-288.

59. Wiech NL, Ursillo RC. Acceleration of despiramine-induced decrease of rat corticerebral beta-adrenergic receptors by yohimbine. *Comm Psychopharmacol* 1980; 4:95-100.

60. Johnson RW, Reisine T, Spotnitz S, Weich N, Ursillio R, Yamamura HI. Effects of despiramine and yohimbine on alpha2 and beta-adrenoreceptor sensitivity. *Eur J Pharmacol* 1980;67:123-127.

61. Lacomblez L, Bensimon G, Isnard F, Dequet B, Lecrubier Y, Puech AJ. Effect of yohimbine on blood pressure in patients with depression and orthostatic hypotension induced by clomipramine. *Clin Pharmacol Ther* 1989;45:241-251.

62. DeSmet PAG, Smeets OSNM. Potential risk of health food products containing yohimbe extracts. *Br Med J* 1994;309:958.

63. Kendler BS. Garlic *(Allium sativum)* and onion *(Allium cepa)*: A review of their relationship to cardiovascular disease. *Prev Med* 1987;16:670-685.

64. Damrau F. The use of garlic concentration in vascular hypertension. *Med Rec* 1941:153:249-251.

65. Piotrowski G. L'Ail en therapeutique. *Praxis* 1948;488-492.

66. Pektov U. Plants with hypotensive, antiatheromatous, and coronarodilating action. *Am J Chinese Med* 1979;7:197-236.

67. Auer W, Eiber A, Hertkorn E et al., Hypertension and hyperlipidemia: Garlic helps in mild cases. *Br J Clin Pract* 1990;69 (Suppl):3-6.

68. Silagy CA, Neil HAW. A meta-analysis of the effect of garlic on blood pressure. *J Hypertension* 1994;12:463-468.

69. Kleijnen J, Knipshild P, Ter Riet G. Garlic, onions, and cardiovascular risk factors. A review of the evidence from human experiments with emphasis on commercially available preparations. *Br J Clin Pharmac* 1989;28:535-544.

70. Bleumink JE, Doeglus HMG, Klokke AH, Nater JP. Allergenic contact dermatitis to garlic. *Br J Dermatol* 1972;87:6-9.

71. Papageorgiou C, Corbet JP, Menezes-Brandao F, Peceguerio M, Benezra C. Allergic contact dermatitis to garlic *(Allium sativum)*: Identification of the allergens. *Arch Dermat Res* 1983;275:229-234.

72. Caporaso N, Smith SM, Eng RHK. Antifungal activity in human urine and serum after ingestion of garlic *(Allium sativum)*. *Antimicrob Agents Chemother* 1983;23:700-702.

73. Arora RC, Arrora S, Gupta RK. The long-term use of garlic in ischemic heart disease: An appraisal. *Atherosclerosis* 1981;40:175-179.

74. Bordia A. Effect of garlic on human platelet aggregation in vitro. *Atherosclerosis* 1978;30:355-360.

75. Rose KD, Croissant PD, Parliament CF, Levin MB. Spontaneous spinal epidural hematoma with associated platelet dysfunction from excessive garlic ingestion: A case report. *Neurosurg* 1990;26:880-881.

76. Cooperative Group for Essential Oil of Garlic. The effect of essential oil of garlic on hyperlipidemia and platelet aggregation. *J Trad Chinese Med* 1986; 6:117-120.

77. Dixit VP, Joshi S. Effects of chronic administration of garlic (*Allium sativum* Linn.) on testicular function. *Ind J Exp Biol* 1982;20:534-536.

78. Bogin E, Abrams M. The effect of garlic extract on the activity of some enzymes. *Food Cosmet Toxicol* 1976;14:417-419.

79. Herik S, Raichle M, Reis D. Spontaneously remitting epidural hematoma in a patient on anticoagulants. *N Engl J Med* 1971;284:1355-1357.

80. Sunter W. Warfarin and garlic. *Pharm J* 1991;246:722.

81. Jackson EK. Diuretics. In: Hardman JG, Limbird LE, Molinoff PB, Ruddon RW. *Goodman & Gilman's The Pharmacological Basis of Therapeutics*. McGraw-Hill Health Professions Division, New York, 1996:685-713.

82. Tyler V. Kidney, urinary tract and prostate problems. In: *Herbs of Choice*, The Haworth Press, Binghamton, NY, 1994:73-86.

83. Pisarik P. Blood pressure-lowering effect of adding grapefruit juice to nifedipine and terazosin in a patient with severe renovascular hypertension. *Arch Fam Med* 1996;5:413-416.

84. Edgar B, Bailey DG, Bergstrand R, Johnsson G, Lurje L. Formulation-dependent interaction between felodipine and grapefruit juice. *Clin Pharmacol Ther* 1990; 47:181, Abstract.

85. Bailey DG, Spence JD, Munoz C, Arnold JMO. Interaction of citrus juices with felodipine and nifedipine. *Lancet* 1991;337:268-269.

86. Edgar B, Bailey DG, Bergstrand R, Johnsson G, Regardgh CG. Acute effects of drinking grapefruit juice on the pharmacokinetics and dynamics of felodipine and its potential clinical relevance. *Eur J Clin Pharmacol* 1992;42:313-317.

87. Bailey DG, Arnold MO, Munoz C, Spence JD. Grapefruit juice-felodipine interaction: mechanism, predictability and effect of naringin. *Clin Pharmacol Ther* 1993;53:637-642.

88. Bailey DG, Arnold JMO, Tran LT, Ahktar J, Spence JD. Marked effects of both erythromycin and grapefruit juice on felodipine pharmacokinetics. *Clin Pharmacol Ther* 1994;55:165, Abstract.

89. Bailey DG, Munoz C, Arnold JMO, Strong HA, Spence JD. Grapefruit juice and naringenin interaction with nitrendipine. *Clin Pharmacol Ther* 1992;51:156, Abstract.

90. Bailey DG, Arnold JMO, Strong HA, Munoz C, Spence JD. Effect of grapefruit juice and naringenin on nisoldipine pharmacokinetics. *Clin Pharmacol Ther* 1993;54:589-594.

91. Hammond TG, Whitworth JA. Adverse reactions to ginseng. *Med J Aust* 1981;1:492.

92. Siegel RK. Ginseng abuse syndrome: Problems with the panacea. *JAMA* 1979;241:1614-1615.

93. Castleman M. Ginseng: Revered and reviled. *The Herb Quarterly* 1990;48: 17-24.

94. Liberti LE, DerMarderosian A. Evaluation of commercial ginseng products. *J Pharmaceutical Sci* 1978;67:1487-1489.

95. Palmer BV, Montgomery ACV, Monteiro JCMP. Ginseng and mastalgia. *Br Med J* 1978;1:1284.

96. Saku K, Hirata K, Zhang B et al., Effects of Chinese herbal drugs on serum lipids, lipoproteins and apolipoproteins in mild to moderate essential hypertensive patients. *J Hum Hypertens* 1992;6:393-395.

97. Takido M, Aimi M, Takahashi S, Yamanouchi S, Torii H, Dohi S. Constituents of aqueous extracts of crude drugs. I. Root of *Scutellaria baicalensis* Georgi (Wogon) (I). *Yakugaku Zasshi* 1975;95:108-113.

98. MacGregor FB, Abernethy VE, Dahabra S, Cobden I, Hayes PC. Hepatotoxicity of herbal remedies. *Br Med J* 1989;299:1156-1157.

99. Weeks GR, Proper JS. Herbal medicines—gaps in our knowledge. *Aust J Hosp Pharm* 1989;19:155-157.

100. Black HR, Ming S, Poll DS et. al., A comparison of the treatment of hypertension with Chinese herbal and western medication. *J Clin Hypertens* 1986;4:371-378.

101. Liu QY, Li B, Gang JM, Karpinski E, Pang PKT. Tetrandrine, a Ca^{++} antagonist: Effects and mechanisms of action in vascular smooth muscle cells. *J Pharmacol Exp Therap* 1995;273:32-39.

102. Lu YM, Forstl W, Dreessen J, Knopfel T. P-type calcium channels are blocked by the alkaloid daurisoline. *NeuroReport* 1994;5:1489-1492.

103. Tyler V. Garlic and other alliums. In *The Honest Herbal*. The Haworth Press, Binghamton, NY, 1993:139-143.

104. Sacks FM, Hebert P, Appel LJ, et al. The effect of fish oil on blood pressure and high-density lipoprotein-cholesterol levels in phase I of the Trials of Hypertension Prevention. *J Hypertens* 1994;12:S23-S31.

105. Appel LJ, Miller ER, Seidler AJ, Whelton PK. Does supplementation of diet with "fish oil" reduce blood pressure? A meta-analysis of controlled clinical trials. *Arch Intern Med* 1993;153:1429-1438.

106. Toft I, Bonaa KH, Ingebetsen OC, Nordoy A, Jenssen T. Effects of *n*-3 polyunsaturated fatty acids on glucose homeostasis and blood pressure in essential hypertension. *Ann Intern Med* 1995;123:911-918.

107. Yetiv JZ. Clinical applications of fish oils. *JAMA* 1988;260:665-670.

108. Morris MC, Sacks F, Rosner B. Does fish oil lower blood pressure? A meta-analysis of controlled trials. *Circulation* 1993;88:523-533.

109. Morris MC, Taylor JO, Stampfer MJ, Rosner B, Sachs FM. The effect of fish oil on blood pressure in mild hypertensive subjects: A randomized crossover trial. *Am J Clin Nutr* 1993;57:59-64.

110. Lungershausen YK, Abbey M, Nestel PJ, Howe PRC. Reduction of blood pressure and plasma triglycerides by omega-3 fatty acids in treated hypertensives. *J Hypertens* 1994;12:1041-1045.

111. Singer P, Melzer S, Goschel M, Augustin S. Fish oil amplifies the effect of propranolol in mild essential hypertension. *Hypertension* 1990;16:682-691.

112. Landmark K, Thaulow E, Hysing J, Mundal HH, Eritsland J, Hjermannn I. Effects of fish oil, nifedipine and their combination on blood pressure and lipids in primary hypertension. *J Human Hypertens* 1993;7:25-32.

113. Howe PRC, Lungershausen YK, Cobiac L, Dandy G, Nestel PJ. Effect of sodium restriction and fish oil supplementation on BP and thrombotic risk factors in patients treated with ACE inhibitors. *J Human Hypertens* 1994;8:43-49.

114. Lee RMKW. Fish oil, essential fatty acids, and hypertension. *Can J Physiol Pharmacol* 1994;72:945-953.

115. Donadio JV, Bergstralh EJ, Offord KP, Spencer DC, Holley KE. A controlled trial of fish oil in IgA nephropathy. *N Engl J Med* 1994;331:1194-1199.

116. Eritsland J, Arnesen H, Seljeflot I, Kierulf P. Long-term effects of *n*-3 polyunsaturated fatty acids on haemostatic variables and bleeding episodes in patients with coronary artery disease. *Blood Coagulation and Fibrinolysis* 1995;6:17-22.

117. Swails WS, Bell SJ, Bistrian BR, et al. Fish-oil-containing diet and platelet aggregation. *Nutrition* 1993;9:211-217.

Chapter 9

Nutraceuticals for Management of Dyslipidemia and Atherosclerosis

Paul W. Jungnickel, PhD

INTRODUCTION

The causal role of an elevated serum cholesterol level in the development of atherosclerosis and its resultant clinical manifestations is now well established.[1] In particular, elevated concentrations of low-density lipoprotein (LDL) cholesterol have been shown to accelerate the development of atherosclerotic lesions.[2] The development of atherosclerotic lesions in the coronary artery wall begins with a fatty streak characterized by the accumulation of cholesterol-laden foam cells below the endothelium in the arterial wall. Fatty streaks subsequently progress to lesions that are larger and more complex through a variety of mechanisms. An important step in the atherosclerotic process involves the oxidation of LDL particles, which makes them more susceptible to macrophage-mediated uptake into foam cells. Oxidized LDL is also more damaging to coronary artery endothelium than is native LDL.[2]

The clinical consequences of atherosclerosis tend to vary based on plaque size and characteristics. Smaller plaques tend to be more unstable and thus prone to rupture or erosion.[3,4] This sets up conditions favorable for thrombus development with resultant arterial occlusion and the initiation of acute coronary syndromes (e.g., myocardial infarction, unstable angina). More highly developed fibrotic plaques tend to be more stable. While less likely to initiate an acute coronary event, they can occlude coronary arteries, resulting in angina pectoris of varying severity.

As shown in recent studies, lowering of elevated LDL cholesterol results in reduced incidence of coronary events in patients with or without clinical evidence of coronary heart disease (CHD).[5-7] In addition, low levels of high-density lipoprotein (HDL) cholesterol are associated with increased CHD risk, while high levels appear to confer protection.[8] Thus, nutraceutical products that produce beneficial modifications of plasma lipoprotein levels may positively impact the atherosclerotic process and the incidence of acute coronary events. Nutraceutical products may also confer benefit by altering other CHD risk factors in a beneficial manner.

CASE STUDY 1: NIACIN

RB is a 42-year-old white male whose father died of sudden cardiac death at age 56. RB is concerned that he might suffer the same fate. He watches his diet closely and recently started taking sustained-release niacin on the advice of a clerk at the local health food store. He is taking two 500 mg capsules three times a day. He had his cholesterol checked three years ago at a health fair and at that time it was 325 mg/dL (he was already on his diet at that time). He wants to go the natural route and has avoided seeing his physician because he does not want to use drugs such as lovastatin (Mevacor) or pravastatin (Pravachol). He tells you that the niacin bothers him a lot, but that is okay because it is a natural vitamin. Discuss the potential benefits and risks of RB's approach.

Discussion

Niacin (nicotinic acid, vitamin B-3) has been used as a lipoprotein modifying agent for over 35 years. Beneficial effects from its use have particularly been seen in patients with existing coronary heart disease. For example, in the Coronary Drug Project,[9] which studied patients who had experienced a previous myocardial infarction, treatment with niacin was found to improve long-term survival when compared to placebo. More recently, angiographic studies have demonstrated beneficial effects of niacin-containing regimens in preventing progression and promoting regression of coronary atherosclerotic lesions.[10,11]

When used as a single agent, niacin can produce substantial modifications in plasma lipoprotein concentrations. At therapeutic doses of 1,500 to 3,000 mg/day, reductions of total cholesterol (15 to 25 percent), LDL cholesterol (15 to 30 percent), and triglycerides (25 to 50 percent) can be achieved. Increases in HDL cholesterol of 25 to 35 percent may occur.[12]

Patients taking niacin often complain of bothersome flushing, pruritus, warmth, and nausea, which prevent many of them from reaching doses that are effective in modifying plasma lipoprotein levels. Strategies that are commonly used to minimize these problems include the initiation of therapy at a low dose (around 100 mg three times daily) with gradual dosage escalation, and pretreatment with aspirin 325 mg prior to each niacin dose.[13,14] Sustained-released (SR) niacin products have also been shown to produce less bothersome adverse effects compared to immediate-release (IR) niacin preparations.[12]

Niacin is widely available without a prescription in pharmacies, health food stores, mail order suppliers, and other retail outlets. The wide availability of niacin without a prescription, and its promotion in publications such as *The 8-Week Cholesterol Cure,*[15] can potentially mislead the public regarding the safety of niacin. However, when used in doses sufficient to modify plasma lipoproteins, niacin should be regarded as a potentially toxic agent.

Hepatotoxicity represents the most severe adverse reaction to niacin. Toxic effects on the liver can range from asymptomatic elevations in hepatic transaminases (AST and ALT), to symptomatic hepatitis. Hepatotoxic reactions appear to be more frequent and severe with SR niacin preparations. In a randomized parallel study McKenney and colleagues[12] found no evidence of hepatotoxicity in 23 patients receiving IR niacin, whereas 12 (52 percent) of 23 patients taking SR niacin had transaminase elevations more than three times the upper limit of normal. Five of these 12 patients had symptoms of hepatic dysfunction (e.g., fatigue, nausea, anorexia). In addition, severe hepatic failure has been reported in three patients who were taking niacin as a lipid-modifying agent.[16-18] Two of these patients had tolerated IR niacin, but developed liver failure after switching to SR niacin formulations.[17,18] Two of the patients recovered with supportive care after niacin was discontinued, while one[17] required liver transplantation. The enhanced toxicity of SR niacin is also highlighted in another report in which three patients were able to tolerate rechallenge with IR niacin after developing hepatitis on SR products.[19] The increased hepatotoxic potential of SR niacin products has led to recommendations discouraging their use.[12,20]

Niacin has also been shown to elevate blood glucose levels.[21] This may result in loss of glycemic control in diabetic patients and development of hyperglycemia in previously normoglycemic patients. Niacin may also elevate blood uric acid levels and lead to the development of gout.[21]

Niacin should be administered cautiously to patients who are receiving the HMG-CoA reductase inhibitor drugs to modify plasma lipid levels, as it may increase the incidence and severity of skeletal muscle toxicity.[22] Currently available HMG-CoA reductase inhibitors include lovastatin (Mevacor), pravastatin (Pravachol), simvastatin (Zocor), fluvastatin (Lescol), and atorvastatin (Lipitor). The clinical picture of myopathy includes elevated creatine kinase (CK) levels with skeletal muscle pain. Patients should be instructed to report all skeletal muscle pain to their physician or pharmacist, and both niacin and the HMG-CoA reductase inhibitor should be stopped.

Although it is easy to regard niacin as an innocuous vitamin, such is not the case when it is used in doses sufficient to modify plasma lipids. Patients receiving niacin in doses of 500 mg/day or greater should be under the care of physicians and monitored for adverse effects, particularly hepatotoxicity and hyperglycemia. Patients should be instructed to report any severe flulike symptoms, and transaminases should be periodically checked to monitor for hepatotoxicity.

CASE STUDY 2: SOLUBLE FIBER

TR is a 54-year-old white male who is trying to modify his lifestyle in order to reduce his risk for cardiovascular diseases. He recently visited his physician and, as part of his routine physical, had a lipoprotein analysis. His values were as follows: total cholesterol 235 mg/dL, LDL cholesterol 175 mg/dL, HDL cholesterol 45 mg/dL, and triglycerides 75 mg/dL. He has no history of hypertension or diabetes, and, other than being a male over 45 years of age, has no risk factors based on the National Cholesterol Education Program (NCEP) guidelines. His physician indicates that he should try to lower his LDL cholesterol to 160 mg/dL, but he does not meet the NCEP criteria for drug therapy (i.e., LDL cholesterol over 190 mg/dL). His physician tells him that he might consider adding substances to his diet that contain high levels of soluble fiber. What substances might be available to TR and how effective are they?

Discussion

A variety of substances containing appreciable amounts of soluble fiber have been recently evaluated for their effects on blood cholesterol levels. Recent studies have demonstrated beneficial effects for oat bran and psyllium-containing substances as well as guar gum. Soluble fibers are thought to lower cholesterol by two mechanisms. Some fibers have been shown to enhance elimination of bile acids in the feces.[23,24] This results in the increased conversion of cholesterol to bile acids by the liver with subsequent upregulation of LDL receptors, resulting in increased removal of LDL from the plasma. Reduction of fat and cholesterol absorption from the gastrointestinal tract has been suggested as an alternative cholesterol-lowering mechanism.[24]

Products containing oat bran have been promoted as having significant cholesterol-lowering effects. Beta-glucan appears to be at least one of the soluble fibers in oat bran with a cholesterol-lowering effect.[25] Various studies have demonstrated differing effectiveness of oat bran as a cholesterol-lowering substance. Some studies have shown significant cholesterol-lowering effects,[23,25,26] while others have demonstrated no effect even when oat bran was consumed in doses up to 90 g/day.[27-29] In reviewing various studies, it is important to critically compare the diets used, as they may have differed in ways other than the mere presence or absence of oat bran. Thus differences seen may not represent an actual effect of oat bran. In a meta-analysis of ten well-designed and controlled trials evaluating oat bran versus a control diet, Ripsin and colleagues[30] found an approximate 6 mg/dL reduction in total blood cholesterol that could be accounted for as a result of the dietary addition of oat bran.

Guar gum is a fiber produced from the endosperm of the seeds of the Indian cluster bean *(Cyamopsis tetragonolobus).*[24] It has been manufactured in a variety of formulations and also is widely utilized by the food industry as a thickening and suspending agent.[31] When taken in doses of 5 to 10 g TID, guar gum produced reductions of 10 to 15 percent in total cholesterol and 15 to 20 percent in LDL cholesterol. Although these initial reductions are quite significant, some studies have found that guar gum's cholesterol-lowering effects may be attenuated over time.

Psyllium is a bulk-forming fiber derived from the plantago *(Plantago ovota)* plant. It is widely used in a variety of laxative products that act by increasing the bulk of the stool. Psyllium was found to produce modest reductions in total and LDL cholesterol in three separate placebo-controlled studies, although none used a crossover design.[32-34] At a dosage of 3.4 g TID, total cholesterol reductions in two studies by Anderson and colleagues[32,33] were 14.8 and 8.2 percent, while LDL cholesterol was re-duced 20.2 and 13.4 percent. Levin and colleagues[34] found more modest total and LDL cholesterol reductions of 5.6 and 8.6 percent respectively with psyllium 5.1 g administered BID.

Products containing soluble fiber have a low potential to produce serious adverse effects. Common adverse effects are gastrointestinal in nature and include flatulence, cramping, bloating, nausea, diarrhea, indigestion, and heartburn. Patients with severe gastrointestinal diseases such as active diverticulitis or inflammatory bowel diseases should be advised against using fiber-containing products.

Patients will obtain varying cholesterol-lowering effects from the consumption of various types of fiber products. The effects are generally modest, but may be important for patients who require some cholesterol reduction in an attempt to reach their goal without the use of conventional drugs. Useful dietary sources of soluble fiber can include guava fruit, barley, dried lentils, peas, and beans, as well as oat bran.[35,36] Soluble fiber products may also be helpful in combination with drug therapy for those patients requiring more substantial lipid modification.

CASE STUDY 3: FISH OIL

SM is a 55-year-old white female who has had type II diabetes for approximately ten years. She is 5 feet 2 inches tall and weighs 215 pounds. She is currently taking glyburide (Diabeta, Micronase, Glynase PresTab) 10 mg daily and metformin (Glucophage) 500 mg three times daily, with her fasting blood glucose levels running between 180 and 220 mg/dL. She had a hysterectomy seven years ago and is receiving hormone replacement therapy with conjugated estrogen (Premarin) 0.625 mg daily. SM is aware that her diabetes greatly increases her risk of heart attack. A recent lipoprotein analysis indicates a significant dyslipidemia (total cholesterol 350 mg/dL, LDL cholesterol 180 mg/dL, HDL cholesterol 40 mg/dL, triglycerides 650 mg/dL). SM has recently heard that consumption of fish oils might reduce her risk of having a heart attack. What are the implications of SM consuming fish oil supplements?

Discussion

Initial interest in fish oils came from a number of studies that reported a low incidence of coronary heart disease in populations consuming large amounts of fish.[37-39] In one study, Greenland Eskimos, who consumed large amounts of fish, were shown to be 13 times less likely to develop CHD when compared to Danes who consumed very little fish.[39] Beneficial effects were also associated with fish consumption in the Zutphen Study.[40] In this study, 852 Dutch men were followed for 20 years. Men who consumed at least 30 g of fish per day were only half as likely to die from CHD compared to men who did not eat fish. Consuming as little as two servings of fish per week was associated with beneficial effects in preventing CHD. However, more recent epidemiological studies have reported different results concerning the beneficial effects of fish consumption. For example, in the Health Professionals Follow-Up Study, Ascherio, Rimm, and Stampfer[41] found that as fish consumption increased there was no additional reduction in the risk of coronary heart disease in men. In contrast, Daviglus and colleagues[42] using data from the Chicago Western Electric Study, found a significant inverse relationship between fish consumption and the 30-year risk of fatal myocardial infarction.

Fish oils produce a number of biological effects due to their content of omega-3 fatty acids. Omega-3 fatty acids differ from the omega-6 fatty acids contained in most vegetable oils (e.g., corn, safflower, and sunflower oils) in that the fatty acids are more unsaturated with the first double-bond located only three carbon atoms away from the terminal methyl group. The common omega-3 fatty acids found in fish oils are eicosapentaenoic acid (EPA) and docosahexanoic acid (DHA). Fish vary greatly in their content of EPA and DHA. As a rule, saltwater fish from colder waters have higher omega-3 fatty acid concentrations than do saltwater fish from warmer waters or freshwater fish. Commercial fish oil products typically contain between 30 percent and 50 percent omega-3 fatty acids.

Fish oils produce many of their biological effects via effects on prostaglandins, thromboxanes, and leukotrienes.[37-39,43] In humans, linoleic acid, the primary dietary omega-6 fatty acid, is converted to arachidonic acid, which is then metabolized via the enzyme cyclooxygenase to form prostaglandins and thromboxanes. Prostaglandin I_2 (PGI$_2$) is particularly important in promoting vasodilation and preventing platelet aggregation. In contrast, thromboxane A_2 (TXA$_2$) has potent vasoconstrictor and platelet-aggregating properties. Thus, PGI$_2$ and TXA$_2$ competition results in different degrees of platelet aggregation and vasoconstriction in various individuals. Fish oil administration results in increased body levels of omega-3 fatty acids. Omega-3 fatty acids are metabolized by cyclooxygenase to PGI$_3$ and TXA$_3$. Individuals consuming fish oil therefore produce PGI$_3$ and TXA$_3$ at the expense of PGI$_2$ and TXA$_2$. PGI$_3$ has activity similar to PGI$_2$, but TXA$_3$ is inactive. Thus, increasing TXA$_3$ levels and decreasing TXA$_2$ levels result in less platelet aggregation and vasoconstriction. Variable increases in bleeding times (prolongation of the activated clotting time by 9 percent in one study) and small reductions in blood pressure (approximately 6 to 8 mmHg) occur. Bleeding times are also increased because omega-3 fatty acids are incorporated into red blood cells with resultant decreased blood viscosity.[38]

Fish oil consumption can also result in altered leukotriene production. Normally, arachidonic acid is metabolized via lipooxygenase to leukotriene B_4, which plays an important role in stimulating inflammation. Supplementation with omega-3 fatty acids results in a shifting of leukotriene production so that some LTB$_5$ is produced at the expense of LTB$_4$. LTB$_5$ is much less potent in stimulating inflammatory responses.

Fish oil supplementation also can produce a variety of effects on plasma lipoprotein levels. Specific effects vary depending on patients' plasma lipoprotein profiles and the fish oil dose used. Phillipson and colleagues[44] reported dramatic decreases in blood cholesterol and triglycerides in patients with severe dyslipidemias who were given diets containing 20 to 30 g/day of omega-3 fatty acids in the form of fish oil capsules or salmon filets. In ten patients with type IIb dyslipidemia, total cholesterol decreased from 285 to 199 mg/dL and triglyceride levels fell from 374 to 137 mg/dL. In ten type V patients, total cholesterol decreased from 373 to 207 mg/dL and triglycerides fell from 1353 to 281 mg/dL.

Less dramatic results were found by Schectman, Kaul, and Cherayil[45] in 16 patients with hypertriglyceridemia. When 15 g/day (9.8 g omega-3 fatty acids) of fish oil was added to their usual diet, triglyceride levels fell from 323 to 163 mg/dL after one month, but rose to 212 mg/dL at the end of three months. The effect of fish oil administration was further attenuated when the dose was decreased to 6 g/day, with mean triglyceride levels increasing to 288 mg/dL by the end of the six-month study. LDL and HDL cholesterol levels were not markedly changed.

Friday, Childs, and Tsunehara[46] evaluated fish oil in eight hypertriglyceridemia noninsulin-dependent diabetic patients. The patients received 15 g/day of fish oil (8 g omega-3 fatty acids) for eight weeks. Average triglyceride levels decreased from 234 to 109 mg/dL, while LDL and HDL levels were unchanged. However in these subjects, fasting blood glucose levels sharply increased from 159 to 193 mg/dL.

Fish oil products may produce a variety of adverse effects.[37-39] The effects of fish oil products on platelet aggregation can potentially make patients more prone to bleeding, although this will be clinically unimportant in most patients. While the previously mentioned Greenland Eskimos had a lower rate of CHD, they also had a higher incidence of hemorrhagic stroke. Fish oils should be used with caution in patients receiving heparin, warfarin (Coumadin), dipyridamole (Persantine), sulfinpyrazone (Anturane), aspirin, and ticlopidine (Ticlid).

Potential adverse effects may occur from fish oil components other than omega-3 fatty acids. Vitamin A and D toxicity is possible if large amounts of cod liver oil are consumed, but is not a problem with other fish oil products. Some concern has been raised about heavy metal toxicity from fish oils, but most commercial products have been purified to the point where this should not be a problem. It should be remembered that fish oils are fats and contain 9 Kcal/g, and patients may unknowingly increase their caloric intake by a significant amount.

Fish oils can potentially reduce the risk of CHD by their beneficial effects on blood pressure, thrombogenesis, and inflammation. The doses necessary to produce these beneficial effects are not well defined but may not be particularly high given the reduced CHD incidence found in populations consuming even small quantities of fish. Fish oils may also prevent CHD by positively influencing plasma lipoprotein levels with the major reductions being in triglycerides. To obtain significant triglyceride reductions, large doses are generally needed and the beneficial effects may be attenuated over time. The effects on LDL and HDL cholesterol are variable. Small, but potentially detrimental, increases in LDL cholesterol may occur.[47]

Despite these limitations, fish oil products may have an important role in the management of severe dyslipidemia. A number of studies have also evaluated the efficacy of fish oils for preventing restenosis of the coronary arteries following angioplasty, and a recent meta-analysis of these studies suggests a small beneficial effect.[48] A minimum daily dosage of 3 g of eicosapentaenoic acid and 1 g of docosahexanoic acid has been recommended.[49]

Individuals desiring to reduce their risk of CHD may achieve benefit from including fish in their diet two to three times per week. Individuals who do not like fish may obtain the same benefit from taking small amounts of fish oil (perhaps 1 to 3 g/day of omega-3 fatty acids).

On the surface, fish oil therapy would seem attractive for a patient such as SM, in that her lipid disorder includes a high triglyceride level. However, it would seem unwise for her to take fish oil products due to the potential to further increase her poorly controlled blood glucose.

CASE STUDY 4: ANTIOXIDANTS

RK is a 44-year-old executive who is concerned about his risk of cardiovascular disease. He has recently quit smoking and started exercising. He also read that antioxidant substances might play a role in helping him to avoid a heart attack. What is the rationale for using antioxidant substances and which of them might RK use to prevent cardiovascular disease?

Discussion

Interest in use of antioxidant substances to prevent atherosclerosis has increased parallel to our increased understanding of the role of oxidized LDL in atherosclerotic plaque formation.[2] Dietary antioxidant substances have little activity in altering plasma lipoprotein levels, but are believed to provide benefit primarily by inhibiting LDL oxidation and thus reducing the development of atherosclerosis.[50,51] Studies supporting beneficial effects of a variety of antioxidant substances have been primarily retrospective; clinical trials have not been performed for most antioxidant substances.

Significant data have accumulated to suggest that vitamin E (alpha-tocopherol) consumption has a beneficial effect in preventing the development of CHD. The Scottish Heart Health Study[52,53] (men and women), Nurses Health Study[54] (women only), and the Health Professions Follow-up Study[55] (men only) have demonstrated significant inverse correlations between vitamin E intake and the relative risk of CHD, although in the Scottish Heart Health Study beneficial effects were not seen in women. The beneficial effects have to date been seen with increasing consumption of vitamin E in the form of supplements rather than from dietary sources. The results from epidemiologic studies suggest that daily consumption of at least 200 IU of vitamin E is necessary to confer any cardiovascular benefit.[51] In the ATBC clinical trial,[56] vitamin E supplementation of 50 IU provided no reduction in cardiovascular mortality in male smokers. However, in the more recently published Iowa Women's Health Study[57] in postmenopausal women, vitamin E consumption from food, but not from supplements, was inversely related to death from coronary heart disease. Consumption of vitamin E appears to be safe, with doses up to 3,200 IU per day being relatively free of adverse effects.[51,58]

Vitamin A is available in a variety of naturally occurring, nutritionally active forms, including retinol, retinyl ester, and carotenoids.[58] Beta-carotene (provitamin A) is converted to retinol, primarily in the intestinal mucosa, and has been the form of vitamin A most studied for its role in the prevention of CHD. In the Scottish Heart Health Study[52,53] an inverse association of undiagnosed CHD and beta-carotene intake was found in men, but not in women. Similar results were found in the Health Professions Follow-up Study,[55] but the risk reduction was limited to current and former smokers and not observed in men who had never smoked. In contrast, Kushi and colleagues[57] found no relationship between vitamin A ingestion and death from CHD in the Iowa Women's Health Study.

Any potential beneficial effects that might be attributed to beta-carotene intake have not been substantiated in clinical trials. In the ATBC study,[56] supplementation with beta-carotene 20 mg daily resulted in an 8 percent increase in mortality compared to placebo, primarily due to increases in deaths from lung cancer and ischemic heart disease. In the recently published Physicians Health Study,[59] 12 years' supplementation with beta-carotene 50 mg every other day produced no significant difference in the incidence of cardiovascular disease when compared to placebo. The Beta-Carotene and Retinol Efficacy Trial (CARET),[60] which compared the combination of beta-carotene 30 mg per day and retinol 25,000 IU per day, was stopped early due to an increased rate of lung cancer in the active treatment group. The participants were men who were exposed to asbestos, and men and women who were heavy smokers. Beta-carotene and retinol treatment also resulted in an increased rate of death from cardiovascular disease, which almost reached statistical significance (relative risk = 1.25, 95 percent confidence interval = 0.99 to 1.61).

The studies to date do not provide sufficient support for the increased intake of beta-carotene or retinol as a means to prevent CHD and suggest that increased cancer risk may occur. The retinol forms of vitamin A are well known for toxicity when consumed in excess, with hepatotoxicity being perhaps the most significant toxic effect.[58] Retinol and retinyl esters also have known teratogenic potential and should not be consumed as supplements by women of childbearing potential. In contrast, beta-carotene is not teratogenic and does not produce classic vitamin A toxicity when consumed in doses of 30 to 180 mg per day. Prolonged consumption of beta-carotene in doses of more than 30 mg per day can produce yellowing of the skin and orange discoloration of the plasma.

Evidence for a beneficial effect of vitamin C is much less convincing, although the results of some epidemiologic studies have suggested it might help prevent CHD. Data from the First National Health and Nutrition Examination Study[61] found an inverse association between vitamin C intake and standardized mortality ratios for all cardiovascular diseases. The association was stronger for men (RR = 0.58, 95 percent CI = 0.41-0.78) than for women (RR = 0.75, 95 percent CI = 0.55-0.99). A similar result was seen in the Scottish Heart Health Study[52,53] with a significant inverse association between vitamin C intake and undiagnosed CHD being found in men but not women. However, other cohort studies have failed to demonstrate such a relationship.[55,62] In the Health Professions Follow-up Study,[55] there was no difference in the risk of coronary disease between those in the highest quintile of vitamin C intake (median = 1162 mg/day) and those in the lowest quintile (median = 92 mg/day). Some studies have suggested that vitamin C consumption may produce beneficial alterations in plasma cholesterol and triglyceride levels, but these findings have not been confirmed by well-controlled studies.[63]

From the above findings, it is not possible to recommend vitamin C supplementation beyond normal recommended daily allowances to prevent CHD. Vitamin C consumption is generally safe at doses up to 4 grams per day.[58] At higher doses precipitation of oxalate, cysteine, or urate renal stones may occur, particularly in individuals with impaired renal function.[51,58]

Flavonoids are antioxidant substances that are found in a variety of dietary components as well as red wine.[64,65] Common flavonoids include quercetin, kaempferol, myricetin, apigenin, and luteolin. Major sources of dietary flavonoids include tea, onions, and apples. In the Zutphen Elderly Study,[65] dietary flavonoid intake was inversely related to coronary disease mortality.

Selenium is an antioxidant substance that has been suggested to have a beneficial effect in preventing CHD. The studies to date have not evaluated selenium intake, but only the relationship between plasma selenium concentrations and the risk of CHD.[51] The findings have been conflicting, and the true effects of selenium on the development of CHD are unknown. Selenium consumption appears to be safe at the recommended maximum intake of 200 mcg per day.

The data to date provide the strongest support for use of vitamin E as an agent to prevent CHD. RK may wish to consider taking vitamin E in a dose of at least 200 mg/day, although doses several times higher are unlikely to pose any significant adverse effect risk. Data are much less supportive for a beneficial effect for vitamin C or selenium, and some evidence suggests that beta-carotene may actually increase CHD and cancer risk.

CASE STUDY 5: GARLIC

RC is a 66-year-old woman who for the past two years has had atrial fibrillation that was resistant to antiarrhythmic drugs. Nine months ago she was placed on warfarin (Coumadin) for stroke prevention. Over the past ten years, RC has tried various natural products in an attempt to improve her health. She has recently read about the use of garlic products as a means to prevent heart disease. What are the benefits and risks associated with RC's use of garlic products?

Discussion

Garlic possesses a number of actions that may be beneficial in the prevention of CHD. These include the modification of plasma lipoprotein levels, inhibition of platelet aggregation, and enhancement of fibrinolysis.[66] Garlic contains a large variety of chemical substances, making it difficult to identify specific garlic constituents that might be responsible for its biological effects. Alliin is the ingredient in garlic which, when it is converted to allicin, is believed to be most responsible for the lipid-modifying and antithrombotic effects.

Fresh garlic contains alliin (inactive) which when crushed interacts with an enzyme called alliinase, which catalyzes the conversion of alliin to allicin. In addition to being responsible for some of the biological actions of garlic, allicin also produces garlic's odor. Garlic is available in a variety of commercially available products, with powdered products being the most common. Dried garlic contains alliin and alliinase, but alliinase is inactivated in the acid environment of the stomach so that little or no allicin is produced.[66] Enteric-coated tablet preparations avoid the acid environment of the stomach and thus enhance allicin production. Allicin is produced, and then binds to cysteine from protein in the diet prior to GI absorption. This reduces the taste and odor of garlic.

Another important issue in the use of powdered garlic relates to the alliin content of various commercial products. Recently some standardization seems to have occurred, with a typical powdered garlic product containing 1.3 percent alliin, which corresponds to a 0.6 percent allicin release.[67]

Oil-based and liquid garlic products are also available. They are unlikely to contain allicin due to stability problems.[66]

The literature contains a large number of studies with conflicting findings about the lipid-modifying actions of garlic. In 1993, Warshafsky, Kamer, and Sivak[68] were only able to identify five of 28 studies as having sufficient scientific rigor for inclusion in a meta-analysis. In these trials, they found a 23 mg/dL (95 percent CI = 17 to 29) net reduction in total cholesterol (about 9 percent), which was produced by garlic consumption equivalent to one-half to one clove of garlic daily. In another meta-analysis, Silagy and Neil[69] reported an approximate 12 percent reduction of total cholesterol. They found no important differences in the effects obtained from powdered garlic in 600 and 900 mg daily doses. Despite the use of standardized powder products, varying results continue to be reported in studies with standardized (1.3 percent alliin) powdered garlic in a daily dose of 900 mg.[67,70,71] Adler and Holub[68] recently reported that the coadministration of garlic powder with fish oil was able to overcome the elevations in LDL cholesterol that occurred with fish oil alone.

Compared to the lipid-modifying effects of garlic, the antithrombotic effects of garlic are more poorly understood. These effects may be obtained by consumption of five to 20 cloves of fresh garlic per day, but doses of garlic powder needed to obtain a clinically useful response have not been documented.[72]

Garlic consumption in fresh or powdered form may alter biological processes in a beneficial manner to positively impact CHD.[73] Aside from garlic's odor, it produces little in the way of adverse effects. Heartburn and flatulence may occur with daily consumption of five or more cloves of fresh garlic.[66] Since RC is receiving warfarin, garlic supplementation may be potentially hazardous in her case due to its antiplatelet and fibrinolytic effects. She need not avoid food where garlic is used as a seasoning, but would be best advised not to consume garlic as a supplement.

OTHER PRODUCTS

A variety of other nutraceutical approaches have been evaluated for potential beneficial impact on dyslipidemia and atherosclerosis. In the Adventist Heart Study,[74] increasing consumption of nuts was associated with reduced rates of nonfatal myocardial infarction and fatal CHD. Although the specific types of nuts consumed were not identified, the most commonly consumed nuts in California, where the study was conducted, are peanuts, walnuts, and almonds. The believed mechanism for CHD risk reduction relates to the fatty acid profile of nuts, which can favorably modify plasma lipoprotein levels.[75]

Beta-sitosterol is a plant sterol that has been used for years to treat hypercholesterolemia. Its chemical structure is similar to cholesterol, and it appears to act by inhibiting cholesterol absorption from the gut. In various studies, doses of 6 g/day produced total cholesterol reductions of 10 to 15 percent and LDL cholesterol reductions of 15 to 20 percent.[76-78]

Alfalfa has been purported to have cholesterol-lowering activity due to its content of fiber and saponins, which inhibit cholesterol and bile acid absorption in the gut.[79,80] In 15 patients with various dyslipidemias, addition of 40 g three times daily of heat-prepared alfalfa seeds to their usual diet resulted in mean reductions of 17 percent in total cholesterol and 18 percent in LDL cholesterol.[81] Alfalfa has significant toxic potential when ingested in doses capable of lowering plasma cholesterol. Two cases of reactivation of systemic lupus erythematosus were reported in women ingesting alfalfa tablets, with the suspected ingredient being L-canavanine, a nonprotein amino acid.[82] A case of pancytopenia, also possibly related to L-canavanine, was seen in a 59-year-old man who on repeated occasions ingested alfalfa seeds 80 to 160 g/day.[83]

Policosanol is a mixture of aliphatic alcohols purified from sugar cane with octacosanol being the primary component. It acts by inhibiting cholesterol synthesis in the liver and increasing the number of hepatic LDL receptors, resulting in increased removal of LDL from the plasma.[84] Much of the clinical research on policosanol has been done in Havana, Cuba. In clinical trials policosanol in doses of 5 to 10 mg/day has produced total cholesterol reductions of 14 to 15 percent, LDL cholesterol reductions of 19 to 24 percent, and HDL cholesterol increases of 0 to 29 percent.[84-86] Policosanol appears to be well tolerated, with little potential for serious adverse effects.

Chromium supplementation has been advocated for its role in lowering blood cholesterol levels as well as enhancing insulin activity, therefore lowering blood glucose levels. Both effects could positively impact the development of CHD. Findings of various clinical studies have supported the presence or absence of activity on blood glucose and/or plasma lipoprotein levels.[87-93] Some of the variations in the findings of these studies may be due to bioavailability differences among the products studied. Picolinic acid forms a stable complex with chromium, which results in improved chromium bioavailability.[88] When administered in a placebo-controlled double-blind crossover study to 28 volunteers, chromium picolinate in a daily dose equivalent to 200 mcg of chromium produced a 7.2 percent reduction in total cholesterol and an 11 percent reduction in LDL cholesterol.[88] Triglyceride and HDL cholesterol levels were unchanged from baseline. Another factor that may account for positive findings in some studies is the low chromium consumption of many individuals. The recommended dietary intake of chromium for adults is 50 to 200 mcg/day, whereas some studies have documented that the typical North American diet contains less than 50 mcg/day.[94,95] Thus, it is difficult to know whether any observed beneficial effects might be due to correction of a chromium deficiency or chromium supplementation beyond the recommended dietary allowance.

CONCLUSION

A number of nutraceuticals appear to have beneficial effects in preventing CHD by modifying plasma lipoprotein levels as well as via other mechanisms. Some have antithrombotic effects and may prevent the development of acute coronary syndromes in patients with existing CHD. While most of these substances are benign, unless consumed in great excess, some adverse effects are possible. When selecting from among the various products, individuals should have a clear understanding of what they are trying to achieve as well as how these products may enhance or adversely impact various aspects of their disease management program. (See Tables 9.1 and 9.2 for summaries of nutraceutical use in the management of dyslipidemia and atherosclerosis.)

TABLE 9.1. Specific Nutraceuticals Used
for the Management of Dyslipidemia and Atherosclerosis

Nutraceutical	Key Points to Remember When Considering for Use
Nicotinic Acid (Niacin)	When taken in therapeutic doses (1500 to 3000 mg/day) provides substantial reductions in total cholesterol, LDL cholesterol, and triglycerides, as well as increases in HDL cholesterol.
	Should be used only under a physician's supervision.
	May elevate blood glucose levels and should be used cautiously, if at all, in diabetic patients.
	Severe hepatotoxicity may occur, especially with SR nicotinic acid products.
	Administration of aspirin prior to nicotinic acid can help prevent flushing, pruritus, and warmth.
Soluble Fiber Products (Oat Bran, Guar Gum, Psyllium, and other dietary sources)	Depending on product and amount consumed, can produce total cholesterol reductions of 5 to 15 percent and LDL cholesterol reductions of 5 to 20 percent.
	Common adverse effects include flatulence, cramping, bloating, nausea, diarrhea, indigestion, and heartburn.
	Low potential for serious adverse effects, but should be avoided in patients with active diverticulitis or inflammatory bowel disease.
Fish Oils	Fish oils contain omega-3 fatty acids, which produce inhibition of platelet aggregation and inflammation via alterations in prostaglandin and leukotriene metabolism.
	Produce substantial lowering of triglyceride levels, particularly when consumed in high doses (20 to 30 grams per day); triglyceride-lowering effects may diminish with continued use.
	Produce variable effects (both decreases and increases) on blood cholesterol levels.
	May increase bleeding risk, particularly when consumed concomitantly with anticoagulant or antiplatelet drugs.

Nutraceutical	Key Points to Remember When Considering for Use
Fish Oils (continued)	Significant reduction in CHD risk may be achieved by weekly consumption of 2 to 3 servings of fish. Individuals who do not like fish may possibly obtain a similar benefit from consuming small amounts of fish oil (equivalent to 1 to 3 grams per day of omega-3 fatty acids).
Vitamin E	Consumption of 200 IU or more per day appears to reduce the risk of CHD. Doses up to 3200 IU per day appear to be safe.
Vitamin A	Studies to date do not provide convincing support for consumption of vitamin A at doses above the RDA as a means of preventing CHD. When consumed in excess, retinol forms of Vitamin A may produce hepatotoxicity. Retinol and retinyl esters are teratogenic and should not be consumed as supplements by women of child-bearing potential. Beta-carotene is not teratogenic and does not produce classic vitamin A toxicity when consumed in doses of 30 to 180 mg per day. Prolonged consumption of beta-carotene in doses over 30 mg per day may cause yellow skin discoloration and orange discoloration of the plasma.
Vitamin C	Studies to date do not provide convincing support for consumption of vitamin C at doses above the RDA as a means of preventing CHD. Vitamin C consumption is generally safe up to a dose of 4 grams per day. At higher doses, precipitation of oxalate, cysteine, or urate stones may occur, particularly in individuals with impaired renal function.
Flavonoids	Have been suggested useful in preventing CHD, but data are not sufficient to support or refute a beneficial effect.
Selenium	Has been suggested useful in preventing CHD, but data are not sufficient to support or refute a beneficial effect.

TABLE 9.1 *(continued)*

Nutraceutical	Key Points to Remember When Considering for Use
Garlic	Standardized powdered garlic products contain 1.3 percent alliin, which corresponds to 0.6 percent allicin release.
	Enteric coated tablets avoid the acid environment of the stomach and enhance allicin release.
	With standardized powder products, doses of 600 to 900 mg/day produce total cholesterol reductions of about 12 percent.
	The antithrombotic effects of garlic, and doses needed to obtain such effects, are not well understood.
	Beneficial lipid-modifying and antithrombotic effects may possibly be obtained by consuming fresh garlic, but the amounts needed to obtain these effects are not known.
Nuts	Fatty acid composition found in nuts may favorably alter plasma lipoprotein levels.
Beta-sitosterol	Reduces total cholesterol by 10 to 15 percent and LDL cholesterol by 15 to 20 percent when taken in a dose of 6 grams/day.
Alfalfa Seeds	Reduced total cholesterol by 17 percent and LDL cholesterol by 18 percent when 40 grams three times daily were consumed.
	May exacerbate systemic lupus erythematosus and produce pancytopenia.
Policosanol	Has produced favorable alterations in total cholesterol, LDL cholesterol, and HDL cholesterol.
	Most research on policosanol has been performed in Cuba.
Chromium	Recommended dietary intake is 50 to 200 mcg/day, but the typical North American diet contains less than 50 mcg/day.
	Chromium picolinate is the most bioavailable chromium form.
	Chromium 200 mcg/day (in picolinate form) reduced total cholesterol by 7.2 percent and LDL cholesterol by 11 percent.

Table 9.2. Overview of Nutraceutical Use
in the Management of Dyslipidemia and Atherosclerosis

Potential mechanisms by which nutraceutical products may inhibit the development of CHD include favorable modification of plasma lipoprotein levels and inhibition of oxidative metabolism of LDL, thus preventing its macrophage-mediated uptake into foam cells and atherosclerotic plaques, and inhibition of thrombosis and inflammation, thus preventing the development of acute coronary syndromes.
When taken in sufficient doses (1500 to 3000 mg/day), niacin produces substantial beneficial modifications of plasma lipoprotein levels. Due to the potential for hepatotoxicity and hyperglycemia, niacin should only be taken by people under the care of a physician. Sustained-release forms of niacin are more hepatotoxic than immediate-release forms and should be used very cautiously, if at all.
A variety of soluble fiber products (e.g., oat bran, psyllium, guar gum) have the potential to modestly lower blood cholesterol levels. These fibers may be combined with conventional cholesterol-lowering drugs, or, for patients requiring only modest lipid modification, may be used in conjunction with diet to prevent the need for conventional drugs.
Fish oils produce substantial triglyceride reduction, particularly when consumed in high doses. Effects on blood cholesterol levels are variable. Alteration of prostaglandin and leukotriene metabolism by omega-3 fatty acids found in fish oils results in beneficial antithrombogenic and anti-inflammatory effects. Individuals may reduce their risk of CHD by consuming 2 or 3 servings of fish per week, or possibly by taking small doses of a fish oil product.
Consumption of antioxidant substances may prevent the development of atherosclerosis by inhibiting LDL oxidation, thus preventing plaque formation. To date, significant evidence suggests that consumption of at least 200 IU per day of vitamin E reduces the risk of CHD. Data are inconclusive for other nutraceuticals, including vitamin A, vitamin C, various flavonoids, and selenium.
Garlic may produce reductions in CHD by modest reductions in cholesterol and poorly understood antithrombotic effects. Beneficial effects may be obtained with fresh garlic or enteric-coated powder formulations.
Nut consumption may reduce CHD risk by favorable modification of plasma lipoprotein levels.
Beta-sitosterol can produce modest reductions in total and LDL cholesterol.
When consumed in large doses, alfalfa seed may produce modest reductions in cholesterol. Its potential toxic effects seem to outweigh any advantages that might be obtained.
Policosanol can produce LDL reductions an average of 20 percent. It is currently being investigated in Cuba.
Chromium can produce modest cholesterol reductions. Administration of chromium as picolinate salt seems to increase bioavailability.

REFERENCES

1. Levine GN, Keaney Jr. JF, Vita JA. Cholesterol reduction in cardiovascular disease: Clinical benefits and possible mechanisms. *N Engl J Med* 1995;332:312-321.

2. Steinberg D, Parthasarthy S, Carew TE, et al. Beyond cholesterol: Modifications of low-density lipoprotein that increase its atherogencity. *N Engl J Med* 1989;320:915-924.

3. Fuster V, Badimon L, Badimon JJ, Chesebro JH. The pathogenesis of coronary artery disease and the acute coronary syndromes. *N Engl J Med* 1992;326: 242-250, 310-318.

4. Burke AP, Farb A, Malcom GT, et al. Coronary risk factors and plaque morphology in men with coronary disease who died suddenly. *N Engl J Med* 1997; 336:1276-1282.

5. Scandinavian Simvastatin Survival Study Group. Randomized trial of cholesterol lowering in 4444 patients with coronary heart disease: The Scandinavian Simvastatin Survival Study (4S). *Lancet* 1994;344:1383-1389.

6. Shepherd J, Cobbe SM, Ford I, et al. Prevention of coronary heart disease with pravastatin in men with hypercholesterolemia. *N Engl J Med* 1995;333:1301-1307.

7. Byington RP, Jukema JW, Salonen JT et al. Reduction in cardiovascular events during pravastatin therapy: Pooled analysis of clinical events of the pravastatin Atherosclerosis Intervention Program. *Circulation* 1995;92:2419-2425.

8. Kannel WB, Castelli WP, Gordon T, McNamara PM. Serum cholesterol, lipoproteins, and the risk of coronary heart disease. *Ann Intern Med* 1971;74:1-12.

9. Canner PL, Berge KG, Wenger NK, et al. Fifteen year mortality in Coronary Drug Project patients: Long-term benefit with niacin. *J Am Coll Cardiol* 1986; 1245-1255.

10. Brown G, Albers JJ, Fisher LD, et al. Regression of coronary artery disease as a result of intensive lipid-lowering therapy in men with high levels of apolipoprotein B. *N Engl J Med* 1990;323:1289-1298.

11. Cashin-Hemphill L, Mack W, Pogoda JM, et al. Beneficial effects of colestipol-niacin on coronary atherosclerosis: A 4-year follow-up. *JAMA* 1990;264:3013-3017.

12. McKenney JM, Proctor JD, Harris S, Chinchili VM. A comparison of the efficacy and toxic effects of sustained- vs immediate-release niacin in hypercholesterolemic patients. *JAMA* 1994;271:672-677.

13. Whelan AM, Price SO, Fowler SF, Hainer BL. The effect of aspirin on niacin-induced cutaneous reactions. *J Fam Pract* 1992;34:165-168.

14. Jungnickel PW, Maloley PA, Vander Tuin EL, et al. Effect of two aspirin pretreatment regimens on niacin-induced cutaneous reactions. *J Gen Intern Med*, 1997; 12:591-596.

15. Kowalski R. *The 8-week cholesterol cure.* New York: Harper & Row, 1987.

16. Clementz GL, Holmes AW. Nicotinic acid-induced fulminant hepatic failure. *J Clin Gastroenterol* 1987;9:582-584.

17. Hodis HN. Acute hepatic failure associated with the use of low-dose sustained-release niacin. *JAMA* 1990;264:181.

18. Mullin GE, Greenson JK, Mitchell MC. Fulminant hepatic failure after ingestion of sustained-release nicotinic acid. *Ann Intern Med* 1989;111:253-255.

19. Henkin Y, Johnson RC, Segrest JP. Rechallenge with crystalline niacin after drug-induced hepatitis with sustained release niacin. *JAMA* 1990;264:181.

20. Jungnickel PW, Maloley PA. Extended-release niacin not problem free. *Am J Hosp Pharm* 1991;48:237-238.

21. Garg A, Grundy SM. Nicotinic acid as therapy for dyslipidemia in non-insulin-dependent diabetes mellitus. *JAMA* 1990;264:723-726.

22. Jungnickel PW, Cantral KA, Maloley PA. Pravastatin: A new drug for the treatment of hypercholesterolemia. *Clin Pharm* 1992;11:677-689.

23. Zhang JX, Hallmans G, Andersson H, et al. Effect of oat bran on plasma cholesterol and bile acid excretion in nine subjects with ileostomies. *Am J Clin Nutr* 1992;56:99-105.

24. Todd PA, Benfield P, Goa KL. Guar gum: A review of its pharmacological properties. *Drugs* 1990;39:917-928.

25. Davidson MH, Dugan LD, Burns JH, et al. The hypocholesterolemic effects of β-glucan in oatmeal and oat bran. *JAMA* 1991;265:1833-1839.

26. Van Horn J, Emidy LA, Liu K, et a l. Serum lipid response to a fat-modified oatmeal-enhanced diet. *Preventive Medicine* 1988;17:277-286.

27. Swain JF, Rouse IL, Curley CB, Sacks FM. Comparison of the effects of oat bran and low-fiber wheat on serum lipoprotein levels and blood pressure. *N Engl J Med* 1991;322:147-152.

28. Leadbetter J, Ball MJ, Mann JI. Effects of increasing quantities of oat bran in hypercholesterolemic people. *Am J Clin Nutr* 1991;54:841-845.

29. Bremer JM, Scott RS, Linton CJ. Oat bran and cholesterol reduction: Evidence against specific effect. *Aust NZ J Med* 1991;21:422-426.

30. Ripsin CM, Keenan JM, Jacobs DR, et al. Oat products and lipid lowering: A meta-analysis. *JAMA* 1992;24:3317-3325.

31. Ma CB, Hart LL. Guar gum in hyperlipidemia. *DICP Ann Pharmacother* 1990;24:480-482.

32. Anderson JW, Zettwoeh N, Feldman T, et al. Cholesterol-lowering effects of psyllium hydrophilic mucilloid for hypercholesterolemic men. *Arch Intern Med* 1988;148:292-296.

33. Anderson JW, Floore TL, Gell PB, et al. Hypocholesterolemic effects of different bulk-forming hydrophilic fibers as adjuncts to dietary therapy in mild to moderate hypercholesterolemia. *Arch Intern Med* 1991;151:1597-1602.

34. Levin EG, Miller VT, Muesing RA, et al. Comparison of psyllium hydrophilic mucilloid and cellulose as adjuncts to a prudent diet in the treatment of mild to moderate hypercholesterolemia. *Arch Intern Med* 1990;150:1822-1827.

35. Jenkins DJA, Wolever TMS, Rao AV, et al. Effect on blood lipids of very high intakes of fiber in diets low in saturated fat and cholesterol. *N Engl J Med* 1993;329:21-26.

36. Singh RB, Rastogi SS, Singh R, et al. Effects of guava intake on serum total and high-density lipoprotein cholesterol levels and on systemic blood pressure. *Am J Cardiol* 1992;70:1287-1291.

37. Gibson RA. The effect of diets containing fish and fish oils on disease risk factors in humans. *Aust NZ J Med* 1988;18:713-722.

38. Holub BJ. Dietary fish oils containing eicosapentaenoic acid and the prevention of atherosclerosis and thrombosis. *Can Med Assn J* 1988;139:377-381.

39. Goodnight Jr SH, Fisher M, FitzGerald GA et al. Assessment of the therapeutic use of dietary fish oil in atherosclerotic vascular disease and thrombosis. *Chest* 1989;95:19S-25S.

40. Kromhout D, Bosschieter EB, Coulander CDL. The inverse relation between fish consumption and 20-year mortality from coronary heart disease. *N Engl J Med* 1985;312:1205-1209.

41. Ascherio A, Rimm EB, Stampfer MJ. Dietary intake of marine *n*-3 fatty acids, fish intake, and the risk of coronary heart disease among men. *N Engl J Med* 1995;332:977-982.

42. Daviglus ML, Stamler J, Orencia AJ, et al. Fish consumption and the 30-year risk of fatal myocardial infarction. *N Engl J Med* 1997;336:1046-1053.

43. Schacky CV. Prophylaxis of atherosclerosis with marine omega-3 fatty acids: A comprehensive strategy. *Ann Intern Med* 1987;107:890-899.

44. Phillipson BE, Rothrock DW, Connor WE, et al. Reduction of plasma lipids, lipoproteins, and apoproteins by dietary fish oils in patients with hypertriglyceridemia. *N Engl J Med* 1985;312:1210-1216.

45. Schectman G, Kaul S, Cherayil GD. Can the hypotriglyceridemic effect of fish oil concentrate be sustained? *Ann Intern Med* 1989;110:346-352.

46. Friday KE, Childs MT, Tsunehara CH. Elevated plasma glucose and lowered triglyceride levels from omega-3 fatty acid supplementation in type II diabetics. *Diabetes Care* 1989;12:276-281.

47. Reis GJ, Silverman DI, Boucher TM, et al. Effects of two types of fish oil supplements on serum lipids and plasma phospholipid fatty acids in coronary artery disease. *Am J Cardiol* 1990;66:1171-1175.

48. Gapinski JP, VanRuiswyk JV, Heudebert GR, Schectman GS. Preventing restenosis with fish oils following coronary angioplasty: A meta-analysis. *Arch Intern Med* 1993;153:1595-1601.

49. Mauro VF, Frazee LA. Use of fish oil to prevent coronary angioplasty restenosis. *Ann Pharmacother* 1992;26:1541-1545.

50. Meyers DG, Maloley PA. The antioxidant vitamins: Impact on atherosclerosis. *Pharmacotherapy* 1993;13:574-582.

51. Odeh RM, Cornish LA. Natural antioxidants for the prevention of atherosclerosis. *Pharmacotherapy* 1995;15:648-659.

52. Bolton-Smith C, Woodward M, Tunstall-Pedoe H. The Scottish Heart Health Study: Dietary intake by food frequency questionnaire and odds ratios for coronary heart disease risk. I. The macronutrients. *Eur J Clin Nutr* 1992;46:85-93.

53. Bolton-Smith C, Woodward M, Tunstall-Pedoe H. The Scottish Heart Health Study: Dietary intake by food frequency questionnaire and odds ratios for coronary heart disease risk. II. The antioxidant vitamins and fiber. *Eur J Clin Nutr* 1992; 46:85-93.

54. Stampfer MJ, Hennekens CH, Manson JE, et al. Vitamin E consumption and the risk of coronary disease in women. *N Engl J Med* 1993;328:1444-1449.

55. Rimm EB, Stampfer MJ, Ascherio A, et al. Vitamin E consumption and the risk of coronary heart disease in men. *N Engl J Med* 1993;328:1450-1456.

56. The Alpha-Tocopherol, Beta Carotene Cancer Prevention Study Group. The effect of vitamin E and beta carotene on the incidence of lung cancer and other cancers in male smokers. *N Engl J Med* 1994;330:1029-1035.

57. Kushi LH, Folsom AR, Prineas RJ, et al. Dietary antioxidant vitamins and death from coronary heart disease in postmenopausal women. *N Engl J Med* 1996; 334:1156-1162.

58. Myers DG, Maloley PA, Weeks D. Safety of antioxidant vitamins. *Arch Intern Med* 1996;156:925-935.

59. Hennekens CH, Buring JE, Manson JE, et al. Lack of effect of long-term supplementation with beta carotene on the incidence of malignant neoplasms and cardiovascular disease. *N Engl J Med* 1996:334:1145-1149.

60. Omenn GS, Goodman GE, Thornquist MD, et al. Effects of a combination of beta carotene and vitamin A on lung cancer and cardiovascular disease. *N Engl J Med* 1996;334:1150-1155.

61. Enstrom JE, Kanim LE, Klein MA. Vitamin C intake and mortality among a sample of the United States population. *Epidemiology* 1992;3:194-202.

62. Riemersma RA, Oliver M, Elton RA, et al. Plasma antioxidants and coronary heart disease: Vitamins C and E and selenium. *Eur J Clin Nutr* 1990;44:143-150.

63. Howard PA, Meyers DG. Effect of vitamin C on plasma lipids. *Ann Pharmacother* 1995;29:1129-1136.

64. Hertog MGL, Hollman PCH, Katan MB, Kromhout D. Intake of potentially anticarcinogenic flavonoids and their determinants in adults in the Netherlands. *Nutr Cancer* 1993;20:21-29.

65. Hertog MGL, Feskens EJM, Hollman PCH, et al. Dietary antioxidant flavonoids and risk of coronary heart disease: The Zutphen Elderly Study. *Lancet* 1993; 342:1007-1011.

66. Tyler VE. *Herbs of choice: The therapeutic use of phytomedicinals.* Binghamton, N Y: The Haworth Press, 1994.

67. Jain AK, Vargas R, Gotzkowsky S, McMahon FG. Can garlic reduce levels of serum lipids? A controlled clinical study. *Am J Med* 1993;94:632-635.

68. Warshafsky S, Kamer RS, Sivak SL. Effect of garlic on total serum cholesterol: A meta-analysis. *Ann Intern Med* 1993;119:599-605.

69. Silagy C, Neil A. Garlic as a lipid lowering agent: A meta-analysis. *J R Coll Physicians—Lond* 1994;28:39-45.

70. Neil HA, Silagy CA, Lancaster T et al. Garlic powder in the treatment of moderate hyperlipidaemia: A controlled trial and meta-analysis. *J R Coll Physicians—Lond* 1996;30:329-334.

71. Simons LA, Balasubramaniam S, von Konigsmark M et al. On the effect of garlic on plasma lipids and lipoproteins in mild hypercholesterolemia. *Atherosclerosis* 1995;113:219-225.

72. Adler AJ, Holub BJ. Effect of garlic and fish-oil supplementation on serum lipid and lipoprotein concentrations in hypercholesterolemic men. *Am J Clin Nutr* 1997;65:445-450.

73. Kleijnen J, Knipschild P, Ter Reit G. Garlic, onions and cardiovascular risk factors. A review of the evidence from human experiments with emphasis on commercially available preparations. *Br J Clin Pharmac* 1989;28:535-544.

74. Fraser GE, Sabate J, Beeson WL, Strahan TM. A possible protective effect of nut consumption on risk of coronary heart disease: The Adventist Heart Study. *Arch Intern Med* 1992;152:1416-1424.

75. Sabate J, Fraser GE, Burke K, et al. Effects of walnuts on serum lipid levels and blood pressure in normal men. *N Engl J Med* 1993;328:603-607.

76. Best MM, Duncan CH, van Loon EJ, Wathen JD. Lowering of serum cholesterol by the administration of a plant sterol. *Circulation* 1954;10:201-205.

77. Best MM, Duncan CH. Modification of abnormal serum lipid patterns in atherosclerosis by administration of sitosterol. *Ann Intern Med* 1956;45:614-622.

78. Richter WO, Geiss HC, Sonnichsen AC, Schwandt P. Treatment of severe hypercholesterolemia with a combination of beta-sitosterol and lovastatin. *Curr Ther Res* 1996;57:497-505.

79. Story JA, White A, West LG. Adsorption of bile acids by components of alfalfa and wheat bran in vitro. *J Food Science* 1982;47:1276-1279.

80. Story JA, LePage SL, Petro MS, et al. Interactions of alfalfa plant and sprout saponins with cholesterol in vitro and in cholesterol-fed rats. *Am J Clin Nutr* 1984;39:917-929.

81. Molgaard J, von Schenck H, Olsson AG. Alfalfa seeds lower low density lipoprotein cholesterol and apolipoprotein B concentrations in patients with type II hyperlipoproteinemia. *Atherosclerosis* 1987;65:173-179.

82. Roberts JL, Hayashi JA. Exacerbation of SLE associated with alfalfa ingestion. *N Engl J Med* 1983;308:1361.

83. Malinow MR, Bardana EJ, Goodnight Jr SH. Pancytopenia during ingestion of alfalfa seeds. *Lancet* 1981;1:615.

84. Pons P, Rodriguez M, Mas R, et al. One-year efficacy and safety of policosanol in patients with type II hypercholesterolemia. *Curr Ther Res* 1994;55:1084-1092.

85. Zardoya R, Tula L, Castano G, et al. Effects of policosanol on hypercholesterolemic patients with abnormal serum biochemical indicators of hepatic function. *Curr Ther Res* 1996;57:568-577.

86. Castano G, Mas R, Fernandez JC, Illnait J. Comparative effects of two once-daily regimens of policosanol in patients with type II hypercholesterolemia. *Curr Ther Res* 1997;58:154-162.

87. Mertz W. Chromium in human nutrition: A review. *J Nutr* 1993;123:623-633.

88. Press RI, Geller J, Evans GW. The effect of chromium picolinate on serum cholesterol and apolipoprotein fractions in human subjects. *West J Med* 1990;152:41-45.

89. Roeback Jr JR, Hla KM, Chambless LE, Fletcher RH. The effects of chromium supplementation on serum high-density lipoprotein levels in men taking beta-blockers. A randomized, controlled trial. *Ann Intern Med* 1991;115:917-924.

90. Wilson BE, Gondy A. Effects of chromium supplementation on fasting insulin levels and lipid parameters in healthy, non-obese young subjects. *Diabetes Res Clin Pract* 1995;28:179-184.

91. Lee NA, Reasner CA. Beneficial effect of chromium supplementation on serum triglyceride levels in NIDDM. *Diabetes Care* 1994;17:1449-1452.

92. Uusitupa MI, Mykkanen L, Siitonen O, et al. Chromium supplementation in impaired glucose tolerance of elderly: Effects on blood glucose, plasma insulin, C-peptide and lipid levels. *Br J Nutr* 1992;68:209-216.

93. Abraham AS, Brooks BA, Eylath U. The effects of chromium supplementation on serum glucose and lipids in patients with and without non-insulin-dependent diabetes. *Metabolism* 1992;41:768-771.

94. Kumpulainen JT, Wolf WR, Veillon C, et al. Determination of chromium in selected United States diets. *J Agric Food Chem* 1979;27:490-494.

95. Anderson RA, Kozlovsky AS. Chromium intake, absorption and excretion of subjects consuming self-selected diets. *Am J Clin Nutr* 1985;41:1177-1183.

Chapter 10

Asthma: A Review of Diagnostic, Pharmacotherapeutic, and Herbal Issues

John G. Prichard, MD
Lucinda G. Miller, PharmD, BCPS

How art thou out of breath, when thou hast breath
To say to me that thou art out of breath? [1]

Out in the Atlantic Ocean great sheets of rain gathered to drift slowly
up the River Shannon and settle forever in Limerick. The rain damp-
ened the city from the Feast of Circumcision to New Year's Eve. It
created a cacophony of hacking coughs, bronchial rattles, asthmatic
wheezes, consumptive croaks. It turned noses into fountains, lungs
into bacterial sponges. It provoked cures galore; to ease the catarrh
you boiled onions in milk blanched with peppers; for the congested
passages you made a paste of boiled flower and nettles, wrapped it
in a rag, and slapped it, sizzling, on the chest. [2]

Juliet's chiding remark to her nurse is, in a sense, emblematic of the state of both our knowledge and treatment of asthma. Such an obvious statement of fact mirrors the wonder one may have that a syndrome as clinically recognizable and dramatic as asthma is not clearly understood and its treatment not universally agreed upon. McCourt's description of the miseries of an Irish winter, and the manner of coping with it, would be familiar in any Western culture.

Asthma is a common, chronic, frightening, appallingly expensive disorder that is disruptive of families and limits work, school, and athletic performance. The illness is made worse by common viral infections. Episodes of breathlessness sometimes occur abruptly, often at night when either self-reliance or an emergency room visit become issues of debate among relations. Treatment is often burdensome, inconsistently prescribed, frequently unmonitored in an objective fashion, and occasionally the illness is confused with other disorders. It is for these reasons, among others, that asthma has been, and remains, an issue of intense interest to "alternative practitioners" of every ilk. Indeed, there is mounting evidence that "alternative practices," including herbal and nutritional therapy, for a variety of chronic disorders, are becoming mainstream—with more than 13 billion dollars expended yearly during and following nearly one half billion visits to those dispensing nontraditional therapy or advice.[3,4]

Evidence exists that asthma incidence is increasing in many countries and deaths due to asthma are, reportedly, accelerating each decade.[5] Further, investigation of asthma deaths indicates that underdiagnosis, under treatment, and under education of patients and families contribute to the majority of them.[6] Data regarding mortality[7] and the contributing role of pharmaceutical agents, beta-2 agonists in particular,[8,9,10] remain contentious. Nonetheless, these issues have recently prompted development of treatment guidelines by the National Institutes of Health.[11]

CASE STUDY 1: MISDIAGNOSIS

A 72-year-old woman was diagnosed with asthma following a three-week bout with dyspnea. She had a long history of perennial rhinitis, eczema, and poorly controlled hypertension. The latter had intermittently been managed by a long-acting beta blocker. Her symptoms were worsened by activity and were particularly marked at night; awakening with severe breathlessness relieved by sitting in front of an electric fan. Wheezing was noted on physical examination. No edema, cardiac murmurs, or gallop sounds were noted. Theophylline was prescribed with slight improvement. After two weeks, however, symptoms worsened. She was seen in an emergency room and found to be in atrial fibrillation and pulmonary edema. The theophylline level was beyond therapeutic range. She was treated for congestive heart failure and theophylline was discontinued, with subsequent resolution of atrial fibrillation.

An inappropriate diagnosis of asthma will inevitably lead to inappropriate therapy. A variety of conditions may have associated symptoms and signs characteristic of the asthmatic syndrome.

This patient's course illustrates a very common difficulty with the diagnosis of asthma. What almost inevitably follows misdiagnosis of asthma is pharmacotherapy that further compounds the initial error. In the foregoing instance, dyspnea and wheezing were attributed to asthma rather than to congestive heart failure due to underlying hypertensive cardiomyopathy. Usual theophylline doses were prescribed and resulted in slight improvement owing to the drug's mild diuretic and, possibly, inotropic effect. Toxic levels eventuated (a common occurrence in congestive failure), resulting in atrial fibrillation. This, in turn, precipitated worsening pulmonary edema.

Asthma is presently defined as an inflammatory disease of the airways causing bronchial hyperreactivity and resulting in limitation of airflow. This is often associated with airway edema, mucus production and, eventually, structural alterations in the smaller airways.[12] Consequently, cough and dyspnea occur on a repetitive basis, often triggered by environmental factors (smoke, volatile chemicals, dust, allergens) and respiratory tract infections. Diagnosis of asthma requires that symptoms are episodic *and* that airflow obstruction is both present and, to some extent, reversible following administration of beta-2 agonists. Additionally, other disorders, often manifesting similar symptoms, should be reasonably excluded.[13] Table 10.1 lists conditions that, among others, may simulate the asthmatic syndrome.

It is rather easy to imagine that asthma is frequently diagnosed or suggested as a unifying rubric to explain episodic cough and/or dyspnea. Given the abbreviated list in Table 10.1, one can well surmise that some of the 15 million Americans with a diagnosis of asthma may not have it, and certainly, some who indeed have asthma may be treated for unrelated conditions.

Additional problems relating to asthma diagnosis is that the disorder is represented by an extraordinary range of severity and may become manifest at any age, with or without a family history.[14,15] As the disease is common, it may be expected to occur in association with other disorders of the cardiopulmonary system, particularly when it evolves in the older patient. It is also evident that some disorders simulating asthma may be, at least transiently, improved by drugs commonly employed in the management of asthma.

PHARMACOTHERAPY

The use of pharmacologic agents to reverse bronchospasm and airway inflammation has become the cornerstone of asthma management. Although rigorous data are lacking, a general consensus has emerged that available agents are frequently not prescribed according to disease severity, in sufficient doses, according to duration of action, or drug delivery systems used are inappropriate to the patient's age.[11]

TABLE 10.1. Disorders That May Mimic Asthmatic Syndrome

Congestive heart failure
Chronic bronchitis
Mechanical obstruction of airways
Chronic cough due to drugs or irritants
Esophageal reflux
Cystic fibrosis
Recurrent upper or lower respiratory tract infection

The medical treatment of asthma has undergone tremendous evolution during the past century. Osler recommended inhalation of amyl nitrate, chloroform, belladonna alkaloids, henbane, stramonium, and lobelia. He noted that some clinicians found inhalation of tobacco smoke, in the form of cigarettes, to be helpful. Injections of morphine, with or without the addition of cocaine, was suggested for terminating an acute attack. It is interesting to note, particularly in light of current debate regarding asthma mortality,[7,16] Osler's observation that ". . . death during an attack of asthma is unknown."[17]

Several agents, remnants from the past century, and from early in the present one, remain in use though are rarely prescribed. Ephedrine is available in over-the-counter (OTC) formulations, and is probably the oldest extant asthma remedy. Epinephrine was introduced for the treatment of asthma about 100 years ago. It remains widely used both in the emergency management of asthma (though not supported by current recommendations) and by OTC metered dose inhalers, tablets, and syrup.

In common use several agents, though not promoted as bronchodilators, are nonetheless used as home remedies for asthma and the persistent, nocturnal cough attendant to it. Eucalyptus oil and camphor *(Cinnamomum camphora),* intended for use in humidifiers, can be found in a variety of OTC formulations. Menthol, a volatile alcohol, is also used as a topically applied "decongestant."

Table 10.2 represents a summary of currently recommended asthma treatments[11] based upon duration and severity of disease and upon the effective duration of the pharmacologic agents.

TABLE 10.2. Pharmacologic Management of Asthma

Disease Severity	Treatment Options	Comments
Mild-Intermittent		
In some patients, attacks are *infrequent though severe*. Intensity of treatment must be increased accordingly.	Inhaled beta-2 agonist used less than three times weekly. Anticholinergics are alternatives (e.g., ipratropium bromide).	Cromolyn or nedocromil may be useful in some patients with predictable exercise or allergin-induced bronchospasm if circumstances can be anticipated.
Mild-Persistent		
Symptoms are persistent but mild, not debilitating but requiring treatment to maintain daily functioning.	Inhaled corticosteroids are foundation of treatment. Cromoglycate or nedocromil may be appropriate as alternatives or addition. Long-acting beta-2 agonists may be useful, particularly if nocturnal symptoms are disruptive.	Some clinicians advocate short half-life theophylline compounds for children with nocturnal symptoms, in addition to inhaled steroids. Long half-life oral beta-2 agonists are sometimes substituted. Leukotriene receptor antagonists may be useful in some patients.
Moderate-Persistent		
Symptoms always present unless treatment undertaken. Peak expiratory flow measurements vary >30 percent.	Higher doses of inhaled steroids and consistent use of long-acting beta-2 agonist.	Long half-life theophylline preparations sometimes used. Numerous drug interactions complicate use in older patients and school/behavioral difficulties may occur in children.
Severe-Persistent		
Without treatment patients will experience constant limitation of activity.	High-dose inhaled steroids. Long-acting beta-2 agonist. Intermittent use of oral corticosteroids. May require intermittent use of short-acting beta-2 agonists.	Some patients may benefit from cromolyn or nedocromil. Sustained duration theophylline is sometimes recommended rather than long-acting beta-2 agonists. Immunosuppressive agents (e.g., methotrexate) may have some value in individual patients.

CASE STUDY 2: INAPPROPRIATE MEDICATION

A 45-year-old construction worker was admitted to the hospital because of a back injury. Excruciating mid-back pain occurred after jumping three feet to the ground from a landing. His past history was unremarkable with the exception of mild asthma, principally manifesting with chest tightness and nocturnal cough once or twice weekly. Neither loss of work nor emergency room visits had been required. Following an episode of bronchitis seven years earlier, a course of prednisone had been prescribed and continued thereafter, at the patient's insistence, as it "kept his asthma away." He felt depressed and lacked energy when the dose was reduced. X rays of the spine showed osteopenia and multiple compression fractures.

Modern pharmacotherapy of asthma is guided both by the duration of action of each agent and disease severity. In the present case, a patient with mild asthma had been managed with a relatively long-acting agent having substantial side effects when prescribed over the long term. His management would have been perfectly satisfactory with the intermittent use of a short-acting beta-2 agonist. Here, reasons beyond the issue of efficacy prompted the patient to continue corticosteroids, with avoidable and likely irreparable complications.

The effectiveness of pharmacologic management should be judged by a number of criteria, including minimal complications deriving from medication use. Additionally, asthma emergencies should ideally no longer eventuate, and there should be little disruption of school, sleep, or athletic activity. Variation of peak expiratory flow rate should remain in target range and, importantly, when it does decline, the patient and/or family should be able to adjust therapy accordingly.

When asthma therapy is manifestly ineffective, a number of issues need be explored. These include adherence to the prescribed regimen, persistent exposure to triggering events, adverse effects of drugs, or detrimental drug interactions.

CASE STUDY 3: NONCOMPLIANCE

A 15-year-old girl was admitted to the hospital because of status asthmaticus. Several hospitalizations had been necessary in the past year, once to the critical care unit. She and her family spoke Spanish but no English. Although she had been referred to an asthma clinic, attendance was rare. Upon discussion with the mother, she admitted to not refilling medications owing to their cost. Instead, a vaporizer was used during attacks and *Siete jarabes,* a patent remedy prepared from botanical oils and honey,[18] was given. A camphor rub was applied to the chest. Both the mother and the patient acknowledged that these remedies were relatively ineffective compared to prescribed medications though, in the absence of the latter, they came to be relied upon.

The foregoing is a common circumstance encountered in a general hospital. Here, the pitfalls of asthma management are chiefly those related to economic factors. In this instance, the family had great faith in the physicians and clinic staff. The difficulties really involved the costs associated with inhaled corticosteroids and long-acting beta-2 agonists, and disruption of work and school involved in clinic attendance. Hence, one will always have to look beyond the specific pharmacologic regimen to gain insight into the reasons for apparent failure of treatment.

HERBAL MEDICINALS

The treatment of asthma with home remedies and herbal prescriptions is long established. The extent to which herbal therapy is undertaken is unknown. Of specific herbal medicinals, none have been studied in a reasonable fashion; hence, their place in asthma therapy is unknown. The variety of herbal and nutritional agents recommended for dietary therapy of asthma is extensive.[19] Understandably, dosage, frequency of use, preparation, and so on are undefined or undisclosed, and benefit is stated though not supported by studies. Benefit has become a matter of testimony though unsupported in a manner that allows experimental repetition or comparative interpretation.

CASE STUDY 4: DISCONTINUED MEDICATION

A 32-year-old woman had moderate, persistent asthma over many years. She had been managed with inhaled corticosteroids and long acting B-2 agonists with rare, though severe, exacerbations that had a rather sudden onset and progressed rapidly. Triggers included marked changes in humidity and tobacco smoke. She moved to California from Arizona with little change in asthma symptoms. After several months, at the encouragement of a friend, she consulted an herbalist who recommended an extract of onion, on a daily basis, as a natural remedy for asthma and allergies. She consumed the onion extract without untoward side effects and continued to feel well. Accordingly she discontinued inhaled corticosteroids and beta-2 agonists once her prescriptions were exhausted. During the following week, easterly winds (typical seasonal, high-velocity winds occurring frequently in southern coastal California) and brush fires occurred. Asthma symptoms recurred, progressed rapidly, and required admission to a critical care unit and mechanical ventilation.

This case illustrates several issues pertinent to both the study of asthma and its clinical management. First, asthma may remit for considerable periods depending upon environmental factors. Second, such remissions, understandably, may be attributed to a variety of unrelated factors (in this instance, onion extract). Also, sudden exacerbations of bronchospasm that progress rapidly represent a particularly dangerous form of asthma. Management of this clinical subset of asthmatic syndromes requires that the patient be well-informed, remain able to self-administer treatment, and have immediate access to medical care. Onion extract had no deleterious effect in this patient, though faith in its effectiveness led to discontinuance of both her usual preventative treatment and a source of continuing care.

Onion *(Allium cepa)* extracts contain thiosulfinates, which inhibit mediators of bronchoconstriction (leukotriene and thromboxane).[20] This has led to the popular notion that onion is helpful in asthma management though no reasonable studies support its use. Similarly, extracts of *Galphimia glauca* (tetragalloyl quinic acid)[21] have shown either reversal or inhibition of bronchoconstriction is limited in vitro. Ginkgo biloba, thought to be the oldest extant tree, is an enormously popular "herbal" medicinal, powder from dried leaves or seeds being consumed in capsules or as tea. Extracts contain flavonoids, which have smooth muscle relaxant effects,[22] perhaps acting via phosphodiesterase inhibition and affecting prostaglandin synthesis. Bronochopulmonary properties have also been attributed to lobeline (secondary to increased epinephrine secretion).[23,24] Again, no meaningful trials have shown benefit in asthma management.

CASE STUDY 5: TYLOPHORA INDICA

AP is a 52-year-old male who presents today in the clinic with increasing shortness of breath and bilateral wheezing. He had previously been diagnosed with asthma and hypertension. His asthma had been well-controlled with flunisolide (AeroBid) inhaler one to two puffs twice daily and albuterol (Ventolin, Proventil) inhaler two to three puffs every six hours. His mild blood pressure had initially been controlled with a low-sodium diet but three months ago had increased and necessitated treatment. He was prescribed amlodipine (Norvasc 5 mg once daily), which adequately controlled his blood pressure. Today, in addition to poor asthma control, his blood pressure has increased to 138/92 mmHg. AP admits to discontinuing flunisolide and albuterol in favor of a new herbal remedy he discovered called *Tylophora indica*. His wife adds that since then he cannot seem to get enough salt and seems to be using an inordinate amount on his food portions. Interpret the findings of the case based on the inclusion of an herbal remedy.

Tylophora indica has been advocated for bronchial asthma based on efficacy first reported by Shivpuri, Menon, and Prakash in 1968.[25] Its active components are believed to be tylophorine and tylophorinine.[26] While the exact mechanism of action has yet to be elucidated, it has been proposed that tylophorine stabilizes mast cell membranes.[27] In this study, mast cells were obtained by lavage of the peritoneal cavity and were examined in 30 albino rats sensitized with sheep red blood cells. Tylophorine was found to antagonize the mast cell degranulating effect of diazoxide, conferring 60 percent inhibition in histamine release. There are no data available comparing tylophorine to other mast cell membrane stabilizers such as cromolyn sodium or ketotifen.

Others have suggested that *Tylophora indica* (alternatively it is also called *Tylophora asthmatica)* may exert its antiasthmatic effect by direct stimulation of the adrenal cortex.[28] The alcoholic extract of finely powdered dried leaves of *Tylophora asthmatica* was administered to albino rats who had been adrenalectomized and dexamethasone-treated and stereotaxically hypophysectomized. They were then assessed for the effects on adrenal weight and function in terms of cholesterol and vitamin C content, and plasma levels of 11-hydroxycorticosteroid. The authors found that *Tylophora indica* adtanozied dexamethasone hypophysectomy-induced suppression of pituitary on adrenal activity and concluded that *Tylophora asthmatica* directly stimulated the adrenal cortex, presumably increasing endogenous corticosteroid levels. The authors further stated that this activity is responsible for the prolonged beneficial effect observed in asthmatics who ingest *Tylophora indica*. This concurs with a crossover, double-blind study of 110 asthmatic patients who were administered *Tylophora indica* leaves or spinach leaves (placebo).[29] At the completion of one week, 62 percent of the *Tylophora*-treated patients had complete to moderate symptomatic relief versus 28 percent in the placebo group; at twelve weeks none of the placebo group had any residual beneficial effects whereas 16 percent of the *Tylophora* group continued to experience beneficial effects. The authors concluded that twelve weeks of benefit following only six days of therapy was significant. There are no studies comparing *Tylophora indica* to corticosteroids (e.g., prednisone, flunisolide).

The number of efficacy studies are limited. In a crossover double-blind study of 195 patients, the dry alcoholic extract of *Tylophora indica* leaves was compared to spinach leaves serving as placebos.[30] Fifty-six percent of patients taking *Tylophora indica* experienced complete to moderate improvement by the end of the first week. (Moderate improvement was described as frequency of attacks reduced to less than half and moderate symptoms during attacks whereas marked improvement was defined as attack frequency less than one-fourth and mild symptoms during attacks.) Thirty-two percent of the placebo group had a similar response, which speaks to either a substantial placebo effect or the variability of the asthmatic conditions.

Two other studies, however, have not been able to replicate these favorable results. There was no significant difference in symptomatic improvement in cough, chest tightness, or wheezing with the *Tylophora* leaf versus the placebo in a study of eight patients.[26] These authors dismissed these findings as indicative of the difficulty in demonstrating efficacy in a condition such as asthma where symptoms vary markedly. In a larger study of 135 patients, *Tylophora indica* was compared to placebo over six days as measured by forced expiratory volume in once second (FEV_1) and peak expiratory flow rates (PEFR).[31] There was no statistically signficant difference between the two groups.

Side effects commonly attributed to *Tylophora indica* include sore mouth, loss of taste for salt, and morning nausea and vomiting continuing for as many days as the preparation was used.[29] These side effects have been reported in approximately 50 percent of patients who had taken *Tylophora indica.*[29] In another study of 195 patients, 16.3 percent experienced nausea, vomiting, mouth soreness, and diminution of taste for salt (versus 6 percent in placebo).[30] The loss of salt taste may account for the increased salt intake of AP but as can been seen, this may adversely affect previously controlled blood pressure. In rat studies, it has been suggested that central nervous system (CNS) depressant effects predominate when high doses of tylophorine are used, potentiating morphine analgesia.[32] Until more definitive data are available, it would be prudent to be cautious in using *Tylophora indica* concomitantly with morphine or any other CNS depressant.

Based on the available data to date, it appears insufficient data exist to support the use of *Tylophora indica* in the treatment of asthma. Because chronic asthma can quickly become acute, the patient is assuming considerable risk in employing an unproven remedy, especially if known effective remedies such as flunisolide and albuterol are discontinued in favor of the herbal remedy. Also, this herb has side effects (e.g, mouth soreness, loss of taste for salt). Not addressed in any of these studies is the issue of standardization. It is unknown if all *Tylorphora indica* leaves contain the same amount of active ingredients. Until proven otherwise, one should assume that lack of standardization exists, hence the same effects cannot be expected from batch to batch.

CASE STUDY 6: ADHATODA VASICA

KR is a 49-year-old male with a long history of chronic severe asthma who presents to the clinic today with vomiting and diarrhea. He has been taking 5 mg of oral terbutaline (Brethine) three times a day, four inhalations of beclomethasone dipropionate (Vanceril) and albuterol (Proventil, Ventolin) two puffs every six hours. He is also taking theophylline (Theodur), 300 mg twice daily. His vital signs are within normal limits but you are concerned that the vomiting and diarrhea may be due to high theophylline levels. You order a level of theophylline which returns at 12 mcg/ml (normal: 10 to 20 mcg/ml). KR admits to experimenting with an herbal product called *Adhatoda vasica*, which he had been told by a friend would potentiate the benefical effects of theophylline. How do you explain KR's findings in view of his herbal use?

Information regarding the use of *Adhatoda vasica* for asthma is extremely sparse. As an Ayurvedic medicinal plant, it has been employed as a liquid extract or syrup, and occasionally the dried leaves are smoked for asthma relief.[33] Isolated chemical constituents include vasicine, vasicinone, anisotine, adhotidine, vasicolinone, vasicoline, and vasicinol.[33] Classified as a quinazoline alkaloid, vasicine has been identified as the active component of *Adhatoda vasica*.[33] It has been associated with vomiting and diarrhea, especially when large doses are employed, which may account for KR's symptoms (0.23 to 0.45 g).[33] When an aqueous solution of vasicinone hydrochloride was studied in mice and dogs (10 mg/kg IV or IM producing peak plasma levels of 9 to 33 mcg/ml), it was found to potentiate the bronchodilatory activity of aminophylline by 150 to 200 percent and that of isoprenaline by 50 to 70 percent.[34] These authors concluded vasicinone had airway smooth muscle relaxant properties.[34] Considerably more study and product standardization is needed before *Adhatoda vasica* can be recommended.

CASE STUDY 7: PICRORHIZA KURROA

BC is a 39-year-old male with mild asthma that has previously been controlled with as-needed use of albuterol (Proventil, Ventolin) inhaler. His chief complaints are headache, abdominal pain, and vomiting. His wife, who has accompanied him to the clinic today, also adds that he has intermittent giddiness, which at times has been embarrassing when it occurs in public. Upon physical examination, his lungs are clear with no wheezing, rales, or rhonchi. BC concurs that his asthma seems to have been well controlled as of late and he has not had to use the albuterol. You ask if he is taking any other medications. His wife volunteers that BC recently began taking a herbal medication, *Picrorhiza kurroa*. Evaluate BC's findings including assessment of his herb use.

Picrorhiza kurroa is an Ayurvedic medicine whose active components and mechanism of action have yet to be elucidated. Its tuberous roots are found in the Himalayan region at altitudes of 3,000 to 5,000 m. In one study, guinea pigs were treated either with *Picrorhiza kurroa* plus the vehicle aloe or control solutions, finding marked inhibitory effects on PAF and allergen-induced bronchial obstruction.[35] The authors hypothesize that *Picrorhiza kurrora* contains androsin, a specific PAF receptor antagonist. Clearly more study is needed.

In a randomized double-blind trial of 72 patients with bronchial asthma, *Picrorhiza kurroa* root powder 300 mg three daily was compared to placebo.[36] Twenty-four patients (29 percent) experienced some clinical benefit but 32 patients (44 percent) deteriorated. Overall there was no significant evidence of reduction in clinical attacks, need for bronchodilatory drugs, or improved lung function as measured by FVC, FEV_1, and PEFR. Significant side effects occurred in ten (20 percent) of subjects, which included vomiting, cutaneous rash, anorexia, diarrhea, itching, and giddiness. In a smaller open trial of ten subjects, short unsustained benefit (as measured by FVC, FEV_1, and PEFR) was seen in six patients, with four patients experiencing significant side effects.[37] These side effects included headache, abdominal pain, vomiting, increased dyspnea, and giddiness. Clearly these symptoms are consistent with BC, who is experiencing headache, abdominal pain, vomiting, and giddiness. Given the spectrum of side effects and lack of clear efficacy, BC should be advised to discontinue *Picrorhiza kurroa* use.

CASE STUDY 8: KHELLIN

KL is a 35-year-old woman who has recently returned from a business trip in Europe. Troubled with mild-to-moderate asthma, KL has been intermittently controlled with cromolyn sodium (Intal) 20 mg four times daily and bitolterol (Tornalate) two to three puffs every six hours. While in Europe she obtained khellin, which she was advised was the same as cromolyn, so she stopped her cromolyn. Is it true that khellin is the same as cromolyn?

Khellin is derived from the plant *Ammi visnaga*. It is purported to dilate coronary arteries and relax smooth muscles throughout the body including those of the bronchi. Studies conducted over 40 years ago assign it bronchodilator activity four to six times greater than that of theophylline.[38] In a study of twelve patients, khellin was administered either intramuscularly (300 mg IM) or orally (50 mg three times daily) in blinded placebo-controlled fashion.[38] Five (42 percent) of the patients improved after the IM and oral administrations as demonstrated by percentage of improvement in the mean expiratory air flow rates. Nausea and vomiting frequently occurred with anorexia, nausea, and dizziness reported in up to 60 percent of cases in which khellin was taken orally. Nausea was frequently noted after the first dose. Cromolyn sodium has been identified as a derivative of khellin; however medicinal chemistry and comparative efficacy data are lacking.

The current fascination with unorthodox therapies is likely to expand. Indeed, what Eisenberg has described as the "invisible mainstream" of herbal therapy, acupuncture, homeopathy, massage therapy, etc., presently accounts for more practitioner visits for advice and treatment than does conventional medicine.[4] Herbal or other "natural" products remain largely untested in terms of efficacy and safety despite the vast amounts consumed for purposes of treatment. As promotion and sales of botanicals and nutraceuticals are successful without licensing, it is doubtful that the burdens of gaining governmental approval, as specific treatments, will be undertaken by manufacturers or alternative practitioners.

Side effects of herbal medicinals such as delirium (*Datura stramonium* or jimsonweed), tachycardia *(Lobelia inflata),* or nausea *(Ginkgo biloba)* may confuse both patients and clinicians and complicate management. For this and other reasons, clinicians are perforce obliged to discover the use of unorthodox medicinals by their patients. Perhaps contrary to intuitive analysis, patients and their families do not seek alternative treatment principally because of dissatisfaction with conventional practitioners.[39,40] In the case of asthma, alternative treatment may be sought because of the disease's chronicity, fear of side effects of orthodox pharmaceuticals, and encouragement from friends and family simply as a consequence of its popularity. A reasonable, nonjudgmental inquiry about use of home remedies, herbal medicinals, or other less than orthodox approaches on the part of our patients would encourage and sustain the therapeutic relationship. (See Table 10.3 for a summary of this chapter's material.)

TABLE 10.3. Summary

Onion extract	Contains thiosulfinates, which may inhibit leukotriene and thromboxane; clinical efficacy unproven.
Galphimia glauca	Contains tetragalloylquinic acid, which may temper bronchial hyperreactivity.
Lobeline	Purportedly increases epinephrine secretion.
Ginkgo biloba	Purportedly has smooth muscle relaxant properties via phosphodiesterase inhibition.
Tylophora indica (asthmatica)	Tylophorine and tylophorinine may stabilize mast cell membranes or may stimulate adrenal cortex; efficacy data inconclusive; side effects include sore mouth, loss of taste for salt, nausea, and vomiting.
Adhatoda vasica	Vasicine and vasicinone may potentiate bronchodilatory activity of theophylline and isoprenaline; lack of conclusive efficacy data.
Picrorhiza kurroa	May contain androsin, a PAF inhibitor; side effects include headache, abdominal pain, vomiting, dyspnea, and giddiness.
Khellin	Isolated from *Ammi visnaga,* is thought to dilate bronchial smooth muscle, may be related to cromolyn; high incidence of GI side effects

REFERENCES

1. Kail AC. *The Medical Mind of Shakespeare.* Williams and Wilkins: New South Wales, 1986:215.

2. McCourt F. *Angela's Ashes.* Scribner: New York, 1996:11-12.

3. Eisenberg DM, Kessler RC, Foster C, Norlock FE, Calkins DR, Delbanco TL. Unconventional medicine in the United States. *N Engl J Med* 1993; 328:246-252.

4. Eisenberg DM. Advising patients who seek alternative medical therapies. *Ann Intern Med* 1997;127:61-69.

5. Beveridge RC, Grunfeld AF, Hodder RV, Verbeek RP. Guidelines for the emergency management of asthma in adults. *Can Med Assoc J* 1996;155:25-37.

6. Goldstein RA, Paul WE, Metcalfe DD, Busse WW, Reece ER. Asthma. *Ann Intern Med* 1994;121:698-708.

7. McFadden ER, Warren EL. Observations on asthma mortality. *Ann Int Med* 1997;127:142-147.

8. Nelson HS. B-adrenergic bronchodilators. *N Engl J Med* 1995;333:499-506.

9. Wanner A. Is the routine use of inhaled B-adrenergic agonists appropriate in asthma treatment? Yes. *Am J Respir Crit Care Med* 1995;151:597-599.

10. Sears MR. Is the routine use of inhaled B-adrenergic agonists appropriate in asthma treatment? No. *Am J Respir Crit Care Med* 1995;151:600-601.

11. *Expert Panel Report II: Guidelines for the Diagnosis and Management of Asthma.* Bethesda, MD: National Asthma Education and Prevention Program; 1997. National Institutes of Health publication 97-4051.

12. Corbridge TC, Hall JB. The assessment and management of adults with status asthmaticus. *Am J Respir Crit Care Med* 1995;151:1296-1316.

13. Patel AM, Axen DM, Bartling SL, Guarderas JC. Practical considerations for managing asthma in adults. *Mayo Clin Proc* 1997;72:749-756.

14. Busse W, Banks-Schlegel SP, Larsen GL. Childhood- versus adult-onset asthma. *Am J Respir Crit Care Med* 1995;151:1635-1639.

15. Sandford A, Weir T, Pare P. The genetics of asthma. *Am J Respir Crit Care Med* 1996;153:1749-1765.

16. Ulrik CS, Frederiksen J. Mortality and markers of risk of asthma death among 1,075 outpatients with asthma. *Chest* 1995;108:10-15.

17. Osler W. *The Principles and Practice of Medicine.* Gryphon Editions: Birmingham, UK, 1978:500.

18. Pachter LM, Cloutier MM, Bernstein BA. Ethnomedical (folk) remedies for childhood asthma in a mainland Puerto Rican community. *Arch Pediatr Adolesc Med* 1995;149:982-988.

19. Pitchford P. *Healing with Whole Foods.* North Atlantic Books: Berkeley, CA, 1993.

20. Dorsch W, Scharff J, Bayer T, Wagner H. Antiasthmatic effects of onions. *Int Arch Allergy Appl Immunol* 1989;88:228-230.

21. Neszmelyi A, Kreher B, Muller A, Dorsch W, Wagner H. Tetragalloylquinic acid, the major antiasthmatic principle of *Galphimia glauca. Planta Medica* 1993; 59:164-167.

22. Shah BK, Kamat R, Sheth UK. Preliminary report of use of *Picrorhiza kurroa* root in bronchial asthma. *J Postgrad Med* 1977;23:118-120.

22. Puglisi L, Salvadori S, Gabrielli G, Pasargiklian R. Pharmacology of natural compounds. I. Smooth muscle relaxant activity induced by a *Ginkgo biloba* L. extract on guinea-pig trachea. *Pharmacol Res Commun* 1988;20:573-589.

23. Cambar PF, Shore SR, Aviado DM. Bronchopulmonary and gastrointestinal effects of lobeline. *Arch Int Pharmacodyn* 1969;177:1-27.

24. Halmagyi DFJ, Kovacs A, Neumann P. Adrenocortical pathyway of lebeline protection in some forms of experimental lung edema of the rat. *Dis Chest* 1958;33:285-286.

25. Shivpuri DN, Menon MPS, Prakash D. Efficacy of *Tylophora indica* in asthma. *J Assoc Physicians India* 1968;16:9

26. Thiruvengadam KV, Haranath K, Sudarsan S, Sekar TS, Rajagopal KR, Zacharian MGM, Devarajan TV. *Tylophora indica* in bronchial asthma. *J Indian Med Assoc* 1978;71:172-176.

27. Gopalakrishnan C, Shankaranarayanan D, Nazimudeen SK, Kameswaran L. Effect of tylophorine, a major alkaloid of *Tylophora indica,* on immunopathological and inflammatory reactions. *Indian J Med Res* 1980;71:940-948.

28. Udupa AL, Udupa SL, Guruswamy MN. The possible site of anti-asthmatic action of *Tylophora asthmatica* on pituitary-adrenal axis in albino rats. *Planta Med* 1991;57:409-413.

29. Shivpuri DN, Menon MPS, Prakahs D. A crossover double-blind study on *Tylophora indica* in the treatment of asthma and allergic rhinitis. *J Allergy* 1969; 43:145-150.

30. Shivpuri DN, Singhal SC, Parkash D. Treatment of asthma with an alcoholic extract of *Tylophora indica:* a crossover, double blind study. *Annals Allergy* 1972;30:407-412.

31. Gupta S, George P, Gupta V, Tandon VR, Sundaram KR. *Tylophora indica* in bronchial asthma—a double blind study. *Indian J Med Res* 1979;69:981-989.

32. Gopalakrishnan C, Shankaranarayanan D, Kameswaran L, Natarajan S. Pharmacological investigations of tylophorine, the major alkaloid of *Tylophora indica*. *Indian J Med Res* 1979;69:513-516.

33. Bhat VS, Nanvati DD, Mardikar BR. *Adhatoda vasica nees*—an Ayurvedic medicinal plant. *Indian Drugs* 1978;15:62-66.

34. Bhalla HL, Nimbkar AY. Preformulation studies III—Vasicinone—A bronchodilatory alkaloid from *Adhatoda vasica nees. Drug Develop Industrial Pharm* 1982;8:833-846.

35. Dorsch W, Stuppner H, Wagner H, Gropop M, Demoulin S, Ring J. Antiasthmatic effects of *Picrorhiza kurroa*. Androsin prevents allergen and PAF-induced bronchial obstruction in guinea pigs. *Int Arch Allergy Appl Immunol* 1991;95:128-133.

36. Doshi VB, Shetye VM, Mahashur AA, Kamat SR. *Picrorhiza kurroa* in bronchial asthma. *J Postgrad Med* 1983;29:89-95.

37. Shah BK, Kamat SR, Sheth UK. Preliminary report of use of *Picrorhiza kurroa* root in bronchial asthma. *J Postgrad Med* 1977;23:118-120.

38. Kennedy MCS, Stock JPP. The bronchodilator action of khellin. *Thorax* 1952;7:43-65.

39. Donnelly WJ, Spykerboer JE, Thong YH. Are patients who use alternative medicine dissatisfied with orthodox medicine? *Med J Aust* 1985;13:539-541.

40. Spigelblatt L, Laine-Ammara G, Pless IB, Guyver A. The use of alternative medicine by children. *Pediatrics* 1994;94:811-814.

Chapter 11

Herbal Medications, Nutraceuticals, and Anxiety and Depression

Teri L. Gabel, PharmD, BCPP

INTRODUCTION

Anxiety is a state of uncertainty and fear, the agitated feeling caused by the anticipation or the realization of danger, and/or an uneasy feeling that something may happen contrary to one's hopes.[1] Anxiety and fear are common occurrences in modern society, serving an adaptive function, driving us to maintain an even balance in our lives. Uncertainty looms in many areas of our lives. Anxiety that results from real situations is healthy and drives us to make adaptive changes that are productive and constructive. Pathologic anxiety or fear concerning unspecified danger interferes with our ability to deal with life as we are unable to develop productive or constructive plans to deal with unknown and possibly unreal dangers.

Throughout the centuries, herbalists have used specific herbs or combinations of herbs to treat the symptoms of psychic distress. The goal of herbal therapy is the perceived underlying imbalance driving the disorder, revitalizing and/or restoring the balance of health in the individual. Many times combinations of specific target herbs are used to increase the effectiveness and modify the potential toxicity of the herbal prescription used. The degree of symptom severity is the deciding factor for whether an herbal remedy is adequate or if treatment with standard allopathic medication is required. Many of these symptoms, such as insomnia, nervousness, fatigue, restlessness, depression, and anxiety, have shown responses to herbal medicines in their mild to moderate forms.

Interestingly, current standard allopathic medicine has been unable to replicate the synergistic effects that are integral to the success of many herbal medicines. In many countries, herbal medicines (e.g., St. John's wort) are as commonly prescribed as traditional medications (e.g., paroxetine [Paxil], nortriptyline [Pamelor]). In the United States, the use of herbal medicines and other alternative approaches to health care are often ridiculed by health professionals. Yet, increasing numbers of U.S. consumers are using alternative forms of treatment/self-treatment for many psychiatric or nervous symptoms.[2]

Several forces underlie the increasing use of herbal medicines by patients with psychiatric disorders. Perhaps highest on the list is frustration with the high cost and the side effect profiles of traditional medications. The cost of physician visits and lack of adequate insurance benefits for these life-long chronic illnesses are also driving this trend. No less important is the wish to escape the continuing stigma of being seen as "crazy." The use of alternate forms of treatment offers an anonymity that many people find desirable. Self-medication has long been a complication of treating mental illness. Alcohol, marijuana, cocaine, and other illicit drugs are commonly used "alternative treatments" for many of these patients. For some patients, herbal medications or nutraceuticals are another potential alternative form of treatment, with the added benefit of little interaction with alcohol for the majority of herbs.

The use of herbal remedies in the United States is one of the fastest-growing segments of the over-the-counter and health food market. With a predicted 13.5 percent annual growth in sales from 1994 to 2001, European sales of herbal remedies are approximately six billion dollars per year.[3] As the use of herbal medicines in this population grows, so does the potential for positive and negative effects of using herbal agents alone and or in combination with traditional medications. Many times the use of herbal medications is not part of the algorithm used in treatment decisions concerning patients at any level. Most physicians and pharmacists do not ask patients about the use of herbal remedies and patients do not volunteer this information, fearing the health care provider will be close minded about their use. This information is important in the proper treatment of a patient and an open mind, the right questions, and correct answers can make the patient comfortable enough to share it.

CASE STUDY 1: GENERALIZED ANXIETY DISORDER

DF is a 40-year-old white female who presents to the clinic with complaints of continually feeling uptight and anxious and of frequent headaches that are like a band around her head. She states she is exhausted at the end of the day and falls asleep almost immediately at night. Her over-the-counter medication use includes a multiple vitamin, triprolidine, and pseudoephedrine (Actifed) if she has a cold, and she uses ibuprofen for occasional headaches. DF admits to drinking two cups of coffee in the morning, denies alcohol or cigarette use, and tells you that her family history is positive for alcohol abuse and she is worried about using traditional medications for her anxiety. She is interested in trying an herbal agent for anxiety.

Discussion

DF suffers from generalized anxiety. As a psychiatric diagnosis, generalized anxiety disorder (GAD) is very common, with a one-year prevalence of about 3 to 8 percent, affecting men twice as often as women. The majority of patients with GAD see their primary care physician or a medical specialist for the physical symptoms of anxiety before seeking psychiatric treatment for the primary problem. On average, only one-third of the patients needing treatment for GAD receive it.[4]

Like DF, many people experience anxiety as a chronic state that, while they have many of the physical and psychological symptoms, is not so disruptive to their lives that it makes them wholly dysfunctional in social and occupational areas. Symptom severity and the degree of dysfunction that results assist in determining whether a person meets the criteria in the *Diagnostic and Statistical Manual for Psychiatric Disorders,* Fourth Edition (DSM-IV) for generalized anxiety disorder (see Table 11.1). Common symptoms of anxiety include headache, difficulty falling asleep, restless unsatisfying sleep, shortness of breath, and excessive worry. Other physical and psychological manifestations of anxiety are listed in Table 11.2. Because stress, anxiety, and their associated symptoms are so prevalent, people commonly treat them with herbal remedies.

Herbal medications that are commonly used in the treatment of anxiety include chamomile, valerian, kava, and passion flower.

Chamomile

There are multiple varieties of chamomile: *Chamaemelum nobile, Matricaria chamomilla,* and *Matricaria recutita* all have been used in related in part to the chemical constituents of the volatile oil. Chamomile flowers contain 1 to 2 percent volatile oil with the ingredients alpha-bisabolol, alpha-bisabolol oxide A and B, and mitricin. Mitricin is then converted to chamazulene. Chamomile also contains bioflavinoids (apigenin, luteolin, and quercetin), which are also considered to be active.[5,6] Apigenin has been found to competitively inhibit the binding of several benzodiazepines.

TABLE 11.1. DSM-IV Diagnostic Criteria for GAD[4]

1. Excessive worry and anxiety occurring more days than not for at least six months, about a number of events or activities.
2. The individual finds it difficult to control the worry.
3. Three or more of the following symptoms are associated with the worry:

feeling on edge	restlessness	irritability
easily fatigued	muscle tension	difficulty concentrating
difficulty		
falling asleep		
staying asleep,		
or unsatisfying sleep		

4. Anxiety or worry is not concerning another primary psychiatric disorder (e.g., schizophrenia) or medical condition.
5. Anxiety, worry, or physical symptoms cause significant impairment in social, occupational, or other important areas of functioning.
6. Anxiety is not substance induced and does not occur exclusively during an episode of another psychiatric disturbance.

Reprinted with permission from the *Diagnostic and Statistical Manual of Mental Disorders,* Fourth Edition. Copyright 1994 American Psychiatric Association.

TABLE 11.2. DSM-IV Physical and Psychological Manifestations of Anxiety

Physical	
Diarrhea	Restlessness
Dilated pupils	Startle easily
Dizziness	Sweating
Hyperreflexia	Syncope
Hypertension	Tachycardia
Muscle tension	Tremulousness
Palpitations	Upset stomach
Paresthesias	
Psychological	
Excessive worry	Difficulty concentrating
Feeling tense	Hypervigilent
	keyed up, or on edge

Reprinted with permission from the *Diagnostic and Statistical Manual of Mental Disorders,* Fourth Edition. Copyright 1994 American Psychiatric Association.

In doses up to 30 mg/kg it appears to have clear antianxiety effects without demonstrating muscle relaxing, sedating, or anticonvulsant activity. At doses between 30 and 100 mg/kg, a mild sedation is produced. Primary uses of chamomile in herbal medicine are the treatment of gastrointestinal spasm or irritation, and as a sedative.[7]

Twelve patients undergoing cardiac catheterization volunteered for a study designed to evaluate the effect of chamomile tea on the heart.[8] Each patient received a six-ounce cup of strong (two tea bags) chamomile tea ten minutes prior to their procedures. The subjects received no other premedication. The authors noted that cardiac catheterization typically elicits a great deal of anxiety in patients, but after drinking the chamomile tea, ten of the 12 patients fell soundly asleep and slept through the procedure. The investigators found chamomile had no cardiac effects, but had strong sedative effects.

Chamomile tea is prepared by pouring boiling water over a heaping tablespoon of dried flowers (or one to two tea bags) and letting it steep covered for five to ten minutes before straining it. The tea can be used at bedtime for sleep or three times a day as a sedative. As a tincture, 0.5 to 1 teaspoon, and if using the encapsulated powder two to three grams are used once to three times a day as above. Doses of chamomile should be taken between meals. Actual therapeutic amounts may vary depending on the effect chamomile has on an individual. Side effects are infrequent.

Valerian (Valeriana officinalis)

Valerian is considered a very potent tranquilizer, antispasmodic, and mild anodyne. Indications for its use include insomnia, mild to moderate anxiety, stress and tension, premenstrual tension, hyperactivity, depression, insomnia, and migraine headaches.[9] The primary active ingredients of valerian remain elusive. Current research is focused on the sesquiterpenes in the volatile oil, and the iridoids or valepotriates. The effectiveness of valerian in anxiety and insomnia may result from interaction with the inhibitor neurotransmitter gamma-amino-butyric acid (GABA). The valerenic acid component may inhibit the breakdown of GABA, thereby enhancing its activity.[10] Valerian has demonstrated the ability to bind to GABA-A receptors, which may be the site of action for its sedating effects.[11] Valerian may also weakly antagonize benzodiazepine receptors.[12] It is possible that a direct relaxing effect on smooth muscle also contributes to valerian's sedating activity.[13] While valerian shares similar mechanisms with allopathic anxiolytics, it has not been associated with dependence.

Two double-blind trials with aqueous extract of valerian (400 to 900 mg) versus a placebo control have confirmed clinically that valerian decreases sleep latency, reduces the number of nighttime awakenings, results in increased dream recall, and improves sleep quality.[14] Valerian is commonly used in combination with lemon balm, passion flower, or other herbs. In a study from Germany, a combination of valerian and lemon balm was compared to triazolam. Both test groups were found to be effective but the herbal group had no daytime sedation or impairment of cognitive function or performance.

Side effects are not reported with valerian, but if used in too large a dose initially, it may cause excitability. It is recommended that the initial recommended dose or any other be decreased if excitability occurs while taking valerian.[15] Valerian does not appear to affect driving ability, potentiate the effects of alcohol, or result in a morning hangover. When used in anxiolytic doses, valerian produces a calm relaxing effect that does not affect the level of arousal or alertness.[16]

Dosing of valerian in the treatment of insomnia is 300 to 400 mg of standardized extract (or two to three grams of herb per cup) at bedtime. The extract should contain at least 0.5 percent essential oil. If valerian is to be used in the treatment of anxiety, a 200 mg to 300 mg dose can be added in the morning.[17] Valerian can be used as a tea, tincture, or capsules. The dosing for the tincture starts at 2.5 ml to 5 ml per dose and is titrated upward to the desired effect.[18] The FDA rates valerian as a GRAS herb (generally regarded as safe).[19]

Passion Flower (Passiflora incarnata)

In 1920, researchers noted that passion flower induced a normal sleep with easy light breathing and little to no mental depression. There was also no confusion on waking. Today passion flower is commonly used for relaxation and sleep.[20]

Active components may be glycosides (harmala compounds and derivatives), maltol and ethyl-maltol, and flavanoids. Chrysin (5,7 dihydroflavone), the primary component of passion flower, has been demonstrated to have demonstrated to have benzodiazepine receptor activity. As a nonnarcotic substance, passion flower is therefore a nonaddicting compound.

A pleasant-tasting tea can be prepared by pouring one cup of boiling water over one teaspoon of dried leaves in a cup and letting it steep for ten to fifteen minutes, then straining. For insomnia, one cup of tea before bedtime is generally helpful in most cases. For the treatment of anxiety, one cup of tea three times a day is the average starting dose. If using the tincture, the dose would be ¼ to 1 teaspoon three times a day. In more severe cases, the potency of the tea can be increased by adding more leaves to the cup with the same amount of water.

Because passion flower has not been evaluated in young children, it is not recommended for children under the age of two, and the use of decreased initial doses is recommended for people older than 65 to allow for possible age-related changes in sensitivity to these compounds. Harmala compounds are uterine stimulants; therefore passion flower is not recommended in pregnant women. It must also be cautioned against confusing *P. incarnata* with *P. caerula,* as the latter contains cyanide.

Kava-Kava (Piper methysticum)

Lehmann and associates studied the effectiveness of kava in the treatment of anxiety in 58 patients with anxiety not considered to be caused by any of the primary mental disorders.[21] The patients were randomized to either placebo or 100 mg kava extract (standardized to 70 mg kavalactones), which was given three times a day for four weeks. After four weeks of treatment, the kava group were statistically improved from baseline on the Hamilton Anxiety Scale (HAM-A), a sixty-item Adjectives Check List, and the Clinical Global Impressions Scale (CGI). The kava group was statistically improved after even one week of treatment with kava. No adverse reactions were reported in the kava group.

Potent sedation, anticonvulsive, antispasmodic, and central muscular relaxant effects have been attributed to kava.[22] The underlying mechanism is not entirely clear. It is possible that kava acts on GABA and benzodiazepine binding sites in the brain.[23] The active constituents of the plant are called kava-pyrones (kawain, dihydro-kawain, methysticin, dihydroyangonin, and yangonin).

The portion of the plant used to produce kava herbal products is the rhizome. Modern methods of producing the plant for the market appear to alter the behavior of the herb slightly.[24] Traditionally, kava is prepared by chewing and spitting the pulp into a container and then letting it ferment. This form of kava has little difference in effect from the more sterile processes used for mass production. Therapeutically, the uses of this herb include anxiety, stress, and restlessness. Because of its CNS depressant profile kava is not recommended for use in patients with depression.

There appear to be no serious side effects to this agent, except, with prolonged use, a temporary yellow coloring of the skin, hair, and nails. Discontinuation of the herb results in the coloring returning to normal over several weeks. Daily ingestion for several months to up to a year or more of kava has been associated with a pellagroid dermopathy. The skin becomes dry and scaly, with the hands, forearms, soles of the feet, shins, and back primarily affected. The rash fades over several months when the use of kava is greatly decreased or ceased altogether.[25] Accommodation difficulties and disturbance of oculomotor equilibrium has been reported. It is not recommended for continued use past three months without medical advice.

It is possible that kava may interact with other CNS depressant agents and it is not recommended that kava be used with other CNS depressants, including alcohol. Additive sedation and lethargy has been reported with the concomitant use of alprazolam (Xanax) and kava in at least one patient.[26] Caution should be used when operating a vehicle and heavy machinery while using kava.

Dosing of kava herbal preparations call for the equivalent of 60 to 120 mg kava pyrones, approximately 100 mg three times a day.

Although current studies have not indicated a concern for the abuse potential of kava in the treatment of anxiety, it has long been reported anecdotally to cause intoxication in large amounts, and has been used in the South Pacific for its intoxicating effect.[27]

Resolution

Our first recommendations for DF would be chamomile, passion flower, or valerian. If DF should decide to try kava, we would recommend caution considering her family history of alcohol abuse. Her use of the herb should be monitored for excessive use. If after a three-month trial there is no significant improvement, DF should discontinue the use of kava.

CASE STUDY 2: ALLERGIES

JW is a 34-year-old female with seasonal allergies to ragweed and other grasses. She is having difficulty at work with resulting anxiety and wants to try chamomile tea. One of her friends warned her that people allergic to ragweed will have allergic reactions to chamomile. JW wants to know if this is true.

Discussion and Resolution

Historic reports of cross allergy between chamomile and ragweed and its relatives are not a clinically relevant concern.[28] Severe allergic reactions to chamomile are rare. JW should be able to safely use chamomile tea for sleep. But if an allergic response develops, she should avoid future use of this agent.

CASE STUDY 3: HOPS

HD is a 65-year-old Hispanic male who presents to your ambulatory clinic with complaints of difficulty sleeping. He states he lies awake for hours before finally falling asleep and then is tired all day. A review of systems and physical exam reveal no physical reason for his insomnia.

Your discussion with him includes a review of sleep hygiene and initial nonprescription alternatives for his insomnia. HD finally shows you the bottle of an herbal sleep remedy he had purchased on his way to the clinic. The label indicates it contains valerian and hops. He asks if it is safe for him to take this product. How do you respond?

Discussion

Hops (Humulus lupulus)

Hops has been used for centuries as a digestive aid and in the treatment of intestinal ailments. Its use as a sedative-hypnotic and a restoring tonic for the nervous system is rather new, merely several hundred years old. The sedative potential of hops came to light when it was discovered that people harvesting the herb became fatigued easily.[29]

Active ingredients in hops include a volatile oil, valerianic acid, estrogenic substances, tannins, bitter principles, and flavonoids. One of the active agents may be 2-methyl-3-butene-2-ol, a constituent that becomes more concentrated as the herb dries. It is suggested by some herbalists that dried, aged herb is best for insomnia.

The sedating effects of hops have been demonstrated to induce sleep. It rapidly induces a soothing, relaxing calm within 20 to 40 minutes.[30]

The use of hops for insomnia is as an infusion or tea. Place two teaspoons of hops in one cup of boiling water and let it infuse for five minutes, then strain and drink. When a tincture is used, 2 ml of the tincture three times a day is used for anxiety and nervous tension; 1.5 ml on a sugar cube is recommended for a nervous stomach. Because hops can be quite sedating, dosage adjustment is usually required.[31] Combinations with other digestive herbs, such as chamomile, peppermint, plantain, and marshmallow are used for irritable bowel syndrome.[32] Hops can also produce sleep via its aroma, and the use of a hops pillow is effective for many people with insomnia.[33]

Side effects are uncommon with hops and large doses have been ingested safely. Direct contact with the hops plant can cause contact dermatitis, and it is therefore recommended that a person use caution when harvesting fresh hops. Because hops does contain substances with estrogenic activity, it is not recommended for pregnant women or women with estrogen-dependent breast cancer.[34] Because hops acts as a mild depressant on higher nerve centers, it is recommended that hops be avoided in depressive states. The use of hops is generally regarded as safe by the FDA.

Resolution

HD could probably use the herbal sleep remedy containing valerian and hops without difficulty. HD should be cautioned of the potential for increased sensitivity to the product due to his age and that the dosing recommendation for a geriatric patient would be lower than that for a younger adult. If he experiences any side effects from the product or is overly sedated he should stop taking the herbal agent and contact the clinic.

CASE STUDY 4: GINSENG AND GOTU KOLA

PI is a 45-year-old male who presents with complaints of daily fatigue and feeling worn out. He describes going to bed at 8:00 p.m. each evening and sleeping soundly until his alarm goes off at 6:00 a.m. He is still exhausted and finds it difficult to get to work on time. At home in the evenings he sits on the davenport eating fast food he picked up on the way home. Sometimes he does not eat at all. PI's lab work is within normal limits, and there are no other symptoms to indicate hypothyroidism or other medical problems. PI's girlfriend recommended he start taking ginseng and gotu kola in addition to a multiple vitamin. Is this wise?

Discussion

Ginseng

Ginseng one of the most popular of the adaptogenic herbs worldwide, and it is number 12 of the 25 top-selling herbs in the United States.[35] By definition, adaptogens increase the body's ability to withstand assault from a variety of toxins, establish normalization of body function, and must be intrinsically harmless. Adaptogens can be stimulating or sedating depending on the needs of the body. Other common adaptogens are listed in Table 11.3.

TABLE 11.3. Adaptogenic Herbs

Tonic Herbs	Chinese Tonic Herbs
Oats	Ginseng
St. John's wort	Dong Quai
Gotu Kola	Fenugreek
Licorice	Astragalus

The primary use of ginseng is to counter damage from emotional and physical stress, prevent the depletion of stress-fighting hormones, and enhance memory.[36] Athletes use ginseng to counter fatigue, increase energy, and improve stamina. In Germany, ginseng is regularly prescribed as a tonic to invigorate and fortify the body.[37]

Ginseng products in the United States may contain one of the three different ginsengs: Chinese or Korean ginseng *(Panax ginseng),* American ginseng *(Panax quinquefolius),* and Siberian ginseng *(Eleutherococcus senticosus),* or combinations of all three. Siberian ginseng is not a true ginseng but is a relative of the ginseng species, containing many of the same active ingredients. Studies with Siberian ginseng have shown it to have clinical activity similar to other ginsengs.

The active ingredients in ginseng are thought to be chemicals called ginsenosides. So far over 13 different ginsenosides have been isolated. Ginseng also contains glycans, and a volatile oil with multiple components yet to be elucidated.[38]

The mechanism of action behind ginseng's activity is unclear, but it is known that ginseng increases the activity of neurotransmitters in the CNS by decreasing their removal from the neuronal synapse.[39] A deficit in the neurotransmitter serotonin (5-HT) is implicated in the mechanism behind many anxiety and depressive disorders and the agents that increase 5-HT in the synapse are useful in the treatment of these disorders. Ginseng may also potentiate the activity of GABA. Ginsenosides have been reported to inhibit c-AMP phosphodiesterase.[40,41,42] Various effects of ginsenosides on corticosteroid secretion run parallel with its effect on c-AMP phosphatase. Whether this activity is helpful in anxiety remains to be explored.

Siberian ginseng has been the focus of 20 years of study in the USSR. Large numbers of subjects were used as well as control groups.[43] The studies concentrated on ginseng's ability to assist the body in resisting stress and maintaining health. In one study of ginseng versus influenza and acute respiratory disease, 180 men were given 0.5 ml of ginseng every other day during the month of March versus the control group. The incidence of influenza and acute respiratory disease in the study group dropped from 17 percent to 12.7 percent.

During the winter, 1,000 factory workers receiving 22 ml of Siberian ginseng daily for two months experienced 2.4 times less incidence of influenza and acute respiratory disease than workers in the control group under similar working conditions.[44] In a two-year study on the reduction of total disease, 1,200 drivers for an automotive plant were given 8 to 12 mg/day of Siberian ginseng extract for two months each year in the spring and autumn. At the end of the experiment, total disease incidence had decreased 20 to 30 percent. In factory-wide open trials occurring over a two-year period, more than 1,300 workers were given two ml of ginseng a day and disease incidence dropped by 30 to 50 percent compared to the control group, which did not receive the ginseng.[45]

Concern about a "ginseng abuse syndrome" appears in some of the U.S. literature. Most articles quote a study of 133 psychiatric patients in which 14 developed an abuse syndrome after using ginseng.[46] Several important issues were not addressed in the article: (1) no diagnoses were given, (2) use of ginseng was not verified (patient report was used), (3) there was no attempt to verify the use of true ginseng versus other herbs thought to be ginseng, (4) there was no control for the use of caffeine by the patients, and finally (5) the dose of ginseng used by these patients was reported at or less than 15 grams a day, well over the recommended daily dose of 2 to 4 grams. Ginseng has not been confirmed to cause an abuse syndrome in other clinical trials.

The side effects of ginseng are typically mild and dose related. Most commonly observed are nervousness, sleeplessness, nausea, and occasionally headache. If these occur and a decrease in dose is not helpful, the agent should be discontinued. Ginseng is also reported to have hormonal effects. Estrogenic effects on women and an increase in testosterone levels in male rats have been reported. Ginseng is also reported to have hypoglycemic activity in mice—therefore it is possible it may interfere with a diabetic's ability to manage the disease if the physician is not aware of the ginseng use.[47] While these data are from small animal studies and case report literature and should be interpreted with caution, the use of ginseng is not recommended in pregnant women and with caution in diabetics. Also, ginseng should not be used by hypertensive patients, patients with cardiac dysrhythmias, clotting problems (ginsenosides inhibit platelet aggregation), acute inflammatory disease, and bronchitis.[48] The stimulating effects of this herb could be problematic in patients suffering from anxiety or nervousness. In healthy adults ginseng appears to have very few side effects and may be beneficial for fatigue and stress.

Dosage recommendations for the use of ginseng vary according to a person's needs. As a tonic 500 mg to 4 grams a day is average. Chronic daily use is not advised, and a two-week break every two months is recommended. The use of excessive doses should also be avoided.

Gotu Kola (Centella asiatica)

Gotu kola is considered a relaxing restorative for the nervous system. Small doses of the herb serve as a tonic while larger doses act as a sedative. Gotu kola does not contain caffeine as it is not a true "kola" nut.[49]

Doses for insomnia are ½ teaspoon in a cup of water. The tea has a bitter taste and honey and lemon are added to make it palatable. It is recommended that it be taken for four to six weeks with a two-week break before reinitiating therapy.

Use of this herb may cause a rash and discontinuation is recommended if the rash develops. The FDA rates it as having undefined safety.[50]

Resolution

PI does not have any of the contraindications for the use of ginseng and could probably use it safely at an initial dose of 500 mg three times daily or a daily dose of between 1.5 and 2 grams regardless of the dosage form. His use should be reassessed after several weeks for efficacy and any side effects. At this time, it cannot be recommended that he take the gotu kola with any certainty of positive results.

CASE STUDY 5: ST. JOHN'S WORT

MJ, a 38-year-old female, is normally an energetic and positive woman, but for the past three weeks she has found herself dreading getting out of bed in the morning, and obtains little joy from her work at the local YMCA. She quit her work golf team and does not go out with her friends anymore. She has lost ten pounds over the past month and finds food unappealing. MJ reads an article in her fashion magazine about nature's miracle cure for the "blues"—St. John's wort. Recognizing many of her symptoms in the description of depression in the article, MJ decides to try St. John's wort, but she comes to the pharmacy to ask your opinion first. What do you recommend?

Discussion

Depression

Depression is the most common psychiatric problem among American adults, with a lifetime prevalence of about 5.8 percent. Furthermore, approximately 10 percent of men and 20 percent of women in the United States will develop major depression (MDE) in their lifetime. The occurrence of milder episodes of depression is much greater. The age of onset for MDE averages the late twenties, but it can occur at any time. It affects women two times more often than men. Almost two-thirds of the 17.6 million Americans suffering from MDE receive no medical treatments. Untreated or undertreated depression is a major cause of morbidity (lost work) and mortality (suicide), and yet depression is one of the most treatable mental illnesses. Costs to the health care system every year as a consequence of depression are in the millions of dollars.

As with general anxiety, many people have depression that does not meet the diagnostic criteria for MDE,[51] but experience many of the symptoms. Symptoms of depression include decreased interest in activities that usually give pleasure, decreased activity levels, or possibly agitation (e.g., pacing, wringing hands), decreased (less often increased) sleep and/or appetite, and inability to concentrate (see Table 11.4).

In severe cases of MDE, suicidal and/or homicidal ideation and possible psychotic symptoms (e.g., voices, delusions) can occur (see Table 11.5). In the more severe cases of depression the patient ceases to function normally in social and occupational arenas, which can result in hospitalization.

TABLE 11.4. Symptoms of Depression

1. Difficulty with sleep, either midnight awakening or early morning awakening, at times hypersomnia.
2. Inability to experience pleasure.
3. Guilt is experienced over typically small and inconsequential issues.
4. Energy is decreased.
5. Ability to concentrate is impaired.
6. Appetite is typically decreased; less often hyperphagia can occur.
7. Psychomotor retardation or agitation.
8. Decreased sexual interest, ability, enjoyment.
9. Crying episodes.
10. Suicidal or homicidal ideation.

TABLE 11.5. DSM-IV Diagnostic Criteria for Major Depressive Episode

Five or more of the following symptoms are present during the same two-week period and represent a change from previous functioning. At least one of the symptoms must be a depressed mood or loss of interest or pleasure.

1. Depressed mood for most of the day, nearly every day.
2. Markedly decreased interest or pleasure in all, or almost all, activities for most of the day, near every day.
3. Significant weight loss (5 percent of body weight in a month) when not dieting, or weight gain, or a decrease in appetite nearly every day.
4. Insomnia or hypersomnia nearly every day.
5. Psychomotor agitation or retardation nearly every day (observed by others).
6. Fatigue or loss of energy nearly every day.
7. Feelings of worthlessness or excessive or inappropriate feelings of guilt nearly every day.
8. Decreased ability to think or concentrate, or indecisiveness, nearly every day.
9. Recurrent thoughts of death, recurrent suicidal ideation with or without a plan, or a suicide attempt.

Symptoms do not meet criteria for another major psychiatric disorder.
Symptoms cause significant distress or impairment in social, occupational, or other important areas of functioning.
Symptoms are not due to the direct effects of a substance or a medical condition.
Symptoms are not better accounted for by bereavement, persist for longer than two months or are characterized by marked impairment in functioning, morbid preoccupation with worthlessness, suicidal ideation, psychotic symptoms, or psychomotor retardation.

The use of St. John's wort *(Hypericum perforatum)* for the treatment of mild to moderate depression is common practice in Germany and other European countries. It is prescribed as a prescription antidepressant, like traditional allopathic antidepressants (fluoxetine [Prozac]), desipramine [Norpramin]).

The presumed active ingredient in St. John's wort is hypericin. Although definitive studies have not been completed, multiple components of the herb may work together to provide the antidepressant activity of St. John's wort. St. John's wort has minor monoamine oxidase inhibiting (MAOI) activity but it is not believed that that mechanism fully accounts for its effectiveness. Current investigations indicate hypericin's ability to inhibit serotonin reuptake may be its primary mechanism of action in the treatment of mild to moderate depression.

Over 25 controlled trials have demonstrated the effectiveness of St. John's wort in the treatment of mild to moderate depression.[52] A recent meta-analysis of 23 randomized trials enrolling 1,757 outpatients diagnosed with mild to moderate depression was conducted. Of the trials, 15 were placebo-controlled and eight compared St. John's wort to positive controls (active medications). Only one of the placebo comparisons and two of the active comparisons used combination products (St. John's wort with another herb such as valerian). The remaining studies used St. John's wort alone. The results of the meta-analysis show that St. John's wort is significantly superior to placebo and is maybe as effective as traditional agents.[53] St. John's wort patients reported fewer side effects than those on placebo and on traditional antidepressants.[54]

The side effects reportedly associated with St. John's wort are fatigue, pruritus, weight gain, and emotional vulnerability. Of concern with the use of St. John's wort is the potential for photosensitivity,[55] a side effect it shares with many traditional antidepressants (e.g., paroxetine [Paxil]). Light-skinned cattle and sheep that have grazed on the agent in large amounts have developed blistering sunburn. This has prompted caution for the use of St. John's wort in fair-skinned people. The use of sunscreen, protective clothing, and avoidance of prolonged exposure to direct sunlight is recommended. No drug-drug or drug-food interactions have been documented despite purported MAOI activity. Patients already taking traditional antidepressants should consult their health care providers before embarking on a trial of St. John's wort. It is not considered effective for the more severe forms of depression. Combinations of traditional antidepressants that block the reuptake of serotonin and St. John's wort should be avoided. Excessive serotonin activity in the brain may lead to the development of serotonin syndrome, which is potentially lethal, with symptoms of restlessness, agitation, confusion, myoclonus, hyperreflexia, autonomic instability, tachycardia, hyperpyrexia, rigidity, and tremor. Initial treatment is the discontinuation of the offending agents with treatment of serious symptomology. If any of the above symptoms should develop when using St. John's wort discontinue use immediately, and seek medical attention.

Due to St. John's wort's low degree of MAO inhibitory activity, the use of a tyramine-free diet (see Table 11.6) is not currently advocated. But the use of excessive amounts of any food or medication on a tyramine-free diet is not recommended. In some situations the combination of an agent that

TABLE 11.6. Examples of MAOI Diet and Drug Restrictions

Excluded Items
Aged meats (salami) and cheeses (blue)
All beer, red wines, and hard liquors
Smoked or pickled items
Broad beans (Italian beans)
Yeast-containing products
Medications Excluded
Meperidine (Demerol)
Decongestants (Sudafed)
Stimulants (Amphetamine)

inhibits MAO and a large amount of tyramine can result in a hypertensive crisis. Symptoms of a hypertensive crisis include increased blood pressure, headache, stiff neck, nausea, vomiting, and clammy skin. If these symptoms develop immediate emergency care is recommended.

Recommended dosing for St. John's wort in the treatment of mild to moderate depression is 900 mg per day in three divided doses.[56] In some cases larger doses may be required (up to 4 grams). Like standard antidepressants, the full antidepressant effect of St. John's wort does not occur for four to six weeks.[57] St. John's wort can be used as a tea or in capsules formulated to contain 300 mg of St. John's wort extract (0.9 mg hypericin).

Resolution

Depression is a serious illness and although MJ's intended use of St. John's wort is probably not harmful, she should be encouraged to discuss her situation with her health care provider. Ruling out potential physical causes of her symptoms (e.g., hypothyroidism), as well as proper assessment of her depression is important for appropriate treatment of her "blues." An open dialogue examining the treatment options available before beginning an herbal remedy for depression is essential. MJ's health care provider can assist her in monitoring the success of therapy, as well as evaluating any side effects that might occur.

Table 11.7 provides several salient points, or "clinical pearls," that clinicians should keep in mind when dealing with patients on, or desiring to use, herbal medications. Other herbal medicines used in the treatment of anxiety, insomnia, and depression are listed in Table 11.8. Data supporting the use of many of these agents are less robust.

TABLE 11.7. Clinical Pearls

- Several herbal products can be useful for mild to moderate symptoms of anxiety, insomnia, and depression.
- Use high-quality standardized herbal products only:

Valerian	0.5 percent essential oil
St. John's wort	0.3 percent or 0.9 mg hypericin
Kava	60 to 120 mg kava pyrones

- Recommended doses:

St. John's wort	300 mg three times a day (depression)
Valerian	300 mg at bedtime (insomnia)
	200 mg twice a day (anxiety)
Kava	100 mg three times a day (anxiety)

Patients over the age of 65 should begin with smaller doses and increase the dose more slowly. Herbal remedies in general are not recommended for children.

- If symptoms do not improve or worsen, contact your health care professional.
- Do not exceed recommended maximum doses.
- Herbal medications are not automatically safer than over-the-counter and prescription medications. Use these agents as recommended only.
- Avoid off-label cure-alls, or products that guarantee 100 percent positive results.

TABLE 11.8. Herbal Sedative Hypnotic and Antidepressant Agents

Black Cohosh *(Cimicifuga racemosa)*
Sedative, relaxing, and restorative for nervous system.
Not for use in pregnancy. Do not exceed stated doses.
California poppy *(Eschscholzia california)*
Gentle and nonaddictive hypnotic, tranquilizer, and anodyne.
Considered safe for children.
Damask rose *(Rosa damascena)*
Gentle sedative, soothing for nerves, antidepressant.
Use only good quality, genuine rose oil medicinally.
Jamaican dogwood *(Piscidia erythrina)*
Sedative, anodyne, good for severe nervous tension, insomnia, and migraine.

TABLE 11.8 *(continued)*

Lavender *(Lavandula spp.)*
Sedative.
Avoid high doses in pregnancy.
Lemon Balm *(Melissa officinalis)*
Antidepressant and restorative for the nervous system.
Linden *(Tilia europaea)*
Reduces nervous tension.
Mugwort *(Artemisia vulgaris)*
A gentle nervine used in mild depression, mild stress, and menopausal tension.
Avoid in pregnancy and breast feeding.
Neroli oil *(Citrus aurantium)*
Sedative and antidepressant, traditionally used for hysteria, panic, and fearfulness.
Pasque flower *(Anemone pulsatilla)*
Nervine and anodyne with sedative action, good for nervous tension.
Use only the dried plant.
Skullcap *(Scutellaria lateriflora)*
Relaxant and restorative for the CNS, good for nervous debility.
Vervain *(Verbena officinalis)*
Relaxing nervine.
Not for use in pregnancy.
Wild lettuce *(Lactuca virosa)*
Sedative, low doses cause sleepiness.
Excess can lead to insomnia.
Wood betony *(Stachys officinalis)*
Sedative and calming for the nervous system, fearfulness, and exhaustion.
Large doses can cause vomiting. Avoid high dose in pregnancy.

REFERENCES

1. *Webster's dictionary.* Kauffman L, Editor. Larchmont, NY, Book Essentials Publications, 1988.

2. Eisenberg DR, Kessler RC, Foster C, Norlock FE, Calkins DR, Delbanco TL. Unconventional medicine in the United States—Prevalence, costs, and patterns of use. *N Engl J Med* 1993;328:246.

3. Grauds CD. Botanical savvy: Consultation tips for pharmacists. *Pharm Times* 1996;62(11):81.

4. American Psychiatric Association. Anxiety Disorders. In *Diagnostic and statistical manual of mental disorders*, Fourth Edition. Washington, DC, American Psychiatric Association, 1994;432.

5. Wicht M. *Herbal drugs and pharmaceuticals*. Boca Raton, FL, CRC Press. 1994.

6. Brown D. Anti-anxiety effects from chamomile compounds. *HerbalGram* 1997;39:19.

7. Ody P. *The complete medicinal herbal.* New York, DK Publishing, 1993.

8. Gould L, Reddy CV, Gomprecht RF. Cardiac effects of chamomile tea. *J Clin Pharmacol* 1973;(November-December):475.

9. Castleman M. *The healing herbs: The ultimate guide to the curative power of nature's medicines.* Emmaus, PA, Rodale Press, 1991;362.

10. Riedel E, Hansel R, Ehrke G. Inhibition of gama-aminobutyric acid catabolism by valerenic acid derivatives. *Planta Med* 1982;46:219.

11. Menninni T, Bernasconi P, Bombardelli E, et al. In vitro study on the interaction of extracts and pure compounds from *Valeriana officinalis* roots with GABA, benzodiazepine and barbiturate receptors. *Fitoterapia* 1993;64:291.

12. Hozl J, Godau P. Receptor binding studies with *Valeriana officinalis* on the benzodiazepine receptor. *Planta Med* 1989;55:642.

13. Houghton PJ. The biological activity of valerian and related plants. *J Ethnopharmacol* 1988;22:121.

14. Leathwood PD, Chauffard F. Quantifying the effects of mild sedatives. *J Psychiat Res* 1982/1983;17(2):115.

15. Castleman M. *The healing herbs: The ultimate guide to the curative power of nature's medicines.* Emmaus, PA, Rodale Press, 1991;362.

16. Cammarata J. *A physician's guide to herbal wellness.* Chicago, Chicago Review Press, 1996:45.

17. Foster S. Herbal medicine: An introduction for pharmacists. *NARD J* 1996; 10:127.

18. Hoffman D. *The herbalist CD rom.* Hopkins Technology, 1993.

19. Castleman M. *The healing herbs: The ultimate guide to the curative power of nature's medicines.* Emmaus, PA, Rodale Press, 1991;364.

20. Mowrey DB. *The scientific validation of herbal medicine.* New Canaan, CT, Keats Publishing, 1986:165.

21. Lehmann E, Kinzler E, Friedemann J. Efficacy of a special kava extract *(Piper methysticum)* in patients with states of anxiety, tension and excitedness of non-mental origin—a double-blind placebo-controlled study of four weeks treatment. *Phytomedicine* 1996;3:113.

22. Singh YN. Kava: An overview. *J Ethnopharmacol* 1992;37:13.

23. Davies LP, Drew CA, Duffield P, Johnston GA, Jamieson DD. Kava pyrones and resin: Studies on $GABA_A$, $GABA_B$, and benzodiazepine binding sites in rodent brain. *Pharmacol Toxicol* 1992;71:120.

24. Singh YN. Kava: An overview. *J Ethnopharmacol* 1992;37:38.

25. Ruze P. Kava-induced dermopathy: A niacin deficiency? *Lancet* 1990;335: 1442.

26. Almeida JC, Grimsley EW. Coma from the health food store: Interactions between kava and alprazolam [Letter]. *Ann Intern Med* 1996;125(11):940.

27. Singh YN. Kava: An overview. *J Ethnopharmacol* 1992;37:13.

28. Hoffman D. *The complete illustrated holistic herbal.* Rockport, MA, Element Books, 1996

29. Castleman M. *The healing herbs: The ultimate guide to the curative power of nature's medicines.* Emmaus, PA, Rodale Press, 1991;213.

30. Mowrey DB. *The scientific validation of herbal medicine.* New Canaan, CT, Keats Publishing, 1986.

31. Ody P. *The complete medicinal herbal.* New York, DK Publishing, 1993;66.

32. Cammarata J. *A physician's guide to herbal wellness.* Chicago, Chicago Review Press, 1996;96.

33. Ibid., p. 47.

34. Castleman M. *The healing herbs: The ultimate guide to the curative power of nature's medicines.* Emmaus, PA, Rodale Press, 1991;212.

35. Grauds CE. Botanical savvy: Consultation tips for pharmacists. *PharmaTimes* 1996;11:81.

36. Bahrke MS, Morgan WP. Evaluation of the ergogenic properties of ginseng. *Sports Med* 1994;18(4):229.

37. American Botanical Council. *Herbs and health series,* Pamphlet. Austin, TX, 1996.

38. Liu C, Xiao P. Recent advances on ginseng research in China. *J Ethnopharmacol* 1992;36:27.

39. Tsang D, Yeung HW, Tso WW, Peck H. Ginseng saponins: Influence on neurotransmitter uptake in rat synaptosomes. *Planta Med* 1985;51(3):221.

40. Bahrke MS, Morgan WP. Evaluation of the ergogenic properties of ginseng. *Sports Med* 1994;18(4):229.

41. Nikaido T, Ohmoto T, Sankawa U, Tanaka O, Kasai R, Shoji J, et al. Inhibitors of cyclic AMP phosphodiesterase in *Panax ginseng* C.A. Meyer and *Panax japonicus* C.A. Meyer. *Chem Pharm Bull* 1984;32(4):1477.

42. Wilkie A, Cordess C. Ginseng—a root just like a carrot? *J Royal Soc Med* 1994;84:594.

43. Hoffman D. *The herbalist. Multimedia CD-Rom,* version 2.0. Hopkins Technology, LLC. Hopkins, MN. 1994.

44. Ibid.

45. Ibid.

46. Seigel RK. Ginseng abuse syndrome: Problems with the panacea. *JAMA* 1979;241:1614.

47. Bahrke MS, Morgan WP. Evaluation of the ergogenic properties of ginseng. *Sports Med* 18(4):243.

48. LaValle J. Ginseng: Ancient Chinese cure-all. *J Retail Pharm* 1997;2(7):42.

49. Mowrey DB. *The scientific validation of herbal medicine.* New Canaan, CT, Keats Publishing, 1986;193.

50. Castleman M. *The healing herbs: The ultimate guide to the curative power of nature's medicines.* Emmaus, PA, Rodale Press, 1991;205.

51. American Psychiatric Association. Mood Disorders. In *Diagnostic and Statistical Manual of Mental Disorders,* Fourth Edition. Washington DC, American Psychiatric Association, 1994;344.

52. Harrer G, Schulz V. Clinical investigation of the antidepressant effectiveness of hypericum. *J Geriatric Psychiatry Neurol* 1994;7(suppl 1):S6.

53. Linde KG, Ramirez CD, Mulrow CD, Pauls A, Weidenhammer W. St. John's wort for depression—an overview and meta-analysis of randomized clinical trials. *Br Med J* 1996;313(8):253.

54. Vorbach EU, Hubner WD, Arnoldt KH. Effectiveness and tolerance of the hypericum extract LI 160 in comparison with imipramine: Randomized double-blind study with 135 outpatients. *J Geriatr Psychiatry Neurol* 1994;7(suppl 1):S19.

55. Ody P. *The complete medicinal herbal.* New York, DK Publishing, 1993;63.

56. Foster S. Herbal medicine. An introduction for pharmacists. *NARD* 1996; 10:138.

57. Hoffman D. *The complete illustrated holistic herbal.* Rockport, MA, Element Books, 1996;104.

Chapter 12

Herbal Medicine and Substance Abuse

Marsha Cline Holleman, MD, MPH

INTRODUCTION

The problem of substance abuse is pervasive and common in our society. Almost one out of four Americans has close ties to someone with a drug dependency problem or alcoholism among family, friends, or co-workers.[1] Among adolescents, the use of marijuana and alcohol has increased since 1992, after a period of decline in the 1980s. In Texas, more than 34 percent of seventh through twelfth graders report using illegal drugs at some point in their lives.[2] Among adults, alcoholism remains a steady problem and the cocaine epidemic of the 1980s is endemic now due to crack cocaine. Crack cocaine users number one to five million, about half of the number of those who use marijuana.[3]

Herbal medicine plays a role in substance abuse in several ways. First, plant materials can be used as psychoactive substances, as has been done for centuries among traditional societies. Second, herbal medicine can play a positive role in the treatment of substance abuse, both as a deterrent and in treating the symptoms of withdrawal. We will see examples of both of these roles in the following cases.

CASE STUDY 1: MORNING GLORY

A girl and her brother, ages 11 and 12, were brought to a family physician's office by their mother for diarrhea accompanied by vomiting. The pair described a three-day bout of watery diarrhea with some vomiting to the point that they were beginning to feel weak and unable to attend school. Their mother could remember no unusual food exposures but pointed out that several other neighborhood children had similar symptoms. The children were prescribed a carbohydrate-rich diet, stool cultures were done that were negative, and the diarrhea resolved spontaneously after a few more days.

The mother called the following week with new information. Her children had confessed to chewing morning glory seeds for the purpose of getting high. While on the Internet, they and their friends had stumbled across the *Growing the Hallucinogens* Web site. Fascinated, they had decided to order morning glory seeds and in the backyard with their friends, had proceeded to chew several hundred seeds each. Along with hallucinations, each one had developed a bout of diarrhea. One of the mothers discovered the seed packet with its warning regarding fungicide treatment. Further investigation at the Web site produced a warning about fungicides producing nausea and diarrhea.

Discussion

Morning glory *(Ipomoea violacea, Ipomoea tricolor)* is a beautifully flowering vine that grows wild throughout much of the United States. The purple or blue blooms of mid- to late summer produce seed-filled pods, and ingesting these seeds produces a hallucinogenic experience. It is produced by a lysergic acid derivative akin to LSD but less potent.[4]

The Internet has several Web sites dedicated to information regarding psychoactive effects of native plants, including *Growing the Hallucinogens: How to Cultivate and Harvest Legal Psychoactive Plants* and *Sputnik Drug Information Zone.* Information formerly passed on by word of mouth and thus less accessible is now easy to find, sometimes with color photographs for easy plant identification. As in this case, Internet users may not pay attention to detail and find themselves sick from side effects or additives.[4]

Commercial seed companies, in part to discourage the misuse of their seeds, sometimes treat morning glory seeds with a fungicide. Treated seed packages are marked with warnings of nausea, vomiting, and diarrhea. Web sites give instructions on avoiding these effects, such as chewing a few seeds to test one's susceptibility to the nausea, or planting the packet of seeds and harvesting the next generation.

Other herbal sources of hallucinogenic substances are shown in Table 12.1.

TABLE 12.1. Hallucinogenic Herbs

Herb	Botanical Source
Catnip	*Nepeta cataria*
Juniper	*Juniperus macropoda*
Kava kava	*Piper methysticum*
Mandrake	*Mandrogora officinarum*
Nutmeg	*Myristica fragrans*
Periwinkle	*Catharanthus roseus*
Thorn apple (jimsonweed)	*Datura stramonium*
Yohimbe	*Corynanthe yohimbe*

Source: Siegel RK. Herbal intoxication: Psychoactive effects from herbal cigarettes, tea, and capsules. *Journal of the American Medical Association* 1976;236(5):473-476.

CASE STUDY 2: VALERIAN

A 41-year-old woman entered a substance abuse treatment center because of hypnotic/sedative abuse. Two years before, her doctor had prescribed codeine after back surgery and since then she had gradually increased her intake. She had no other drug dependencies. At peak usage she was taking 600 mg per day. She realized her problem when she began doctor hopping for the purpose of obtaining prescriptions of the medication and decided to seek treatment.

Initially she underwent detoxification and then entered a residential treatment program. She did well except for difficulty sleeping, which impaired her daytime productivity. She was given valerian liquid extract 1.0 ml at bedtime, which helped her fall to sleep quickly. She completed her program with great success. One year later she attributed her sobriety to the pivotal effect of obtaining sleep at a crucial point in her treatment program. She had not continued to need valerian after two weeks of use.

Discussion

Valerian, also known as garden heliotrope, has been ascribed sedative properties for several centuries. It produces a shortened sleep latency, less wake time after sleep, lower frequency of waking, and reduced nighttime motor activity,[5] although EEG effects on sleep did not reach significance.[6] For a chemically dependent patient, its sedative properties are ideal, as it is considered not to be addicting.[7] Although valerian is generally safe, one of its components is cytotoxic,[8] but no evidence of liver damage was found among those who took large doses.[9]

A goal of substance abuse treatment is to become independent of medications and substances of any kind, except for those that are medically indicated, and instead to become able to handle stresses behaviorally and cognitively. Valerian may help in this regard by relieving withdrawal symptoms of insomnia without exposing the patient to the risk of addiction.

Table 12.2 lists several other herbal ingredients with sedative properties.

TABLE 12.2. Herbal Ingredients with Sedative Properties

Calamus	Nettle
Celery	Passion Flower
Chamomile, German	Sage
Couchgrass	Scotch Broom
Elecampane	Skullcap
Ginseng	Shepherd's Purse
Goldenseal	St. John's wort
Hops	Valerian
Hydrocotyle	Wild Carrot
Jamaica Dogwood	Wild Lettuce

Sources: Newall CA, Anderson LA, Phillipson JD. *Herbal Medicines: A Guide for Health-Care Professionals.* London: Pharmaceutical Press, 1996:261. Siegel RK. Herbal Intoxication: Psychoactive effects from herbal cigarettes, tea, and capsules. *Journal of the American Medical Association* 1976;236(5):473-476.

CASE STUDY 3: GOLDENSEAL

Counselors at a drug treatment facility occasionally collected random urine drug screening samples from clients to determine client compliance with the program's rules of abstinence. One counselor asked a teenager sent to the facility by his parole officer to give a urine sample. The sample had a dark amber-brown appearance and the result was negative for substances, including marijuana, amphetamines, cocaine, opiates, and benzodiazepines. Later, however, the teenager admitted to his counselor that he had been smoking marijuana on his weekend passes. He had successfully hidden his relapses by drinking goldenseal tea, which had resulted in a false negative urine drug screen.

Discussion

Goldenseal, sometimes known as yellow root, has been ascribed antibiotic, immunostimulant, and anticonvulsant properties, among others.[10] Another use, well known among some supplying urine specimens for drug testing, is as an adulterant that can produce a false negative urine screen.[11,12] Goldenseal either may be taken by mouth as a tea or in liquid form or can be added to the urine after voiding. The mechanism of action is not well understood, but may involve the alkaloids present in goldenseal. (Other well-known adulterants include lemon, Drano, and bleach, the last two being used by drenching the hands in these substances and then urinating on the hands into the urine cup!) One way to know if urine has been contaminated by goldenseal is the urine color, which becomes a darker amber or more brown than usual.[12]

Toxicities of goldenseal are infrequent but at high doses include nausea, anxiety, depression, seizures, paralysis, and death.[10] Other herbs might be used for the purpose of altering urine drug screens. These are listed in Table 12.3.

TABLE 12.3. Herbal Ingredients with Diuretic Activity

Agrimony	Dandelion	Shepherd's Purse
Cornsilk	Elder	Squill
Couchgrass	Pokeroot	Yarrow

Source: Newall CA, Anderson LA, Phillipson JD. *Herbal Medicines: A Guide for Health-Care Professionals.* London: Pharmaceutical Press, 1996:281.

CASE STUDY 4: KUDZU

A 52-year-old man with alcohol dependence has been sober for three weeks. He had decided to quit drinking when he began having difficulty with his memory, job attendance, wife, and finances. He began attending Alcoholics Anonymous at the recommendation of a friend and gradually decreased his alcohol intake to zero. He was currently having tremendous urges to drink, however, especially while watching sports on television.

He consulted his family physician, who recommended naltrexone as an effective medication both to decrease alcohol craving and to decrease the mood-elevating aspects of alcohol intake. The patient decided instead to try a kudzu preparation from the health food store that a friend in one of his Alcoholics Anonymous groups had recommended. The folk medicine worked well. While watching a football game he could not resist having a beer, but drank no more than one before he began having flushing, sweating, nausea, vomiting, and headache. The reaction lasted several hours. After this experience, he has remained sober for three years.

Discussion

Kudzu root, or *Radix puerariae,* from the vine that has overgrown many southern U.S. forests, has been used for alcohol aversion therapy in China for centuries.[13] In the last few years, its mechanism of action has been clarified in a U.S. laboratory, where it has been shown that the extract contains two potent, reversible inhibitors of human alcohol dehydrogenase iso-zymes, diadzein and genistein.[14] When injected into alcoholic hamsters, the hamsters ingested 50 percent less alcohol than baseline. It works much like disulfiram (Antabuse), although disulfiram inhibits a different alcohol dehydrogenase isozyme that may have broader actions.[15] Researchers hope that producing another alcohol dehydrogenase inhibitor based on kudzu, which is more potent and specific, may reduce some of disulfiram's side effects, such as drowsiness, and make for a better-tolerated medication to reduce alcohol intake among humans.

CASE STUDY 5: ANGEL'S TRUMPET

A 14-year-old boy was brought to the emergency room by his parents, who reported he had come home from a friend's house acting strangely. He talked incessantly about the beautiful sunset and occasionally struggled to leave the room. On exam, his pulse was 110, temperature 99.6, and respiratory rate 22. His pupils were dilated, his mouth was dry, and bowel sounds were absent.

He underwent gastric lavage, which produced plant materials including seeds and leaves, and he received activated charcoal. After an overnight stay in the intensive care unit, he regained normal mental status and physical exam. He revealed to his parents that he had ingested angel's trumpet seeds for use as a hallucinogen.

Discussion

Several plant and herbal agents produce anticholinergic effects, including angel's trumpet *(Brugmansia candida* or *Datura candida)*. Patients with these effects are commonly described as "hot as a hare, dry as a bone, red as a beet, blind as a bat, and mad as a hatter." Effects occur within minutes of seed ingestion and several hours of leaf and flower ingestion.[16] Besides the symptoms of the patient in this case, others include urinary retention and muscular weakness.

Treatment ranges from observation only to full support depending on the dosage ingested. Patients do best when treated in a calm manner with little extraneous noise and light. Gastric lavage may be attempted up to 24 or 48 hours after ingestion since the anticholinergic effect may have slowed gastric emptying. Overdosage may result in respiratory depression and circulatory collapse.[17] Physostigmine, a cholinesterase inhibitor, may be given to patients who have severe symptoms, including seizures or severe hypertension.

A related plant, jimsonweed, or *Datura stramonium,* has also been described as commonly used for hallucinogenic experiences due to its anticholinergic effect. (Originally known to American colonists as the Jamestown weed, its current name is a contraction of the original name.)[18] Its seeds are ingested most commonly, but it has also been available in a cigarette form.[19] Mandrake is another herb that produces its hallucinogenic effects anticholinergically. Additional herbal ingredients with psychoactive properties are listed in Table 12.4. See also Table 12.5 for a summary of this chapter's material.

TABLE 12.4. Additional Herbal Ingredients with Psychoactive Properties

Ingredient	Source	Effect
California Poppy	*Eschscholtzia californica*	Mild euphoriant
Cinnamon	*Cinnamomum camphora*	Mild stimulant
Damiana	*Turnera diffusa*	Mild stimulant
Hydrangea	*Hydrangea paniculata*	Stimulant
Kola Nut	*Cola* species	Stimulant

TABLE 12.4 *(continued)*

Ingredient	Source	Effect
Lobelia	*Lobelia inflata*	Mild euphoriant
Ma huang	*Ephedra sinica*	Stimulant
Mate	*Ilex paraguayensis*	Stimulant
Mormon Tea	*Ephedra nevadensis*	Stimulant
Passion Flower	*Passiflora incarnata*	Mild stimulant
Prickly Poppy	*Argemone mexicana*	Narcotic-analgesic
Snakeroot	*Rauwolfia serpentina*	Tranquilizer
Wormwood	*Artemisia absinthium*	Narcotic-analgesic

Sources: Siegal RK. Herbal intoxication: Psychoactive effects from herbal ciga-rettes, tea, and capsules. *Journal of the American Medical Association* 1976;236(5):473-476. Eliason GC, Kruger J, Mark D, Rasmann DN. Dietary sup-plement users: Demographics, product use, and medical system interaction. *Journal of the American Board of Family Practice* 1997;10(4):265-271.

TABLE 12.5. Summary

Valerian has nonaddicting sedative properties that can be helpful in withdrawing from opiates, alcohol, and cocaine.
Goldenseal is used to produce false negative urine drug screen results. It often turns the urine a brown color.
Kudzu root is effective in alcohol aversion therapy.
The anticholinergic effects of angel's trumpet and jimsonweed include a psychoactive effect.
The Internet sites *Grow the Hallucinogens* and *Sputnik Dug Information Zone* give information on herbal preparations that produce psychoactive effects.
Many naturally occurring plant parts can serve as psychoactive substances, including periwinkle and yohimbe. See Tables 11.1, 11.2, and 11.4.

REFERENCES

1. The nation's substance abuse problem. 1995 National Survey: Fact Sheet. Join Together via Internet: her.org/JTO/issues/National_Survey/facts.html.

2. Teen drug use still on upswing. *New View.* Texas Commission on Alcohol and Drug Abuse. 1996; December: 6-7.

3. Gawin FH, Khalso ME, Ellinwood E. Stimulants. In: Galanter M, Kleber HD, eds. *Textbook of Substance Abuse Treatment.* Washington, DC: American Psychiatric Press; 1994:111.

4. Micke MM. The case of hallucinogenic plants and the Internet. *Journal of School Health.* 1996;66(8):277-280.

5. Newall CA, Anderson LA, Phillipson JD. *Herbal Medicines: A Guide for Health-Care Professionals.* London: Pharmaceutical Press; 1996:261.

6. Leathwood PD, Chauffard F. Quantifying the effects of mild sedatives. *Journal of Psychiatric Research* 1982-1983;17(2):115-122.

7. Nebelkopf E. Herbal therapy in the treatment of drug use. *International Journal of the Addictions* 1987;22(8):695-717.

8. Lindahl O, Lindahl L. Double blind study of a valerian preparation. *Pharmacology, Biochemistry and Behavior* 1989;32(4):1065-1066.

9. Chan TY, Tang CH, Critchley JA. Poisoning due to an over-the-counter hypnotic, Sleep-Qik (hyoscine, cyproheptadine, valerian). *Postgraduate Medical Journal* 1995;71:227-228.

10. Newall, Anderson, Phillipson, op. cit., pp. 151-152.

11. Wu AH, Forte E, Casella G, et al. CEDIA for screening drugs of abuse in urine and the effect of adulterants. *Journal of Forensic Sciences* 1995;40(4):614-618.

12. Mikkelsen SL, Ash KO. Adulterants causing false negatives in illicit drug testing. *Clinical Chemistry* 1988;34(1):2333-2336.

13. Kudzu extract shows potential for moderating alcohol abuse. *American Journal of Health-Systems Pharmacy* 1994;51:750.

14. Keung WM. Biochemical studies of a new class of alcohol dehydrogenase inhibitors from *Radix pueurariae. Alcoholism, Clinical and Experimental Research* 1993;17(6):1254-1260.

15. King QM, Vallee BL. Daidzin: A potent, selective inhibitor of human mitochondrial aldehyde dehydrogenase. *Proceedings of the National Academy of Science USA* 1993;90:1247-1251.

16. Greene GS, Patterson SG, Warner E. Ingestion of Angel's Trumpet: An increasingly common source of toxicity. *Southern Medical Journal* 1996;89(4): 365-369.

17. Olin BR, editor-in-chief. *Drug Facts and Comparisons,* 1995 edition. St. Louis, MO: Facts and Comparisons; 1995:1705.

18. Klein-Schwartz W, Oderda GM. Jimsonweed intoxication in adolescents and young adults. *Am J Dis Child* 1984;138:737-739.

19. Siegel RK. Herbal intoxication: Psychoactive effects from herbal cigarettes, tea, and capsules. *Journal of the American Medical Association.* 1976;236(5):473-476.

Chapter 13

Common Herbal Products Used in Cancer Prevention and Treatment

Timothy R. McGuire, PharmD

INTRODUCTION

Before discussing the common herbal remedies that have been used in the prevention and treatment of cancer, it is useful to discuss the underlying motivations that leads cancer patients to herbal remedies and other complementary therapies. The characteristics of patients who use alternative medicines include those who are young to middle aged, those who are in the upper socioeconomic class, and those who have a chronic medical condition. The use of complementary therapies in the management of cancer is high, estimated at about 16 percent in one study. This level of use likely results from the fear surrounding the toxicities of allopathic treatment of cancer and the fear of a painful death.[1]

The next several paragraphs review the pathophysiology of cancer and how this may relate to the high use of complementary therapies. The limitation of studies evaluating diet in the prevention of cancer is also discussed. Dietary studies serve as a good model to demonstrate the limitations of the herbal literature as the use of herbs can be considered a specialized form of dietary management. A distinction can be made between general dietary management and the use of herbal remedies in that herbs have been used to treat cancer while diet has not been applied in the treatment of cancer.

Cancer claimed the lives of more than half a million Americans in 1997.[2] The rates of cancer are increasing for reasons that are not entirely understood. Possible explanations given are greater exposure to chemical carcinogens, greater viral oncogenesis, and variables of lifestyle including diet, excercise, and stress. Because treatment of the common cancers (colorectal, lung, breast, and prostate) remains less than optimal, a greater emphasis has been placed on cancer prevention. The common cancers are not curable in an advanced stage, and large numbers of patients with metastatic disease who have no curative treatment options are searching for nonconventional therapy. Metastatic cancer patients are a vulnerable population willing to utilize nontraditional methods of treatment despite limited information on their value and an unknown toxicity profile. A survey performed in the early 1990s reported that a high percentage of cancer patients use some source of alternative medicine.[3] The lack of effective allopathic treatment options results in the use of alternative therapies that have not been proven effective by controlled trials.

Methods of preventing cancer are not clearly defined but generally have focused on maintaining a low-fat diet and consuming sufficient fruits and vegetables for micronutrient balance.[4] The data supporting a correlation between cancer and diet have largely been case control studies that are open to many interpretations. The uncertainty of case control studies results from the lack of controls; thus, the contribution of unidentified confounding variables cannot be adequately assessed. These studies have generally shown that lower fat intake reduces the risk of developing several common cancers.[5]

The difficulty in intrepreting this data is best illustrated by the work that has been performed on breast cancer. The case control studies that determined a correlation between fat intake and breast cancer in women have major limitations since there is no low-fat group in the United States, where the average fat intake exceeds 30 percent. This is significantly higher than in Asian countries where fat accounts for less than 25 percent of caloric intake. For compliance reasons, cohort studies that prospectively evaluate the relationship between dietary fat and breast cancer have to be performed in societies where the normal everyday diet is lower in fat than in the United States. Because of the inability to maintain a low-fat diet, group cohort studies performed in the United States have had difficulty finding a relationship between fat and breast cancer.[6,7]

China has become the laboratory for studies to determine the role of dietary fat and breast cancer.[7] Since the Chinese have low dietary fat intake, it is a matter of placing the study group on a high-fat diet and having the low-fat control group maintain their normal diet. The difficulty of demonstrating cause and effect is illustrated by the confounding variables in this population. The usual low-fat diet in China is high in fiber and soy content. There is increasing evidence that the higher soy diet and not the lowered fat content offers protection from breast cancer. Soy is high in phytoestrogens, which are naturally occurring estrogen antagonists that can lower estrogenic activity.

Estrogen has been long thought to function as a promotional agent for the development of breast cancer; thus women who have greater estrogen exposure are at higher risk for breast cancer. The role of estrogen is supported by observational data showing that early menarche and late menopause increases breast cancer risk, and lower estradiol levels as a result of early pregnancy lowers a woman's risk for breast cancer. In addition, postmenopausal estrogen replacement increases the risk of breast cancer. This relationship between soy and estrogen antagonism complicates the interpretation of the proposed relationship between fat and breast cancer risk.[7,8] The reduction in breast cancer associated with a low-fat diet may be explained by high phytoestrogen consumption.

Not all of the established causes of cancer are identified as a result of controlled investigation. Sometimes the weight of circumstantial evidence developed from case control studies is so great that an association cannot be reasonably denied. To date the most important preventable lifestyle cause of cancer is smoking. The type of data supporting cigarette smoking as the predominant cause of lung cancer is from case control and animal work. The limitations of this type of data allowed tobacco companies to deny a causal link for decades. The controlled trials that would have established cause and effect were too expensive, and since lung cancer develops over thirty years, too long a follow-up time is required to be practical. The sheer weight of laboratory and epidemiologic evidence, however, was convincing to any objective scientist. The fact that the epidemiology of lung cancer had been collected for more than 50 years on millions of Americans who smoked allowed for a level of certainty that cannot be reproduced with other potential risk factors.

The above discussion illustrates the complexity of interpreting the epidemiologic data evaluating environmental causes of cancer.[8] The data remains weak on dietary causes of breast cancer, consisting of either epidemiologic studies or in vitro mechanistic data. Similar to the case of diet and cancer, there are no data conclusively showing that herbal remedies reduce the risk of cancer. Unlike smoking and cancer, no large body of literature exists that supports the value of herbal remedies in cancer prevention.

When assessing the value of herbal remedies in the prevention and treatment of cancer one is faced with great uncertainty. There is seldom clinical data supporting the usefulness of a given herbal remedy. When there is such data, it has been generated from a small number of patients and responses are nearly always reported as partial responses, often with inadequately reported methods of assessing tumor volume. The quality of this data is not compelling given the small percentage of patients who have spontaneous partial responses and the difficulty of accurately measuring partial responses. In addition, data on the usefulness of these substances is anecdotal at best, and often no rational mechanism exists for their proposed use.

The support for the use of herbal remedies in the prevention and treatment of cancer often includes a statement that these agents cause no harm. If one considers the cost of herbal and related remedies it often causes significant financial hardship (e.g., shark cartilage costs $50 for two weeks of therapy) and may be toxic to the point of causing increased mortality (e.g., laetrile). In addition, case control data has suggested that herbal remedies may increase the risk of nasopharyngeal cancer in the Philippines.[9] Many of the traditional herbal remedies used in the Philippines will increase cellular growth, which may serve as a promotional step in causing this cancer, which is endemic to the Philippines. The ability of many of these herbal remedies to stimulate the immune system may have negative consequences in autoimmune diseases and in transplant patients. The case at the end of this chapter demonstrates the potential deleterious effects of herbal remedies on transplant patients. These examples would counter the view that herbal remedies may at worst be neutral. This level of financial and health risk is certainly acceptable if there is benefit from herbal remedies in the prevention and treatment of cancer. Unfortunately, the prevention data is sparse and what is available is mostly in vitro or in animals.

HERBALS AND NATURAL PRODUCTS

In the following sections, the individual herbal or natural product remedies that have commonly been used in the prevention and treatment of cancer are discussed. The lack of data on the clinical usefulness of these agents and the underlying proposed mechanism of action will be emphasized. The mechanisms of action will be evaluated in light of the underlying pathophysiology of cancer and any clinical data relevant to prevention and treatment. In addition to the traditional herbal remedies, shark cartilage, a natural product treatment for cancer, will be evaluated because it has received significant attention over the last several years and its proposed mechanism of action may be common to several of the herbal remedies. In addition, it illustrates the difficulty of administering natural products in a form that is bioavailable.

SHARK CARTILAGE

While shark cartilage is not an herbal product, its recent use illustrates many of the difficulties associated with consuming herbal remedies. Shark cartilage has activity against various tumors via an antiangiogenic effect.

Cartilage is an avascular tissue with vessel growth being inhibited by the proteoglycans in cartilage. Proteoglycan inhibition of angiogenesis may result from several mechanisms including inhibition of migration and proliferation of endothelium, which is required for new vessel formation. When vessel growth is inhibited, the growing tumor lacks the oxygen and nutrients required for survival and the tumor becomes necrotic. This inhibition of angiogenesis may be the mechanism of action of tumor necrosis factor alpha, a cytokine released from macrophages, and is the proposed mechanism of action of several herbal remedies reported to have antitumor activity.

An article in the mid-1980s and a recently published article[10,11] identified the active component of shark cartilage to be a heat-stable protein with a molecular weight below 10,000 daltons. Shark cartilage is administered orally and is commonly used by cancer patients. Given that proteins are not absorbed across the gut wall intact, it is doubtful that the biologically active components of shark cartilage are bioavailable, and therefore it is unlikely to be useful in the treatment of cancer.

The popularity of this natural product began in the 1980s when, in a set of uncontrolled experiments, a cancer clinic in Cuba reported a series of partial responses in patients with terminal solid tumors after treatment with high doses of shark cartilage. Shark cartilage was administered as a retention enema. This data, which was widely reported in the lay press, has yet to be published and is suspiciously optimistic. However, this publicity led to public pressure for more controlled studies in the United States. After reviewing the world's experience with shark cartilage, the NCI has declined to perform a controlled trial because of the lack of evidence of activity.

CYTOKINE MECHANISMS

Several of the herbal products that have been advertised as being useful in the prevention and treatment of cancer have been shown in vitro to stimulate macrophage function and release inflammatory cytokines. Cytokines are chemicals released from cells, particularly cells of the immune system, that serve as chemical messengers to other cells. They can both activate and suppress the immune system. Cytokines released from activated macrophages are more specifically called monokines and are responsible for stimulating immune function and are involved in inflammation. Cancerous changes in cells are not an uncommon event but host immunity destroys cells that have undergone malignant transformation. This tumor surveillance function of the immune system results from the generation of natural killer cells and cytotoxic T-lymphocytes under cytokine stimulation. Stimulation of this arm of the immune system aids in tumor surveillance and protects against the development of clinical cancer.

Among the cytokines involved in the generation of antitumor lymphocytes are TNF-alpha, IL-1, and interferon. Each of the cytokines has been identified in mononuclear cell culture after treatment with several herbal remedies. The release of these inflammatory cytokines has been proposed as a mechanism for anticancer activity of these immunostimulatory herbs. If these agents work solely by this mechanism, the clinical value of these herbal products must be questioned, given that all these cytokines can be produced in large quantities by recombinant methods. These cytokines have been ex-tensively evaluated in the treatment of cancer, often with disappointing results. Since they can be produced in large quantities it makes more sense to administer the pure cytokine, which can be dosed to toxicity and antitumor effect, rather than an herbal remedy that does not have standardized activity. Herbs that may work via macrophage stimulation and cytokine release will have the same limitation as the pure cytokines, being associated with severe toxicity syndromes. For example, TNF-alpha produces fever and a severe wasting syndrome, IL-1 produces fever and capillary leak syndrome, and interferon-alpha produces fever and a chronic flulike syndrome.

Unless the herbal components are able to release the cytokines only at the tumor site and keep systemic concentrations low, it is unlikely that they can be used clinically because of high toxicity. Agents whose activity has been proposed to be mediated via cytokine release should have toxicity of fever and chills. In general, when one evaluates the individual agents that have generally been considered immunostimulants, one is struck by the lack of systemic side effects such as fever. The lack of cytokine-mediated toxicity certainly leaves significant doubt regarding the proposed mechanism of any antitumor effect demonstrated by these herbal remedies.

Aloe vera has been studied and used clinically in feline leukemia, a fatal disease in cats that is caused by the feline leukemia virus. Acemannan is a major carbohydrate component of aloe vera and is reported to have both an anticancer and antiviral activity and to stimulate macrophage function.[12] The proposed mechanism of action of acemannan is the release of macrophage-derived cytokines that have antitumor activity (TNF-alpha and interferon). Acemannan has been shown to clinically stabilize and prolong the survival of cats with feline leukemia.[13]

Feline leukemia virus is a retrovirus that has similarity to HIV. Similar to the feline leukemia virus, HIV is an oncogenic virus, which explains the higher rates of leukemia and lymphoma in AIDS patients than in the general population. The usefulness of this remedy in AIDS patients for the prevention and treatment of cancer has not been determined. However, it is unlikely to be practical if it works via the generation of cytokines, given that part of the detrimental effect of AIDS, including a wasting syndrome, is a result of increased release of macrophage-derived cytokines. In addition, elevations in interferon systemically may predict for progression of AIDS.[14] There is more of an a priori reason to believe aloe vera would be detrimental to AIDS patients than helpful.

Clinically, a randomized placebo-controlled study was performed in AIDS patients on AZT or ddI. Patients on these antiretroviral drugs were randomized to acemannan or placebo. Acemannan had no effect on disease parameters but it was well tolerated.[15] This clinical trial was initiated because of in vitro work reporting synergistic antiviral activity between acemannan and AZT.[16] As is often the case, in vitro observation was not repeated by clinical assessment. The fact that acemannan was well tolerated suggests a lack of cytokine release. An alternative mechanism of action has been suggested and supported by a recent in vitro study that showed an increase in activity of cytotoxic T-lymphocytes.[17] This has renewed interest in this agent but will require further clinical investigation to determine if this in vitro activity translates into antiviral or antitumor activity.

Echinacea has been proposed to have immunostimulatory activity. In vitro it activates macrophages and increases their activity against tumor cells.[18] The cytokines that have been identified include TNF and IL-1.[18,19] The component of the echinacea product that increases cytotoxicity is a polysaccharide. The polysaccharide component isolated from echinacea protected immunosuppressive mice from *Candida albicans* and *Listeria monocytogenes* infections.[19] This anti-infective activity may correlate with increased cell-mediated immunity after administration of the polysaccharide. This improvement in cell-mediated immune response may translate into increased antitumor effects. In addition to generating cytotoxic T-lymphocytes and monokines in cell culture, in normal subjects physiologic changes occurred which were consistent with increased neutrophil and monocyte activity. This in vivo data was consistent with cytokine activation of the cell-mediated immune system.[20] The polysaccharide component of echinacea was administered to these normal subjects by the intravenous route, and there is no data on whether it is absorbed orally, which is the usual route of administration of the herbal product.

Mistletoe is a potent inducer of cytokines in vitro, stimulating the release of interleukin-1 and TNF-alpha. Presumably it is this immunostimulation that explains tumor regression reported in mice.[21] Given the toxicity of these inflammatory cytokines, it is unlikely that this will be a very useful agent for the prevention of cancer in humans. However, mistletoe has been used in the treatment of cancer. Iscador, a mistletoe preparation, has been given intravenously to 20 breast cancer patients and found to increase natural killer cells and cell-mediated immunity. Activation of these elements of the immune system may lead to enhanced tumor cell kill.[22]

ANTIOXIDANT MECHANISMS

Antioxidants are useful agents for the prevention of several cancers. There are data demonstrating benefit in preventing colorectal cancer and lung cancer. These agents may prevent carcinogenesis by inhibiting the initiation of cancer by reactive radicals. Not only are antioxidants capable of preventing oxidative damage by carcinogens, they are able to reduce the formation of carcinogens such as nitrosamine. Nitrosamines are carcinogens formed in the stomach as a result of nitrites reacting with amino groups on proteins. Nitrosamines are potent carcinogens and are a recognized cause of various gastrointestinal cancers. The antioxidant activity may reduce the incidence of gastrointestinal cancer by reducing nitrosamine formation in the gut. In addition to the potential beneficial effects of antioxidants on the gastrointestinal mucosa, antioxidant vitamins such as vitamin A and E may reduce the risk of lung cancer by reducing the amount of smoking-related exposure to free radicals.[23]

Allium herbs/vegetables include plants in the garlic and onion family. These herbs and vegetables contain anticancer organosulfur compounds that include diallyl disulfides. These organosulfur compounds can inhibit H-Ras-transformed tumors by inhibiting the association of the gene product with the cell membrane. Chronic administration of garlic also has been reported to increase the activity of natural killer cells toward lymphoma cells. While some of the biochemical activities described above may be important in treating cancer, the largest body of literature exists on the use of allium plants in preventing cancer. In addition to increased tumor surveillance, garlic has demonstrated the ability to decrease nitrosamine formation in the GI tract. Epidemiologic data from China demonstrated a large reduction in gastric cancer with the high intake of allium vegetables, possibly as a result of the antioxidant properties of the thiol-containing compounds in these vegetables.[24]

Green tea is a fairly well-studied herb. Catechins, isolated from green tea, have antioxidant properties. Catechins are polyphenolic compounds that not only are potent antioxidants but will also inhibit nucleoside transport. While the inhibition of nucleoside transport is unlikely to be beneficial in cancer prevention, it may have therapeutic value in the treatment of cancer when used in conjunction with antimetabolites.[25] There are contradictory epidemiologic studies on cancer incidence and green tea consumption. The epidemiologic data largely exists on the ability of green tea to prevent cancer. One of the working theories is that the polyphenols in green tea inhibit the formation of nitrosamines by a mechanism similar to the allium herbs and vegetables and thus would likely reduce the risk of digestive cancers.

In a review of epidemiological evidence on tea and cancer there is a general impression that green tea produces a small reduction in the risk of gastrointestinal cancer.[26] In addition to the antioxidant activity, the polyphenols in green tea may inhibit protein kinase C activation. Protein kinase C regulates cellular growth by phosphorylating target proteins involved in cell progression through the cell cycle. Generally, stimulating cellular growth is a tumor promotion step. If the inhibition of protein kinase C is found to be an important mechanism for the chemopreventive effect of green tea, its preventive effect may extend beyond the gastrointestinal tract.

Chaparral has anticancer activity that is mediated by the antioxidant nordihydroguaiaretic acid. It has been used to treat cancer in humans but has produced only partial responses, and because of the uncertainty of measuring a partial response the activity of this remedy remains in question. The lack of data demonstrating anticancer activity coupled with a growing body of literature reporting the severe toxicity associated with chaparral places this remedy in the unproven and dangerous category. A recent review of chaparral-induced toxicity reported on 18 cases. Adverse events reported to the FDA between 1992 and 1994 found 13 cases of hepatotoxicity. In four cases, there was progression to cirrhosis and in two individuals there was liver failure requiring transplantation.[27] Given the lack of established activity and the severe liver toxicity associated with the use of chaparral, this herbal remedy should be avoided. If an antioxidant effect is desired several medications with low toxicity can be recommended.

In addition to the general antioxidant activity of chapparal it contains substances that inhibit the cyclooxygenase enzyme. Because cyclooxygenase is responsible for the oxidative conversion of procarcinogens to carcinogens, inhibition of this enzyme may be a method to prevent cancer. Cyclooxygenase in the GI epithelium may activate carcinogens and may explain the epidemiologic evidence which suggests that chronic aspirin and NSAID users have a reduced risk of colorectal cancer.[28] Rather than using an unproven hepatotoxic herb, a judicious use of NSAIDS may be more reasonable, if the initial findings of colorectal cancer risk reduction can be confirmed.

MISCELLANEOUS MECHANISMS

The following herbs may exert their antitumor effect by several diverse mechanisms. One potential mechanism is protein kinase C (PKC) inhibition, which is a relatively well-documented method of inhibiting the growth of cancer cells. Protein kinase C operates to accelerate cellular growth. The inhibition of PKC by tamoxifen may explain the drug's activity in vitro against tumors other than breast cancer. Several of the other herbs listed below have been reported to have a direct cytolytic effect on cancer in cell culture. It is doubtful that this activity operates in vivo given that the toxicity syndromes such as bone marrow suppression and hair loss have not been reported with the use of these herbs and would be expected if they directly killed rapidly growing cancer cells. Another set of herbs may work via an inhibition of angiogenesis and thus may inhibit cancer cell metastasis.

Ginseng use in a case control study produced a 50 percent reduction in the risk of cancer. In an experimental animal model ginseng decreased the risk of cancer in animals given various carcinogens. None of these data are particularly compelling and a proposed mechanism for the preventive activity of ginseng remains unclear. Duda and colleagues did suggest an interaction with the estrogen receptor, and thus ginseng may serve as an antiestrogen in estrogen-receptor-positive breast cancer.[29] This proposed effect in breast cancer does not explain a more general inhibition of carcinogenesis advertised in the lay literature. Any general anticancer activity may result from natural killer cell generation, although the data is very preliminary.[30]

Benzaldehyde is a volatile oil found in large amounts in almond oil. It is also a component of laetrile. Benzaldehyde has been shown to have static activity against several tumor cell lines. In addition, a benzaldehyde component was investigated in over 90 patients with advanced cancer, of which 57 were evaluable. Approximately 50 percent of patients had either a complete or partial response. The majority of these patients had only a partial response, which may be reasonably discounted because these were uncontrolled studies with poor demonstration of partial responses. What was interesting was that ten patients were reported to have achieved a complete remission. This is an amazing complete response rate in these uniformly fatal tumors and must be viewed with significant skepticism.[31] Other studies have not confirmed these overly optimistic results.[32] Further work is needed to assess the activity of these natural compounds and a potential mechanism needs to be proposed.

Berbamine and Berberine are chemicals isolated from goldenseal, Oregon grape root, and barberry root, which may have activity in the prevention and treatment of various cancers. In cell culture these agents are able to antagonize the effect of several promotional agents and thus potentially prevent carcinogenesis. In cell culture, berberine had activity against malignant brain tumors equivalent to carmustine (BCNU) and may be able to potentiate BCNU activity. In rats with brain tumors BCNU and berberine combinations had activity superior to either alone.[33] Given the poor prognosis of patients with brain cancer, this combination may have future application in CNS tumors. Its proposed mechanism is to stimulate macrophage activity leading to increased cytostatic effect on tumor cells. A concern is the severe toxicity associated with other agents that stimulate macrophage function, which was discussed earlier. Generally, agents that work via a cytokine mechanism have had limited clinical utility because of toxicity syndromes.

Bromelain is a proteolytic enzyme complex isolated from the stem of pineapple. It has been shown to inhibit metastases of lung cancer in mice. In addition, bromelain has been reported to cause differentiation of various leukemias in cell culture. It has also been reported to cause regression of tumor when used alone and combined with standard chemotherapeutics.[34]

Coumarin is a component of several medicinal plants including sweet clover and red clover. Laboratory data suggests that coumarin has direct effects on tumor cells as well as a monocyte/macrophage stimulatory effect. A reputable report in 45 patients with metastatic renal cell carcinoma, a tumor with poor treatment options, supported coumarin activity. There was an objective tumor response rate (50 percent or greater reduction in tumor size) of 33 percent and surprisingly three patients had a complete response. There were no significant toxicities from coumarin.[35]

Cloud fungus is a source of protein-bound polysaccharide that survives oral administration and is approved as a drug in Japan. This herbal remedy works via an immunostimulatory mechanism. Patients receiving curative resection of colorectal cancer were randomized to protein-bound polysaccharide or placebo. Patients who received protein-bound polysaccharide had a significant reduction in cancer recurrence.[36]

CONCLUSION

A long history of using herbal remedies can be found in the prevention and treatment of cancer. Sufficient data has shown the value of antioxidants in the prevention of cancer, and herbs that work via this mechanism may have chemopreventive value. Currently, no data support the use of herbal remedies in the treatment of cancer. It is important to encourage patients with cancer who are using herbal products, to discuss their use of herbs with their oncologists. As a general recommendation, patients using antioxidant herbs may be counseled to increase their consumption of cruciferous vegetables, garlic, and onion rather than more expensive herbal products. See Table 13.1 for a summary of this chapter's material.

TABLE 13.1. Summary

Shark cartilage	Antiangiogenic effect; doubtful oral bioavailability of biologically active components.
Aloe vera	Acemannan may stimulate macrophage function stimulating release of TNF-alpha and interferon, which have antitumor activity; may have deleterious effects in patients with AIDS.
Echinacea	Proposed to have immunostimulatory activity; unknown if effective orally.
Mistletoe	Potent inducer of cytokines stimulating release of TNF-alpha and interleukin-1; iscador IV increased natural killer cells in patients with breast cancer.
Antioxidant vitamins	Vitamins A and E may reduce risk of lung cancer by reducing formation of free radicals.
Allium	Garlic and onion, containing diallyl disulfides inhibit H-Ras transformed tumors; may decrease nitrosamine formation in GIT.
Green tea	Catechins have antioxidant properties and inhibit nucleoside transport; may inhibit protein kinase C; contradictory epidemiologic studies regarding efficacy in cancer.
Chaparral	Nordihydroguaiaretic has antioxidant properties; hepatotoxic; unproven and dangerous.
Ginseng	Antiestrogen properties may be of benefit in breast cancer; preliminary data suggest natural killer cell generation; much more data needed.
Laetrile	Benzaldehyde may have tumor static activity.
Goldenseal, Oregon grape root, barberry root	Berbamine/berberine may prevent carcinogenesis; may potentiate carmustine activity; use may be limited by toxicity.
Pineapple	Bromelain may cause tumor regression; more study needed.
Sweet and red clover	Coumarin stimulates macrophage activity.
Cloud fungus	Japanese herbal remedy with immunostimulatory activity may reduce cancer recurrence.

CASE STUDY

JJ is a 21-year-old Asian American female who is three months s/p renal transplant and presents to her nephrologist with decreased urine output.

Physical Exam: Unremarkable

Laboratory

140	105	2.1/60	CBC: WNL
5.2	24	110	

Past Medical History

Patient was found to be in chronic renal failure on routine physical examination two years prior to the current admission. Despite restricting protein intake the patient went onto hemodialysis over the course of the following six months. Patient was maintained on twice-weekly hemodialysis for the next fifteen months without complications. Patient underwent living related transplant which was uneventful except for a slight rejection episode six weeks after transplant, which responded to pulse steroid therapy. Patient was stable until the current major rejection episode.

Medications

Neoral 5 mg/kg/day (level on admission 250 ng/ml —monoclonal TDx)
Prednisone 20 mg/day (taper)
Azathioprine 25 mg/day

Clinical Course

Over the course of the next week the patient became aniuric, requiring reinstitution of hemodialysis. History taken by the physician was unremarkable. The patient and mother were considered good historians and both indicated that the patient never missed her immunosuppressive doses. Compliance was supported by a therapeutic cyclosporine level. During morning rounds the patient was drinking a pungent tea; when asked the patient gave a history of consuming the herbal remedy over the last three weeks because her mother was told by her pharmacist in Chinatown that it would protect her daughter from infection. The patient was told to stop the tea and was placed on three days of high-dose steroids followed by a taper. Over the next several months the patients kidneys returned to baseline.

Evaluation

While a cause and effect cannot be proven, since many of the Chinese herbal products that protect against infections stimulate the immune system, the herbal tea may have initiated this atypical severe rejection episode. This was a well-matched living related kidney with a very low risk of acute graft loss. Stimulating cell mediated immunity increases alloreactivity and may explain this unusual event. Once the rejection episode occurred the tea was stopped and standard immunosuppressive rescue protocols instituted.

REFERENCES

1. Downer SM, Cody MM, McCluskey P, Wilson PD, Arnott SJ, Lister TA, Slevin ML. Pursuit and practice of complementary therapies by cancer patients receiving conventional treatment. *B Med J* 1994;309:86-89.

2. Parker SL, Tong T, Bolden S, Wingo PA. Cancer statistics, 1997. *CA Cancer J Clin* 1997;47:5-27.

3. Eisenberg DM, Kessler RC, Foster C, Norlock FE, Calkins DR, Delbanco TL. Unconventional medicine in the United States. *N Engl J Med* 1993;328:246-252.

4. Kohlmeirer L, Mendez M. Controversies surrounding diet and breast cancer. *Proc Nutr Soc* 1997;56:369-382.

5. Kaaks R, Riboli E. The role of multi-center cohort studies in studying the relation between diet and cancer. *Cancer Lett* 1997;114:263-270.

6. Hunter DJ, Spiegelman D, Adami HO, Beeson L, van den Brandt PA, Folsom AR, et al. Cohort studies of fat intake and the risk of breast cancer—a pooled analysis. *N Engl J Med* 1996;334:356-361.

7. Prentice RL. Measurement error and results from analytic epidemiology: Dietary fat and breast cancer. *J Natl Cancer Inst* 1996;88:1738-1747.

8. Wu AH, Ziegler RG, Horn-Ross PL, Normura AM, West DW, Kolonel LN, et al. Tofu and risk of breast cancer in Asian Americans. *Cancer Epidemiol Biomarkers Prev* 1996;901-906.

9. West S, Hildesheim A, Dosemeci, M. Non-viral risk factors for nasopharyngeal carcinoma in the Philippines: Results from a case-control study. *Int J Cancer* 1993;55(5):722-727.

10. Lee A, Langer R. Shark cartilage contains inhibitors of tumor angiogenesis. *Science* 1983;221:1185-1187.

11. McGuire TR, Kazakoff PW, Hoie EB, Fienhold MA. Antiproliferative activity of shark cartilage with and without TNF-alpha in human umbilical vein endothelium. *Pharmacotherapy* 1996;237-244.

12. Zhang L, Tizard IR. Activation of a mouse macrophage cell line by acemannan: The major carbohydrate fraction from aloe vera gel. *Immunopharmacology* 1996;35:119-128.

13. Sheets MA, Unger BA, Giggleman GF, Tizard IR. Studies of the effect of acemannan on retrovirus infections and clinical stabilization of feline leukemia virus infected cats. *Mol Biother* 1991;3:41-45.

14. Piasecki E, Ledwon TK, Inglot AD, Knysz B, Simon K, Inglot M, et al. Interferon and TNF responses of HIV positive patients as markers for monitoring of the AIDS progression. *Arch Immunol Ther Exp Warz* 1994;42:439-445.

15. Montaner JS, Gill J, Singer J, Raboud J, Arseneau R, McLean BD, Schechter MT, et al. Double-blind placebo-controlled pilot trial of acemannan in advanced human immunodeficiency virus disease. *J Acquir Immune Defic Syndr Hum Retrovirol* 1996;12:153-157.

16. Kahlon JB, Kemp MC, Yawei N, Carpenter RH, Shannon WM, McAnalley BH. In vitro evaluation of the synergistic antiviral effects of acemannan in combination with AZT and acyclovir. *Mol Biother* 1991;3:214-216.

17. Womble D, Helderman JH. The impact of acemannan on the generation and function of cytotoxic T-lymphocytes. *Immunopharmacol Immunotoxicol* 1992;14:63-77.

18. Stimpel M, Proksch A, Wagner H, Lohmann-Matthes ML. Macrophage activation and induction of macrophage cytotoxicity by purified polysaccharide fraction from the plant *Echinacea purpurea*. *Infect Immun* 1984;46:845-849.

19. Steinmuller C, Roesler J, Grottrup E, Franke G, Wagner H, Lohmann-Matthes ML. Polysaccharides isolated from plant cell cultures of *Echinacea purpurea* enhances the resistance of immunosuppressed mice against systemic infections. *Int J Immunopharmacol* 1993; 15:605-614.

20. See DM, Broumand N, Sahl L, Tilles JG. In vitro effects of echinacea and ginseng on natural killer cell and antibody dependent cell cytotoxicity in healthy subjects and chronic fatigue syndrome or AIDS patients. *Immunopharmacology* 1997;35:229-235.

21. Kuttan G, Kuttan R. Immunological mechanisms of action of the tumor reducing peptide from mistletoe extract (NSC 635089) cellular proliferation. *Cancer Lett* 1992;66:123-130.

22. Hajto T, Lanzrein C. Natural killer and antibody-dependent cell-mediated cytotoxicity activities and large granular lymphocyte frequencies in *Viscum album* treated breast cancer patients. *Oncology* 1986;43:93-97.

23. Greenwald P, Cullen JW, Kelloff G, Pierson HF. Chemoprevention of lung cancer: Problems and progress. *Chest* 1988;96:14S-17S.

24. Zheng W, Blot WJ, Shu XO, Gao YT, Ji BT, Ziegler RG, Fraumeni JF Jr. Diet and other risk factors for laryngeal cancer in Shanghai, China. *Am J Epidemiol* 1992;136:178-191.

25. Zhen Y, Cao S, Xue Y, Wu S. Green tea extract inhibits nucleoside transport and potentiates the antitumor effect of antimetabolites. *Chin Med Sci J* 1991;6:1-5.

26. Blot WJ, Chow WH, McLaughlin JK. Tea and cancer: A review of the epidemiological evidence. *Eur J Cancer Prev* 1996;5:425-438.

27. Sheikh NM, Philen RM, Love LA. Chaparral associated hepatotoxicity. *Arch Intern Med* 1997;157:913-919.

28. Sheng H, Shao J, Kirkland SC, Isakson P, Coffey RJ, Morrow J, et al. Inhibition of human colon cancer cell growth by selective inhibition of cyclooxygenase-2. *J Clin Invest* 1997;99:2254-2259.

29. Duda RB, Taback B, Kessel B, Dooley DD, Yang H, Marchiori J, et al. pS2 expression induced by American ginseng in MCF-7 breast cancer cells. *Ann Surg Oncol* 1996;3:515-520.

30. Yun YS, Lee YS, Jo SK, Jung IS. Inhibition of autochthonous tumor by ethanol insoluble fraction from *Panax ginseng* as an immunomodulator. *Planta Med* 1993; 59:521-524.

31. Kochi M, Takeuchi S, Mizutani T, Mochizuki K, Matsumoto Y, Saito Y. Antitumor activity of benzaldehyde. *Cancer Treat Rep* 1980;64:21-23.

32. Tanum G, Tveit KM, Host H, Pettersen EO. Benzylidene-glucose: No effect after all? *Am J Clin Oncol* 1990;13:161-163.

33. Zhang RX, Dougherty DV, Rosenblum ML. Laboratory studies of berberine used alone and in combination with BCNU to treat malignant brain tumors. *Chin Med J Engl* 1990;103:658-665.

34. Barkin S, Taussig SJ, Szekerezes J. Antimetastatic effect of bromelain with or without its proteolytic and anticoagulant activity. *J Can Res Clin Oncol* 1988; 114:507-508.

35. Marshall ME, Mendelsohn L, Butler K, Riley L, Cantrell J, Wiseman C, et al. Treatment of metastatic-renal cell carcinoma with coumarin and cimetidine: A pilot study. *J Clin Oncol* 1987;5:862-866.

36. Torisu M, Hayashi Y, Ishimitsu T, Fujimura T, Iwasaki K, Katano M, et al. Significant prolongation of disease free period gained by oral polysaccharide administration after curative surgical operations of colorectal cancer. *Cancer Immunol Immunother* 1990;31:261-268.

Chapter 14

Herbal Medicinals
for Dermatologic Uses

Stephen Gillespie, PhD

INTRODUCTION

Inclusion of herbal drugs in this chapter is primarily based upon endorsed uses by European drug regulatory agencies such as the German Commission E or upon published clinical trials. Other herbs with traditional reputations but without official endorsements are included to more fully inform the reader of the repertoire of claims.

Skin, the largest organ of the body, is a complex organ that functions primarily as a protective barrier between the body and the environment. It is composed of three regions, epidermis, dermis, and hypodermis, with a number of interdependent cell types and appendages (hair follicles, sebaceous glands, and sweat glands). The homeostasis between skin cells may be affected by external physical (temperature, humidity), chemical (detergents, solvents), and radiation (sunlight) conditions, by xenobiotics such as drugs, and by internal disorders such as lupus erythematosus. Skin manifestations of these factors result in diverse pigmentation, benign and malignant, acute and chronic inflammatory, and infectious disorders.

The epidermis is composed of stratified epithelial cells in five layers. The innermost layer, the stratum germinativum, consists of keratinocytes, which divide and move upward. Above the basal layer is the stratum spinosum, which contains prickle cells, keratinocytes, Langerhans cells, melanocytes, and melanin granules. The outermost layer, the stratum corneum, is the body's primary barrier to the environment, and is composed of keratinized tissue that is constantly desquamated. The dermis lies below the epidermis and consists of collagen and elastin in a mucopolysaccharide matrix, nerves, capillaries, hair follicles, sebaceous glands, sweat glands, fibroblasts, and mast cells. The hypodermis, or subcutaneous tissue, lies below the dermis and is composed of loose connective tissue and adipose tissue, providing pliability, thermal control, and cushioning.

Inflammatory Dermatoses

Inflammatory dermatoses may be acute (days to weeks) or chronic (months to years). Acute lesions may include erythema, pruritis, and edema. Chronic lesions often show altered epidermal growth, atrophy, or hyperplasia.

ATOPIC DERMATITIS

Atopic dermatitis, or eczema, is a type of eczematous dermatitis occurring primarily in children and young adults. Etiology is unknown, but a family history of eczema, hay fever, or asthma is a predisposing factor. It may be exacerbated by irritants, allergens, or temperature and humidity extremes. Most patients report deterioration of their condition in fall and winter. The evidence for food reactivity in atopic dermatitis is conflicting. Pruritis is the primary symptom. Erythematous plaques are seen on the face and in flexural areas. The moisture content of the stratum corneum is lower than normal skin.[1,2]

Management of eczema is empirical. Treatment of inflammatory dermatoses involves first removing potential irritants and allergens from the environment. Frequent bathing is discouraged, as it promotes dry skin. Acute weeping or oozing lesions should be dried; wet compresses and colloidal oatmeal baths may be used. Topical corticosteroids in an oil-in-water base may be applied. Chronic, dry lesions should be treated by hydrating the skin. Bath oils, emollients applied to damp skin, and water-in-oil ointments with or without topical corticosteroids may be used.[3]

A recent survey in Norway revealed that 51 percent of 444 patients with atopic dermatitis and 42 percent of 506 patients with psoriasis used one or more alternative medical treatments, primarily homeopathy, dietary intervention, and herbal remedies. The atopic patients commonly cited lack of effective treatment by physicians as a motivating factor.[4] Clinicians should remain aware of patients' behavior and monitor efforts to document the effects of alternative therapies.

Many herbal treatments are recommended for treatment of atopic dermatitis. Although many recent articles have appeared about the use of traditional Chinese medicine in eczema, the remedies are complex mixtures that are not standardized.[5,6] This chapter will therefore primarily be concerned with herbal monopreparations.

Herbal treatment of atopic dermatitis involves use of astringent solutions to dry acute weeping lesions, topical application of anti-inflammatory herbal preparations, or internal use of a fixed oil containing a high percentage of γ-linolenic acid.

CASE STUDY 1: MOIST COMPRESSES

Patient History

A three-year-old female presents in January with dry skin accompanied by prurigo, lichenification, and eczematous lesions, characterized by erythema and edema but few exudative lesions. Lesions are seen on the face and back of the neck and on flexural areas inside the elbows and behind the knees. The most marked areas of involvement are in flexural areas. Severe pruritis is present and the patient exhibits intense scratching. The patient is restless and anxious. The patient lives in a high altitude, semiarid region. The patient's father has asthma and multiple food allergies. The parents wish to treat her condition with natural medicines.

Clinical Considerations

The patient's history is consistent with atopic dermatitis. Conservative, prophylactic measures to be suggested include use of humidifiers and avoidance of excessively warm room temperatures. Removal of irritants from the patient's environment, such as tobacco smoke, harsh soaps, and wool clothing, may be suggested. Chronic physical trauma caused by ill-fitting clothing should be eliminated. Removal of potential sources of allergens such as pets and house plants may also be suggested.

Herbal therapy should initially be directed at drying any exudative lesions. The use of loosely fixed moist compresses can be recommended. The compresses are applied three to four times daily for one to two hours. Compresses should be changed every ten to 20 minutes, as soon as they become warm and dry.[7] Following are several herbal drugs that have been used with these compresses.

Oak Bark

The dried inner bark of *Quercus alba* L. (Fagaceae), the white oak, was an official drug in the *United States Pharmacopoeia* (USP) from 1820 to 1916, and in the *National Formulary* (NF) from 1916 to 1936. It was used as an astringent. In Europe the barks of *Q. robur* L., the British or common oak, and of *Q. petraea* (Matt.) Leibl, the sessile or winter oak, are sources of cortex (bark). The bark is from younger branches and twigs.[8]

Oak bark contains 8 to 20 percent condensed tannins: catechins, oligomeric proanthocyanidins, and some ellagitannins.[8] Tannins have astringent properties; they cause the precipitation of proteins, rendering them resistant to proteolysis. The precipitated proteins form a protective coat, beneath which new tissue regeneration may take place. Moist tannin-containing compresses cool the skin and cause vasoconstriction. Percutaneous penetrability of tannins is low.[3,9] Oak bark tannins are said to be well tolerated by the skin, causing no irritation, and are recommended by Weiss, German physician and author of a well-known text of medical herbalism, as the foremost drug for weeping eczema.[7]

For external use a decoction is prepared from one to two tablespoons of the chopped bark or from two teaspoons (6 g) of the coarsely powdered bark boiled for 15 minutes in 500 ml water. The liquid is then strained, cooled, and used undiluted.[7,10]

Commission E considers oak bark an astringent and virostatic agent useful for external use in inflammatory skin conditions, for internal use in nonspecific, acute cases of diarrhea, and as a gargle for mild inflammation of the gums and mucous membranes. External use or baths for exudative lesions covering large areas is contraindicated. For external use and as a gargle recommended duration of use is not longer than two to three weeks. No known side effects are reported. For storage, protection from light and moisture is recommended. The amount of extractable tannins decreases with time.[11]

Walnut Leaf

The dried leaves of the English walnut, *Juglans regia* L. (Juglandaceae) are also used as an astringent based on their content of about 10 percent ellagitannins.[12] Commission E considers aqueous extracts of walnut leaves an astringent for inflammation of the skin. A decoction is prepared from 5 g (5 teaspoons) of the chopped drug in 200 ml water.[13]

Witch Hazel Leaves

The dried leaves of *Hamamelis virginiana* L. (Hamamelidaceae) were an official drug in the USP from 1882 to 1916, and in the NF from 1916 to 1955. The drug was used as an astringent. Witch hazel leaves contain 3 to 10 percent tannins, a mixture of gallotannins, condensed catechins, and proanthocyanidins.[14]

Distilled witch hazel extract was official in the USP from 1905 to 1926, and in the NF from 1888 to 1905 and from 1926 to present. It is considered a safe and effective astringent by the FDA. It is prepared by steam distillation of twigs followed by addition of alcohol to give a 14 to 15 percent solution. Only a trace amount of volatile oil is extracted, as tannins are not extracted by this distillation. Any astringent action is due to the alcohol content. This is the only common commercially available product in the United States.

Like oak bark and walnut leaves, a tannin-containing aqueous extract of witch hazel leaves is a useful initial treatment for weeping eczema and is used similarly. Commission E considers aqueous extracts of witch hazel leaves an astringent for inflammation of the skin and mucous membranes. A decoction for external use and as a gargle is prepared from 5 to 10 g of the chopped drug in 250 ml water. No contraindications or side effects are noted. Storage considerations are the same as for oak bark.[15] When used internally for diarrhea, witch hazel preparations are reported to cause occasional stomach upset in susceptible individuals, and liver damage due to witch hazel tannins in rare cases.[14]

Mallow

Weiss recommends moist compresses of mallow as an alternative to oak bark for treatment of weeping eczema.[7] The dried leaves or flowers of *Malva sylvestris* L. (Malvaceae), common mallow, or of *M. neglecta* Wallr., dwarf mallow, may be used. Therapeutic activity is due to 8 to 10 percent mucilage that yields arabinose, glucose, rhamnose, galactose, and galacturonic acid upon hydrolysis.[16] A 10 percent decoction can be used in the same manner as the tannin-containing herbs above. Commission E considers mallow a demulcent for irritation of the mucous membranes of the mouth and throat. No contraindications or side effects are noted.[17]

Wild Pansy

The aerial parts of *Viola tricolor* L. (Violaceae) are used in Europe to treat acute and chronic eczema. The drug contains about 10 percent mucilage yielding glucose, galactose, arabinose, and rhamnose upon hydrolysis, and numerous other phytochemicals including flavonoids, carotenoids, and small amounts of saponins.[18] Commission E recommends infusions or decoctions of wild pansy for external treatment of seborrheic dermatitis (seborrhea) and seborrhea of the scalp of nursing infants.[19] The galenical preparation is made from 1.5 g (1 teaspoon) finely chopped drug and 150 ml water. Along with the compresses, the tea can also be consumed orally three times daily.[7,18]

CASE STUDY 2: TOPICAL PREPARATIONS

Patient History

A 13-year-old male presents in October with pruritis, lichenification, prurigo, scratch marks, and crusting. The skin is dry; lesions are on the face, neck, and flexural areas. The patient has a history of hay fever. What herbal remedies might he try?

Clinical Considerations

The location and type of lesions, time of year, and hay fever are consistent with adolescent phase atopic dermatitis. The time of year may also reflect the emotional stress of school, which may have a negative effect on the condition at puberty.

The conservative measures recommended in Case Study 1 should be instituted first. Since no exudative lesions are present, topical therapy should include skin hydration and control of itching. Topical hydrocortisone and other corticosteroids may help to control pruritis in lichenified plaques; these plaques may take many months to resolve. Herbal therapy of chronic or dry lesions involves topical use of anti-inflammatory products. Several alternatives to topical OTC and prescription corticosteroids may be tried. Following are herbs used for this purpose.

Chamomile

Preparations of the dried flowers of the chamomiles are used in Europe to treat a variety of inflammatory conditions of the skin and mucosa.[20-22] The term chamomile is used for two distinct plants: *Matricaria recutita* L. (Asteraceae) is known as German or Hungarian chamomile, or matricaria, and *Chamaemelum nobile* L. (Asteraceae) is known as Roman or English chamomile. The constituents of the two plants are not identical but both are used similarly.[20-22]

Terpenoid (α-bisabolol, matricin, chamazulene) and flavonoid (apigenin, luteolin) constituents of German chamomile have anti-inflammatory actions.[23-25] The in vivo skin penetration of α-bisabolol in mice and of apigenin and luteolin in humans has been demonstrated.[26,27] Creams containing matricaria extract have demonstrated beneficial effects in the treatment of eczema.[28] Infusions contain only 10 to 15 percent of the terpenoid-containing volatile oil, but do contain the flavonoids.[20,29] The use of products prepared from standardized hydroalcoholic extracts is more effective.[30] A German product,

Kamillosan, containing 400 mg of a solid extract, is standardized to a minimum content of 7 mg α-bisabolol and 0.4 mg chamazulene per 100 g ointment.[22]

Commission E recommends 3 to 10 percent infusions of chamomile for use in external compresses and rinses prepared by covering the container and allowing to stand for ten minutes. As a bath additive, an infusion prepared from 50 g drug in 10 L water is used; 1 tablespoon ≅ 2.5 g. No side effects are noted, but patients are warned not to use the infusion near the eyes.[31] Chamomile hypersensitivity is rare.

For nonexudative lesions, semisolid external formulations (creams and ointments) of chamomile are probably the most desirable dosage forms, as their application two to three times daily is less troublesome than preparation and application of compresses. Bathing using a bath additive can be recommended. Commercial, standardized semisolid formulations are not generally available in the United States at this time.

Yarrow

The dried aerial parts of *Achillea millefolium* L. (Asteraceae) are used similarly to chamomile. Like chamomile, yarrow contains the anti-inflammatory constituents, including chamazulene. The drug is used externally for its antipruritic activity in skin inflammations.[32-34] Compresses can be prepared from infusions prepared from 2 g of the drug (1 teaspoon ≅ 1.5 g) and 150 ml boiling water or from equivalent doses of hydroalcoholic extracts. A bath additive may be prepared from 100 g yarrow to 20 L water. Commercial semisolid preparations for external use are available in Europe. Hypersensitivity to yarrow and other Asteraceae is contraindicated.[32]

Licorice Root

Licorice consists of the dried roots and rhizome of *Glycyrrhiza glabra* L. (Fabaceae). It is one of the most popular herbs in Chinese medicine, with many traditional uses including treatment of inflammatory skin conditions.[35] Licorice is widely used in Europe to heal peptic ulcers.[36] The most important constituent of licorice root is glycyrrhizin, a triterpenoid saponin glycoside with expectorant and anti-inflammatory activities.[37] Glycyrrhetic acid (GA), the aglycone of glycyrrhizin, has also been shown to be a potent inhibitor of 11βb-hydroxysteroid dehydrogenase (11β-OHSD), thus potentiating the action of cortisol by inhibition of its metabolic inactivation to cortisone.[38]

Evans reported that topical application of ointments containing active isomers of GA has anti-inflammatory action in a variety of subacute and chronic dermatoses, with no rebound phenomenon noted. In a comparison trial of GA ointment and hydrocortisone that was not blinded, randomized, or placebo-controlled, Evans stated that hydrocortisone was superior in acute and infantile eczemas, while GA ointment was superior in chronic conditions characterized by inflammation and pruritis. The concentrations of the hydrocortisone preparations were not reported. In a second uncontrolled trial of GA ointment very good results were reported in treatment of contact dermatitis, eczema of the extremities, seborrheic eczema, and psoriasis. GA ointment was not reported to cause sensitization.[39]

Teelucksingh and colleagues studied the possibility of enhancing the local glucocorticoid activity of hydrocortisone by inhibiting 11β-OHSD with GA.[40] The enzyme was demonstrated to be present in human epidermis from biopsies of normal volunteers and from patients with eczema and psoriasis. Using the Stoughton-McKenzie bioassay of glucocorticoid anti-inflammatory activity,[41] the in vivo response of normal skin to hydocortisone acetate, beclomethasone dipropionate, GA (20 mg/ml), and a mixture of GA (20 mg/ml) and hydrocortisone acetate in 95 percent ethanol was measured. Beclomethasone caused the greatest response. GA and ethanol alone had no effect. Hydrocortisone showed weak activity, but the addition of 2 percent GA greatly increased its activity, to about half the activity of beclomethasone at the highest concentrations (10 mg/ml and 10 µg/ml, respectively). Patients with eczema or psoriasis were not studied.[40]

As with chamomile, licorice root, or GA ointments are probably the most desirable dosage form, but are not generally available in the United States. Compresses could be prepared from infusions or decoctions prepared from 1 teaspoon of the finely chopped drug and 150 ml water; 1 teaspoon ≅ 3 g.

Fenugreek

The seeds of fenugreek, *Trigonella foenum-graecum* L. (Fabaceae), is endorsed by Commission E for external use as an emollient to treat local inflammations and eczema. Several anti-inflammatory steroidal saponins are present in the seeds, as well as a high content of mucilage. A paste for use with compresses is prepared by stirring 50 g of the powdered drug in 250 ml boiling water for five minutes. Warm compresses are applied several times daily. Repeated external use may cause undesirable skin reactions, according to Commission E.[42]

Gamma-Linolenic Acid

Recent studies have shown that adults and children with atopic dermatitis have elevated plasma phospholipid levels of *cis*-linoleic acid (LA), the main dietary essential fatty acid, and lower levels of its metabolites γ-linolenic acid (GLA), dihomo-γ-linolenic acid (DGLA), and arachidonic acid (AA).[43,44] A defect in the function of δ-6-desaturase (D6D), the enzyme that catalyzes the conversion of LA to GLA, has been postulated as a major factor in the development of atopic dermatitis.[44] This defect leads to decreased production of prostaglandins E1 (PGE 1), a metabolite of DGLA, and of E2 (PGE 2), a metabolite of AA, and the subsequent alterations in cell-mediated and humoral immunity and increased disposition to inflammation in atopic skin.[45] Oral administration of GLA is proposed to increase levels of D6D metabolites of LA by bypassing the D6D defect and may therefore improve the clinical symptoms of atopic dermatitis.

$$D6D \qquad\qquad \rightarrow AA \rightarrow PGE\ 2 \rightarrow PGE\ 1$$
$$LA \rightarrow GLA \rightarrow DGLA$$

Products containing GLA-rich seed oils are available in the United States Evening primrose oil (EPO) is obtained from the seed of *Oenothera biennis* L. (Onagraceae), a plant native to North America. The fixed oil is composed of about 70 percent LA and about 9 percent GLA. The seed of *Ribes nigrum* L. (Grossulariaceae), the European black currant, yields a fixed oil with 14 to 19 percent GLA. Borage seed oil, containing 20 to 26 percent GLA, is obtained from the seed of *Borago officinalis* L. (Boraginaceae). There is concern that borage seed oil may contain low levels of hepatotoxic unsaturated pyrrolizidine alkaloids.[46]

A number of studies have been published concerning the clinical utility of GLA supplementation in atopic dermatitis and other dermatoses, but interpretation of the results remains controversial. Results from a meta-analysis of nine controlled trials in eight centers of Epogam (Searle, U.K.) in the treatment of atopic eczema showed improvements almost always significantly better than those of placebo. Three hundred eleven patients, ages 1 to 60 years, took part in the trials. Both physician and patient scores in the four parallel studies showed Epogam significantly better than placebo. Similar results were obtained from the five crossover trials, but the doctor scores did not reach significance. There was no effect of placebo on pruritus, but a highly significant response to Epogam. Improvements in clinical condition were positively correlated to rises in DGLA and AA levels.[47]

The meta-analysis has been criticized on the basis of study design.[45] The nine trials had differences in dose of EPO (from 2 to 12 500 mg Epogam capsules/day), treatment periods (from 4 to 12 weeks), and evaluation criteria. Onset of activity and the dose-response relationship for EPO were not established.

Results of newer trials are mixed. In a controlled study of 51 children with a mean age of 4.2 years, high dose EPO (0.5 g/kg/day; 15 capsules of Epogam for a 15 kg child) significantly improved overall severity of atopic dermatitis compared to placebo.[48] A controlled study of 39 patients with chronic hand dermatitis, ages 19 to 75 years, given 12 capsules of Epogam daily for 16 weeks, failed to find a statistical difference between treated and placebo groups.[49] Additional trials are being conducted and planned. Based on the concept of defect in D6D and generally positive results so far, some investigators believe GLA supplementation is worth considering as a treatment of first choice, before the use of steroids.[50]

No adverse effects of EPO have been reported. Chronic toxicity and carcinogenicity studies of EPO in rats, mice, and dogs revealed no important adverse effects or tumor differences.[51,52]

Treatment of patients with acute or chronic atopic eczema with EPO appears to hold promise, although there is not yet consensus. Patients with childhood eczema may benefit the most, primarily due to the ability of EPO to relieve pruritis and the possibility of reducing or minimizing the use of steroids. A minimum four-week trial should be made.

PSORIASIS

Psoriasis is a disorder of epidermal cell kinetics. It is a common chronic inflammatory dermatosis characterized by a relapsing nature and variable clinical features. It affects 1 to 2 percent of people in the United States, exhibits onset at any age with a peak incidence in the third decade of life, is equally common in males and females, and shows a genetic predisposition, with one-third of patients reporting some relative with the disease. Psoriasis is frequently localized to the elbows, knees, lumbosacral area, intergluteal cleft, and the scalp. Typical lesions of psoriasis vulgaris, the most common form, are well-demarcated pink plaques covered by loosely adherent silvery-white scales; small blood droplets rapidly appear after removal of scales (Auspitz sign). The scaly lesions may persist for months to years. Other forms of psoriasis, such as psoriatic erythroderma, may be more generalized in distribution, and can cause total-body erythema and scaling. Pruritis is a significant symptom. Pain is a complaint when the palms, soles, and intertriginous areas are involved. There is an increased incidence of arthritis and myopathy associated with the disease. Psoriasis may be provoked by physical trauma (Koebner's phenomenon) such as abrasions, adhesive tape, pressure, shaving, and vaccinations. Infection, stress, and certain drugs (antimalarials, lithium, beta-adrenergic blockers, and abrupt withdrawal of systemic and possibly of topical corticosteroids) may trigger manifestations of psoriasis. The cause of psoriasis is unknown.[3,53]

Treatment of psoriasis is empirical. Prescription drug treatment for psoriasis includes topical anthralin and high-potency corticosteroids, systemic psoralens plus UVA phototherapy, and systemic corticosteroids, methotrexate, etretinate, and cyclosporine. The FDA recommends that only mild cases of psoriasis be self-treated and lists only coal tar preparations, salicylic acid, and topical hydrocortisone as Category I OTC products.[3]

A recent survey in North Carolina of 317 psoriasis patients reports 51 percent of respondents used one or more alternative treatments including dietary intervention, herbal remedies, and vitamin therapies. Twenty-one percent of males and 25 percent of females reported past or present use of herbal remedies. Use of these treatment modalities was associated with greater psoriasis severity but not with greater intensity of conventional medical treatment. The authors suggest that the subpopulation that uses alternative medicine may be less inclined to use intensive conventional medical treatment, or, alternatively, that patients requiring intensive conventional medical treatment may have previously used alternative treatments and found them relatively ineffective.[54]

A variety of herbal medicines have been used to treat psoriasis. Several are also used for atopic dermatitis and were discussed above. Reports concerning traditional Chinese medicine and a Hungarian mixture of several plant extracts known as oleum horwathiensis[55] exist in the literature, but for reasons cited above will not be discussed. Weiss mentions saponin drugs for treatment of psoriasis.[7] Licorice root is such a drug and can be used externally as for eczema, either alone or as a potentiator of topical hydrocortisone. Preparations of chamomile for external use may also be used for anti-inflammatory actions.

CASE STUDY 3: MILD PSORIASIS

Patient History

A 34-year-old female presents with a complaint of dry, scaly red patches on her elbows and knees. She states that the condition began appearing sporadically in her twenties and has become worse since she separated from her husband. She has received some relief from topical OTC hydrocortisone but says that lesions reappear when the medication is discontinued. What herbal medicinals might she try?

Clinical Considerations

The location and type of the patient's lesions and the patient's age and the relationship of the disease to stress are consistent with psoriasis vulgaris. Gentle rubbing removes the scales from the symmetrical plaques, subsequently revealing the Auspitz sign. The localized lesions are not extensive. A trial of herbal therapy does not appear to be unwarranted in this mild case. External licorice root may be tried, as rebound effects have not been noted.[39] Using a chamomile bath additive may also be tried.

Very little information about treatment of psoriasis with EPO has appeared in the scientific literature. A trial of 37 patients with chronic, stable psoriasis given 12 capsules daily containing a combination of 430 mg EPO and 107 mg fish oil found no significant difference between treated and control groups, however.[56] Dietary supplementation with fish oils containing large amounts of essential fatty acids is reported to have some limited utility in the treatment of psoriasis. Doses of both the fish oil and EPO were smaller than used in previous trials of fish oil alone for psoriasis or of EPO alone for eczema.

Capsaicin

Capsaicin is the pungent principle in the fruit of various species of *Capsicum* (Solanaceae). It causes depletion of substance P from sensory nerve terminals. Substance P, a peptide transmitter, is involved in pain transmission, in cutaneous vasodilation, and in the inflammatory process. Based on the concept that substance P is implicated in the pathophysiology of psoriasis, capsaicin has been investigated to treat psoriasis. Topical capsaicin cream has shown some utility in the treatment of psoriasis.[57,58]

In a study of 44 patients with moderate to severe psoriasis vulgaris (at least 10 percent body surface involvement), 22 were treated with 0.01 percent capsaicin cream and 22 were treated with 0.025 percent capsaicin on one side of the body. Both groups applied vehicle to the other side of the body. Creams were applied four times daily for six weeks. Highly significant greater reduction in scaling and erythema was observed on treated sides than on vehicle-treated sides. Effectiveness of the two concentrations was nearly identical. Eighteen patients experienced burning, stinging, and itching of the skin on the treated side. Such sensations were more common with the 0.025 percent cream. These reactions generally diminished with time but resulted in discontinuance of therapy during the study by eight patients.[57]

In a larger study 0.025 percent capsaicin cream was evaluated in patients with stable, plaque-type psoriasis of moderate severity (5 to 10 percent body surface involvement). Ninety-eight patients were treated topically with capsaicin four times daily and 99 patients were treated with vehicle for six weeks. The treated group showed significantly greater improvement by physicians' global scores at week four and week six and significantly greater relief of pruritis at week four and week six by patients' ratings. Fifty-four patients in the capsaicin group experienced burning or stinging at sites of application; this diminished or disappeared during the study in most patients. Thirty-six patients in the treated group withdrew during the study, primarily due to adverse effects, and 22 in the vehicle group withdrew, mostly due to treatment failure.[58]

Nervous System

Some alternative medicine providers advocate treating nervous conditions that may exacerbate psoriasis. Along with topical and systemic herbal treatments, separate nervine tonics are recommended.[59] Preparations of valerian (*Valeriana officinalis* L.) and passion flower (*Passiflora incarnata* L.) for oral use are suggested as calming agents. St. John's wort (*Hypericum perforatum* L.) preparations for oral use are suggested if signs of depression are associated with chronic psoriasis.[60] Information about these herbs is found in Chapter 11.

INTERNAL TREATMENT
OF ATOPIC DERMATITIS AND PSORIASIS

Herbal medicine providers generally promote internal "metabolic stimulation," herbs that stimulate bile production, and diuretics as necessary treatment for external skin disorders, based on the concept that many skin manifestations reflect systemic imbalances. Weiss recommends metabolic teas containing diuretic and laxative herbs, as well as chamomile.[7] Sarsaparilla (*Smilax* spp.), figwort (*Scrophularia nodosa* L.), and licorice root have also been recommended for internal treatment of eczema and psoriasis.[59-62] Figwort contains triterpenoid saponins but also contains cardiac glycosides that may be potentially toxic. Chamomile and licorice root have demonstrated anti-inflammatory activity but no clinical studies support internal use for skin disorders. It should be noted that Commission E recommends that duration of internal use of licorice root in an average daily dose equivalent to 200 to 800 mg glycyrrhizin be limited to four to six weeks due to sodium and water retention and depletion of potassium.

There are no objections to daily ingestion of doses up to an equivalent of 100 mg glycyrrhizin as a flavoring.[63]

Sarsaparilla

Sarsaparilla was an official drug in the USP from 1820 to 1955 and in the NF from 1955 to 1965. A poorly controlled two-year study published in 1942 reported oral treatment of 75 psoriasis patients with sarsasaponin (a water-soluble glycoside of sarsasapogenin, from sarsaparilla) tablets of unspecified dosage. The treatment was said to have a "decided and beneficial" effect on 62 percent of patients, with chronic, plaque-type psoriasis responding the most favorably. No untoward cardiovascular, renal, GI, or hematopoietic effects were noted.[64] In an article from 1931, oral consumption of a daily dose of an aqueous sarsaparilla extract, prepared by soaking 15 g of the dried root in 1 L of water overnight followed by boiling for 20 minutes the next morning, was reported to reduce scaling and red patches with no adverse effects.[65]

The *British Herbal Compendium* (BHC) lists psoriasis and eczema as indications for sarsaparilla.[61] The dosage is 2 to 4 g of the dried root three times daily. Decoctions of 2 to 4 ml of a 1:1 extract with 50 percent ethanol may also be used. Commission E lists skin diseases and psoriasis as applications for sarsaparilla, but does not endorse its therapeutic use, cautioning that efficacy for psoriasis is not proven. The Commission E monograph lists gastric irritation and temporary renal impairment as side effects and notes that several drug interaction risks exist; *Digitalis* glycoside and bismuth absorption is increased and elimination of hypnotics is accelerated.[62]

Other Herbs

Burdock

Preparations of dried burdock leaves and roots, from *Arctium lappa* L. (great burdock), or from *A. minus* (Hill) Bernh. (common burdock) (Asteraceae), are listed in the BHC or by Commission E for both internal and external use in eczema and psoriasis.[66,67] No recent pharmacological work has been reported, however, and Commission E does not endorse therapeutic use of burdock for the claimed applications.[67] Adulteration with the roots of *Atropa belladonna* L. (deadly nightshade) is possible due to the very similar appearance of the roots, and cases of atropine poisoning from adulterated commercial samples originating in Eastern Europe have been reported.[67,68]

Clivers, Lady's Bedstraw

Preparations of clivers, or cleavers, the dried aerial parts of *Galium aparine* L. (Rubiacae), are used in Britain both internally and externally to treat psoriasis and other skin diseases.[59,69,70] A related plant, lady's bedstraw (*G. verum* L.), is used in Germany internally as a diuretic and externally for damage to the skin, but is not endorsed for any specific indication.[70] No contraindications are noted.

Fumitory

Preparations of the dried aerial parts of fumitory, *Fumaria officinalis* L. (Fumariaceae), are used internally in Britain and Europe for chronic eczema and psoriasis.[59,71,72] Commission E endorses fumitory for its spasmolytic activity in the upper GI tract and for biliary complaints but not for therapy of dermatoses.[72] BHC lists pregnancy and lactation as contraindications.[71]

ACNE VULGARIS

Acne vulgaris is a common, self-limited chronic inflammatory dermatosis involving the pilosebaceous unit. Onset occurs primarily during adolescence, although it may start as early as 6 to 8 years of age or may not appear until age 20 or later. Duration is of several years followed by spontaneous remission. Acne affects both males and females, although males tend to have more severe disease. Etiology is unknown, but keratinous material in the follicle becomes more dense, and sebaceous glands are larger and produce more sebum in acne patients. *Propionibacterium acnes,* an anaerobe present in the follicle of acne patients, is thought to produce highly irritating fatty acids by breakdown of sebaceous oils. *P. acnes* also secretes chemotactic factors that may contribute to the inflammatory response.

The primary site of acne is the face and to a lesser extent the back, chest, and shoulders. Several types of lesions are present. Noninflammatory lesions are open or closed comedones, slightly elevated lesions with visible (open) or difficult to visualize (closed) impactions of keratin and lipid. Inflammatory lesions vary from small papules to pustules to large nodules. Scars may be present, appearing as sharp, punched-out pits.

Treatment of acne is directed toward correcting the altered pattern of follicular keratinization, decreasing sebaceous gland activity, decreasing the *P. acnes* population, and producing an anti-inflammatory effect. Topical vitamin A, benzoyl peroxide, and antibiotics as well as systemic antibiotics and, for severe acne, systemic glucocorticosteroids and isotretinoin are used in treatment.[73]

CASE STUDY 4: ACNE VULGARIS TREATMENT

Patient History

A 16-year-old male presents with mild to moderate inflammatory lesions on the face. He complains that the 5 percent benzoyl peroxide he uses topically causes itching and scaly, dry skin. He wants to try a natural medicine, stating that synthetic drugs are toxic. Inspection of the patient's lesions reveals open and closed comedones as the predominant lesions with moderate involvement of inflamed papules and a few inflamed pustules.

Clinical Considerations

Signs and symptoms are consistent with acne vulgaris. The patient's complaint about irritant effects of benzoyl peroxide (BP) is common. A variety of herbal products have been used to treat acne. Most are used topically for their anti-inflammatory or antibacterial actions.

Tea Tree Oil

The leaves of a native Australian tree, *Melaleuca alternifolia* (Maiden and Betche) Cheel (Myrtaceae), yield about 2 percent of a pale yellow oil upon steam distillation. Tea tree oil, as it is known, contains up to 60 percent of terpinen-4-ol, a terpenoid with antibacterial activity.[74]

A clinical trial of tea tree oil for treatment of acne has shown some promise. Sixty-one acne patients were treated with topical commercially available 5 percent water-based BP. Fifty-eight patients were treated with a 5 percent water-based gel preparation of Ateol tea tree oil from Australian Plantations Pty Ltd. Efficacy was assessed by counts of inflamed and non-inflamed lesions monthly for three months. Skin tolerance was also assessed on this schedule. Reduction of number of inflamed lesions by both products was significant at one, two, and three months, but BP was significantly superior to tea tree oil at all assessment times. Reduction of number of noninflamed lesions by both products was also significant at one, two, and three months, with no significant difference between the two products at any stage. Skin scaling, pruritis, and dryness were significantly greater in the BP group at one and/or two months. Skin oiliness was significantly different at all stages, the BP group showing increasingly less oiliness. Overall, 79 percent of the BP group and 44 percent of the tea tree oil group reported unwanted side effects.[75]

Arnica

Tyler states that arnica, the dried flower heads of *Arnica montana* L. (Asteraceae) and other *Arnica* species, has a long-standing reputation for the external treatment of acne, bruises, sprains, muscle aches, and as a counter-irritant.[76] The constituent helenalin is anti-inflammatory but may also induce contact dermatitis.[76] Commission E considers arnica anti-inflammatory when used topically, but cautions that prolonged treatment of damaged skin quite often causes edematous dermatitis and can lead to eczema; preparations of high concentration may cause vesicle formation or necrosis.[77] The most commonly used form of arnica is a 1:10 tincture prepared with 70 percent ethanol. The tincture is diluted three to ten times with water for use in compresses. Ointments and creams with a maximum 20 to 25 percent of the tincture or with a maximum of 15 percent arnica oil prepared from one part drug and five parts vegetable oil may also be used. Commercial arnica creams and ointments are widely available in Europe.[76] Arnica allergy is a contraindication and internal use should be avoided due to cardiac toxicities.[77]

Other Herbs

Burdock

Burdock leaf and root has been traditionally used both internally and externally for acne, but proof of efficacy is lacking.[67] In France burdock root is accepted for its traditional uses both internally and externally for therapy of mild cases of acne.[66]

Nettle

The dried leaves or aerial parts of *Urtica dioica* L. (Urticaceae) are accepted for traditional use both internally and externally for mild cases of acne.[78] Nettle is also used for seborrhea of the scalp. Commission E considers nettle a supportive treatment for irrigation of the urinary tract but does not endorse its therapeutic use in skin conditions.[79]

For a summary of herb use in dermatologic conditions, see Table 14.1.

TABLE 14.1. Herbs Used in Dermatologic Conditions

Atopic Dermatitis	Psoriasis	Acne Vulgaris
Useful Herbs*		
Exudative Phases:		
Oak Bark	Licorice Root	Tea Tree Oil
Walnut Leaves	Chamomile	Arnica
Witch Hazel	Capsaicin	
Mallow		
Wild Pansy		
Dry Lesions:		
Chamomile		
Yarrow		
Licorice Root		
Fenugreek		
γ-Linolenic Acid		
Traditional Use*		
Sarsaparilla	Sarsaparilla	Burdock
Fumitory	Burdock	Nettle
	Clivers	
	Fumitory	

*Herbal drug has an endorsement from Commission E or clinical trials show support for the indication.

**Herbal drug has folk or traditional reputation but no endorsement or support for the indication.

MEDICINAL AND NATURAL PRODUCTS CHEMISTRY

The following descriptions include the purported active constituents but are not exhaustive accounts of all known constituents.

A. **Tannins.** Tannins are widely distributed, complex mixtures of polyphenols. True tannins are polymeric substances with molecular weights of about 1,000 to 5,000. Simpler, low molecular weight phenolics are often found with tannins, including gallic acid, catechins, and chlorogenic acid. Tannins are classified as hydrolyzable and nonhydrolyzable or condensed tannins. Hydrolyzable tannins are readily hydrolyzed by acids and are composed of gallic and ellagic acid derivatives esterified with glucose. Condensed tannins, also called proanthocyanidins, require hot acid to break bonds, and are related to the flavonoid pigments, yielding anthocyanidins. They appear to be condensation products of catechins and flavan-3,4-diols.[80,81]

B. **Mucilages.** Gums and mucilages are plant hydrocolloids that are anionic or nonionic polysaccharides or their salts and are usually hetero-geneous in composition. Mucilages are said to form a slimy mass in water.[82]

C. **Chamomile.** Matricaria contains 0.3 to 1.5 percent essential oil, containing the sesquiterpene α-bisabolol, the sesquiterpene lactone matricin (prochamazulene), chamazulene (from matricin via hydrolysis, dehydration, and decarboxylation), and other constituents. the drug also contains flavones and flavonols, coumarins, and mucilage.[30] Roman chamomile contains 0.4 to 2.4 percent essential oil, consisting mainly of aliphatic esters, n-butyl angelate predominating. Sesquiterpene lactones, mainly nobilin, and different than matricaria, are present. Flavonoids including apigenin and luteolin are also present.[83,84] Roman chamomile should be stored in glass containers and protected from light and moisture.[84]

D. **Yarrow.** Yarrow contains 0.21 percent essential oil consisting of up to 50 percent chamazulene depending on the origin, with oxygenated monoterpenes including linalool and camphor also present. Sesquiterpene lactones including achillicin (a major prochamazulene) and millefin are present. Flavonoids include apigenin and luteolin.[32-34] Yarrow should be stored in glass containers and protected from light and moisture.[32]

E. **Licorice Root.** Licorice root contains 2 to 5 percent triterpenoid saponins, mainly glycyrrhizin, a glycoside that yields two glucuronic acids and the pentacyclic triterpenoid glycyrrhetic acid upon hydrolysis. About 1 percent flavonoids are also present.[36,85] Licorice root should be protected from light and moisture in storage.[85]

F. **Fenugreek.** Fenugreek contains 45 to 60 percent mucilaginous polysaccharides, 20 to 30 percent protein, and 6 to 10 percent of a fixed oil. Several steroidal saponins are also present, including foenugraecin, a tripeptide ester of diosgenin.[42]

G. **Gamma Linolenic Acid.** GLA is a polyunsaturated fatty acid; 18:3 (6Z, 9Z, 12Z). Epogam is a capsule preparation containing 500 mg of the seed oil from a hybridized variety of *Oenothera biennis* selected and bred to yield oil of constant composition. The oil consists of 8.9 percent GLA, 74.7 percent LA, 6.8 percent palmitic acid, and 7.7 percent oleic acid. Efamol is an equivalent product of Serono OTC, Milan.[86]

H. **Capsaicin.** Capsaicin is the vanillyl amide of isodecenoic acid. It is a component of the oleoresin of *Capsicum* species and is present at about 0.02 percent in the dried, ripe fruit. Capsaicin topical preparations must be applied four or five times daily for at least four weeks for sufficient depletion of substance P to occur.[87]

I. **Sarsaparilla.** Sarsaparilla contains 1 to 3 percent steroidal saponins, based on the isomeric aglycones sarsasapogenin and smilagenin. Sitosterols, stigmasterol, and about 50 percent starch are also present.[61]

J. **Tea Tree Oil.** Besides the major constituent, terpinen-4-ol, tea tree oil also contains pinene, 1,8-cineole, p-cymene, linalool, α-terpinene, γ-terpinene, α-terpineol, and terpinolene.[74,88]

K. **Arnica.** Depending on the species, arnica contains 0.2 to 1.5 percent sesquiterpene lactones, principally helenalin and its derivatives, arnifolins, and chammisonolides. Flavonoids and an essential oil are other constituents.[77]

See Table 14.2 for a summary of treatments suggested in this chapter.

TABLE 14.2. Summary

Acute Atopic Dermatitis	1. Dry lesions with compresses of astringent (tannin) or demulcent (mucilage) herbal preparations. 2. Apply topical preparations of anti-inflammatory or emollient herbs after lesions are dried—creams, ointments, compresses, or baths may be used. 3. Internal use of gamma-linolenic acid may be useful.
Chronic Atopic Dermatitis	1. Apply topical preparations of anti-inflammatory or emollient herbs—creams, ointments, compresses, or baths may be used. 2. Internal use of gamma-linolenic acid may be useful.
Psoriasis	1. Apply topical preparations of anti-inflammatory or emollient herbs—creams, ointments, compresses, or baths may be used. 2. Topical capsaicin preparations may prove beneficial.

TABLE 14.2 *(continued)*

Acne Vulgaris	1. Apply topical preparations of tea tree oil, or 2. Topical preparations of arnica.
Cautions	1. Asteraceae hypersensitivity—arnica, burdock, chamomile, and yarrow may cause allergic contact dermatitis. 2. Internal use of arnica should be strictly avoided. 3. Prolonged, high-dose internal use of licorice root has adverse cardiovascular effects.

REFERENCES

1. Rajka G. *Essential Aspects of Atopic Dermatitis.* Springer-Verlag, Berlin, 1989.

2. Leung DYM, Rhodes AR, Geha RS, Schneider L, Ring, J. Atopic dermatitis (atopic eczema). In: *Dermatology in General Medicine,* Fourth Edition. Fitzpatrick TB, Eisen AZ, Wolff K, Freedberg IM, Austen KF, eds., McGraw-Hill, New York, 1993, pp. 1543-1564.

3. West DP, Nowakowski PA. Dermatologic Products. In: *Handbook of Nonprescription Drugs,* Eleventh Edition. American Pharmaceutical Association, Washington, DC, 1996, pp. 537-568.

4. Jensen P. Use of alternative medicine by patients with atopic dermatitis and psoriasis. *Acta Derm Venereol* 1990;70:421-424.

5. Latchman Y, Banerjee P, Poulter LW, Rustin M, Brostoff J. Association of immunological changes with clinical efficacy in atopic eczema patients treated with traditional Chinese herbal therapy (Zemaphyte). *Int Arch Allergy Immunol* 1996; 109:243-249.

6. Sheehan MP, Stevens H, Ostlere LS, Atherton DJ, Brostoff J, Rustin MH. Follow-up of adult patients with atopic eczema treated with Chinese herbal therapy for 1 year. *Clin Exp Dermatol* 1995;20:136-140.

7. Weiss RF. *Herbal Medicine.* AD Arcanum, Gothenburg, Sweden, 1988, pp. 328-338.

8. Frohne D. Quercus cortex. In: *Herbal Drugs and Phytopharmaceuticals.* Bisset NG, ed., medpharm, Stuttgart, 1994, pp. 402-403.

9. Tyler VE, Brady LR, Robbers JE. *Pharmacognosy,* Ninth Edition. Lea & Febiger, Philadelphia, 1988, pp. 77-81.

10. Tyler VE. *Herbs of Choice: The Therapeutic Use of Phytomedicinals.* The Haworth Press, Binghamton, NY, 1994, pp. 151-170.

11. Oak Bark. *Bundesanzeiger,* no. 22a. Cologne, Germany, February 1, 1990.

12. Willuhn G. *Juglandis folium.* In: *Herbal Drugs and Phytopharmaceuticals.* Bisset NG, ed., medpharm, Stuttgart, 1994, pp. 281-282.

13. Walnut leaf. *Bundesanzeiger,* no. 101. Cologne, Germany, June 1, 1990.

14. Czygan FC. *Hamamelidis folium.* In: *Herbal Drugs and Phytopharmaceuticals.* Bisset NG, ed., medpharm, Stuttgart, 1994, pp. 245-247.

15. Oak Bark. *Bundesanzeiger,* no. 154. Cologne, Germany, August 21, 1985.

16. Wichtl M. *Malvae flos.* In: *Herbal Drugs and Phytopharmaceuticals.* Bisset NG, ed., medpharm, Stuttgart, 1994, pp. 313-316.

17. Mallow. *Bundesanzeiger,* no. 43. Cologne, Germany, March 2, 1989.

18. Willuhn G. *Violae tricoloris herba.* In: *Herbal Drugs and Phytopharmaceuticals.* Bisset NG, ed., medpharm, Stuttgart, 1994, pp. 527-529.

19. Wild Pansy. *Bundesanzeiger,* no. 50. Cologne, Germany, March 13, 1986.

20. Tyler VE. *Herbs of Choice: The Therapeutic Use of Phytomedicinals.* The Haworth Press, Binghamton, NY, 1994, pp. 57-59.

21. Chamomile. *British Herbal Compendium,* Vol. 1. Bradley PR, ed., British Herbal Medicine Association, Bournemouth, U.K., 1992, pp. 154-157.

22. Mann C, Staba EJ. Chamomile. In: *Herbs, Spices, and Medicinal Plants: Recent Advances in Botany, Horticulture, and Pharmacology,* Vol. 1. Craker LE, Simon JE, eds., Oryx Press, Phoenix, 1986, pp. 233-288.

23. Isaac O. Therapy with chamomile—Experiences and verifications. *Dtsch Apoth Ztg* 1980;120:567-570.

24. Della Loggia R. Lokale antiphlogistche Wirkung der Kamillen-Flavone. *Dtsch Apoth Ztg* 1985;125(suppl I):9-11.

25. Della Loggia R. Chamomile extracts exerted anti-inflammatory effects when applied topically in animal models of inflammation. *Planta Med* 1990;56: 657-658.

26. Hahn B, Holz J. Absorption, distribution and metabolism of [14C]-levomenol in the skin. *Arzneimittel Forschung* 1987;37:716-720.

27. Merfort I, Heilmann J, Hagedorn-Leweke U, Lippold BC. In vivo skin penetration studies of camomile flavones. *Pharmazie* 1994;49:509-511.

28. Patzelt-Wenczler R. Erfahrungen mit Kamillosan® Creme unter Praxisbedingungen. *Dtsch Apoth Ztg* 1985;125(suppl I):12-13.

29. Tyler VE, Brady LR, Robbers JE. *Pharmacognosy,* Ninth Edition. Lea & Febiger, Philadelphia, 1988, pp. 466-467.

30. Willuhn G. *Matricariae flos.* In: *Herbal Drugs and Phytopharmaceuticals.* Bisset NG, ed., medpharm, Stuttgart, 1994, pp. 322-325.

31. Chamomile. *Bundesanzeiger,* no. 228. Cologne, Germany, December 5, 1984.

32. Willuhn G. *Millefolii herba.* In: *Herbal Drugs and Phytopharmaceuticals.* Bisset NG, ed., medpharm, Stuttgart, 1994, pp. 342-344.

33. *British Herbal Compendium,* Vol. 1. Bradley PR, ed., British Herbal Medicine Association, Bournemouth, U.K., 1992, pp. 227-229.

34. Chandler RF. Yarrow. *Can Pharmaceutical J* 1989;122:41-43.

35. Leung AY. Licorice. In: *Encyclopedia of Common Natural Ingredients Used in Food, Drugs, and Cosmetics.* John Wiley & Sons, Toronto, 1980, pp. 220-223.

36. Chamomile. *British Herbal Compendium,* Vol. 1. Bradley PR, ed., British Herbal Medicine Association, Bournemouth, U.K., 1992, pp. 145-148.

37. Chandler RF. Licorice, more than just a flavor. *Can Pharmaceutical J* 1985;118:420-424.

38. Valentino R, Stewart PM, Burt D, Edwards CRW. Liquorice inhibits 11β-hydroxysteroid dehydrogenase in the rat. *J Endocrinol* 1987;112(suppl):260.

39. Evans FQ. The rational use of glycyrrhetinic acid in dermatology. *Br J Clin Pract* 1958;12:269-274.

40. Teelucksingh S, Mackie ADR, Burt D, McIntyre MA, Brett L, Edwards CRW. Potentiation of hydrocortisone activity in skin by glycyrrhetinic acid. *Lancet* 1990;335:1060-1063.

41. Barry BW, Woodford R. Activity and bioavailability of topical steroids. In vivo/in vitro correlations for the vasoconstrictor test. *J Clin Pharmacol* 1978; 3:43-65.

42. Willuhn G. *Foenugraeci semen.* In: *Herbal Drugs and Phytopharmaceuticals.* Bisset NG, ed., medpharm, Stuttgart, 1994, pp. 203-205.

43. Manku MS, Horrobin DF, Morse N, Kyte J, Jenkins K, Wright S, Burton JL. Reduced levels of prostaglandin precursors in the blood of atopic patients: Defective delta-6-desaturase function as a biochemical basis for atopy. *Prostaglandins Leukotrienes Med* 1984;9:615-628.

44. Strannegard IL, Svenerholm L, Stranegard Ö. Essential fatty acids in serum lecithin of children with atopic dermatitis and in umbilical cord serum of infants with high or low IgE levels. *Int Arch Allergy Appl Immunol* 1987;82:422-423.

45. Kerscher MJ, Korting HC. Treatment of atopic eczema with evening primrose oil: Rationale and clinical results. *Clin Investig* 1992;70:167-171.

46. Tyler VE. *Herbs of Choice: The Therapeutic Use of Phytomedicinals.* The Haworth Press, Binghamton, NY, 1994, pp. 137-139.

47. Morse PF, Horrobin DF, Manku MS, Stewart JCM, Allen R, Littlewood S, Wright S, Burton J, Gould DJ, Holt PJ, Jansen CT, Mattila L, Meigel W, Dettke T, Wexler D, Guenther L, Bordon A, Patrizi A. Meta-analysis of placebo-controlled studies of the efficacy of Epogam in the treatment of atopic eczema. Relationship between plasma essential fatty acid changes and clinical response. *Br J Dermatol* 1989;121:75-90.

48. Biagi PL, Bordoni A, Hrelia S, Celadon M, Ricci GP, Cannella V, Patrizi A, Specchia F, Masi M. The effect of gamma-linolenic acid on clinical status, red cell fatty acid composition and membrane microviscosity in infants with atopic dermatitis. *Drugs Exp Clin Res* 1994;20:77-84.

49. Whitaker DK, Cilliers J, de Beer D. Evening primrose oil (Epogam®) in the treatment of chronic hand dermatitis: Disappointing therapeutic results. *Dermatology* 1996;193:115-120.

50. Horrobin DF, Morse PF. Evening primrose oil and atopic eczema. *Lancet* 1995;345:260-261.

51. Everett DJ, Greenough RJ, Perry CJ, MacDonald P, Bayliss P. Chronic toxicity studies of Efamol evening primrose oil in rats and dogs. *Med Sci Res* 1988; 16:863-864.

52. Everett DJ, Perry CJ, Bayliss P. Carcinogenicity studies on Efamol evening primrose oil in rats and mice. *Med Sci Res* 1988;16:865-866.

53. Christophers E, Sterry W. Psoriasis. In: *Dermatology in General Medicine,* Fourth Edition. Fitzpatrick TB, Eisen AZ, Wolff K, Freedberg IM, Austen KF, eds., McGraw-Hill, New York, 1993, pp. 489-514.

54. Fleischer AB, Feldman SR, Rapp SR, Reboussin DM, Exum ML, Clark AR. Alternative therapies commonly used within a population of patients with psoriasis. *Cutis* 1996;58:216-220.

55. Lassus A, Forsström S. A double-blind study comparing oleum horwathiensis with placebo in the treatment of psoriasis. *J Int Med Res* 1991;19:137-146.

56. Oliwiecki S, Burton JL. Evening primrose oil and marine oil in the treatment of psoriasis. *Clin Exp Dermatol* 1994;19:127-129.

57. Bernstein JE, Parish LC, Rapaport M, Rosenbaum MM, Roegnigk HH. Effects of topically applied capsaicin on moderate and severe psoriasis vulgaris. *J Am Acad Dermatol* 1986;15:504-507.

58. Ellis CN, Berberian B, Sulica VI, Dodd WA, Jarratt MT, Katz HI, Prawer S, Krueger G, Rex IH, Wolf JE. A double-blind evaluation of topical capsaicin in pruritic psoriasis. *J Am Acad Dermatol* 1993;29:438-442.

59. Hoffman D. *The Holistic Herbal.* Element Books, Longmead, England, 1988, pp. 73-82.

60. Stelling K. Psoriasis: An integrated approach for phytotherapy. *Br J Phytotherapy* 1991/1992;2:133-137.

61. *British Herbal Compendium,* Vol. 1. Bradley PR, ed., British Herbal Medicine Association, Bournemouth, U.K., 1992, pp. 194-195.

62. Licorice. *Bundesanzeiger,* no. 164. Cologne, Germany, September 1, 1990.

63. Licorice. *Bundesanzeiger,* no. 90. Cologne, Germany, May 15, 1985.

64. Thurmon FM. The treatment of psoriasis with a sarsaparilla compound. *N Engl J Med* 1942;227:128-133.

65. Philippsohn A. Ekzem- und Psoriasbehandlung nach eigener Methode. *Dermat Wchnschr* 1931;93:1220-1223.

66. *British Herbal Compendium,* Vol. 1. Bradley PR, ed., British Herbal Medicine Association, Bournemouth, U.K., 1992, pp. 48-49.

67. Burdock. *Bundesanzeiger,* no. 22a. Cologne, Germany, February 1, 1990.

68. Tyler VE. *The Honest Herbal,* 3rd Edition. The Haworth Press, Binghamton, NY, 1993, pp. 63-64.

69. *British Herbal Compendium,* Vol. 1. Bradley PR, ed., British Herbal Medicine Association, Bournemouth, U.K., 1992, pp. 61-62.

70. Wichtl M. *Galii veri herba.* In: *Herbal Drugs and Phytopharmaceuticals.* Bisset NG, ed., medpharm, Stuttgart, 1994, pp. 225-227.

71. *British Herbal Compendium,* Vol. 1. Bradley PR, ed., British Herbal Medicine Association, Bournemouth, U.K., 1992, pp. 102-104.

72. Fumitory. *Bundesanzeiger,* no. 173. Cologne, Germany, September 18, 1986.

73. Strauss JS. Sebaceous glands. In: *Dermatology in General Medicine,* Fourth Edition. Fitzpatrick TB, Eisen AZ, Wolff K, Freedberg IM, Austen KF, eds., McGraw-Hill, New York, 1993, pp. 709-726.

74. Tyler VE. *Herbs of Choice: The Therapeutic Use of Phytomedicinals.* The Haworth Press, Binghamton, NY, 1994, p. 160.

75. Bassett IB, Pannowitz DL, Barnetson R St. C. A comparative study of tea-tree oil versus benzoyl peroxide in the treatment of acne. *Med J Aust* 1990;150: 455-458.

76. Tyler VE. *Herbs of Choice: The Therapeutic Use of Phytomedicinals.* The Haworth Press, Binghamton, NY, 1994, p. 157.

77. Willuhn G. *Arnica flos.* In: *Herbal Drugs and Phytopharmaceuticals.* Bisset NG, ed., medpharm, Stuttgart, 1994, pp. 83-87.

78. Bulletin Officiel No. 90/22 bis. Avis aux fabricants concernant les demandes d'authorisation de mise sue le marché des médicaments à base de plantes. Ministére des Affaires Sociales et de la Solidarité: Direction de la Pharmacie et du Médicament, Paris, 1990.

79. Nettle. *Bundesanzeiger,* no. 76. Cologne, Germany, April 23, 1987.

80. Trease GE, Evans WC. *Pharmacognosy,* Twelfth Edition. Baillière Tindall, London, 1983, pp. 376-378.

81. Robbers JE, Speedie MK, Tyler VE. *Pharmacognosy and Pharmacobiotechnology.* Williams & Wilkins, Baltimore, 1996, pp. 139-141.

82. Ibid., pp. 40-41.

83. *British Herbal Compendium,* Vol. 1. Bradley PR, ed., British Herbal Medicine Association, Bournemouth, U.K., 1992, pp. 191-193.

84. Willuhn G. *Chamomillae romanae flos.* In: *Herbal Drugs and Phytopharmaceuticals.* Bisset NG, ed., medpharm, Stuttgart, 1994, pp. 140-142.

85. Willuhn G. *Liquiritae radix.* In: *Herbal Drugs and Phytopharmaceuticals.* Bisset NG, ed., medpharm, Stuttgart, 1994, pp. 301-304.

86. Brenner RR. The oxidative desaturation of unsaturated fatty acids in animals. *Mol Cell Biochem* 1974;3:41-52.

87. Robbers JE, Speedie MK, Tyler VE. *Pharmacognosy and Pharmacobiotechnology.* Williams & Wilkins, Baltimore, 1996, pp. 134-135.

88. Carson CF, Riley TV. Antimicrobial activity of the major components of the essential oil of *Melaleuca alternifolia. J Appl Bacteriol* 1995;78:264-269.

Chapter 15

Gynecological and Obstetric Concerns Regarding Herbal Medicinal Use

Larry Kincheloe, MD, FACOG

Herbal medicinals for obstetrical and gynecological concerns includes a very wide spectrum of conditions. These include gynecological disorders such as menstrual irregularities, premenstrual syndrome, menopause, sexually transmitted diseases, and to enhance sexual experience.[1] Herbals have also been used to treat male and female infertility disorders as well as pregnant and postpartum patients. The discussion could fill volumes for any of these areas. This chapter, however, will be limited to the herbal medicinals with the most solid research behind them and for which the strongest recommendations can be made.

HISTORY

Herbs have been used since the beginning of time for gynecological and obstetric conditions and have been found throughout all cultures. In some cases herb use has been recorded, as in Chinese and European writings. Because many native cultures transmit knowledge by oral traditions, many of these herbs are only now being identified and studied.

Some herbs from the Amazonian jungles and tropical islands such as the native herbs of Tonga are being used by shamans for infertility, menometrorrhagia, postpartum hemorrhage, dysmenorrhea, and breast pain. It is felt that there are tremendous avenues for future studies for new pharmaceuticals in these and many other yet-to-be identified native plants.[2,3] Van Payvelde found the potential for many medicinals in a study of 25 plants of Rwanda. Sixteen entities had activity against *Neisseria gonorrhea* and *N. meningitis* and six had activity against *Streptococcus pyogenes* and *Staphyl-*

ococcus aureus.[4] The antimicrobial action of the plant extracts was determined by the disk diffusion method. Agar plates were inoculated with a suspension of the microorganisms to obtain a uniform inoculum. Disks were then impregnated with 2 mg of each plant extract and applied to the surface of the inoculated plates. Next, the degree of inhibition of bacterial growth was measured. Again, these preliminary studies indicate bountiful areas for future research.

In the middle ages, some people believed that wearing belts of human skin facilitated labor and helped with its pain or that ingesting an extract of ground-up mummified bodies would help delay menstruation.[5] Some authors try to mystify the area of herbal medicine with claims that herbs can bring the menstrual tides into synchronicity with the lunar tides. Others feel that taking herbs at certain phases of the moon will facilitate their healing properties or that the shape of a plant (Doctrine of Signatures) will reveal something about its properties.[6,7]

In discussing the use of herbal medicine in obstetrics, a higher standard is required than when dealing with gynecological concerns. If adults choose to use medicinal herbs, they can make a reasonably informed choice about their acceptance of the risks and benefits of these preparations. When dealing with an unborn fetus who is a passive member in this decision making process, it is imperative to have more solid data when making recommendations for the use of herbal medications, or any medications for that matter, to be taken during pregnancy. Bunce, in an article on the use of herbal preparations in pregnancy, made the disclaimer, "Because the author is not licensed to directly or indirectly dispense medical advice, if you use the information contained herein, without the advice of a physician, you are prescribing for yourself and the author assumes no responsibility."[8] As a physician, I cannot make recommendations and then make these types of disclaimers. I must have data and studies to support recommendations and it was with this ethical responsibility in mind that I reviewed the following studies.

CASE STUDY 1: PREMENSTRUAL SYNDROME

A 22-year-old female presents with complaints of bloating and severe nervous tension that occur two weeks before her menstrual cycle. A complete history and physical exam fail to reveal any pathological process. She requests treatment for her symptoms. After recording her symptoms for three cycles, her charts indicate a five- to seven-pound weight gain as well as a subjective increase in nervous tension and crying spells.

Discussion

Premenstrual syndrome (PMS) has no universally accepted definition but usually is considered to be a set of symptoms that appear during the luteal phase, which decrease or resolve at the time of menses.[9] The symptoms or behaviors must also be of a degree that interferes with one's ability to function on a daily basis. A medical and psychological exam should be completed to rule out other physical or psychiatric disorders and a daily rating of symptoms should be completed for two to three cycles before making the diagnosis of PMS.[10] The most commonly described symptoms include abdominal bloating, anxiety/depression, breast tenderness, water retention, fatigue, weight gain, and appetite changes.

Valerian

Approximately 200 species of valerian *(Valeriana officinalis)* exist throughout the world and it has been well-known as a treatment for nervous tension and sleep disorders for more than 1,000 years.[11-17] The fresh drug comes from the dried rhizomes and roots of the perennial herb *Valeriana officinalis*. It does not have a significant odor but one does develop over time secondary to enzyme hydrolysis of herbal compounds. Isovaleric acid is the compound imparting to valerian its distinctive "dirty sock" odor.[15,17] Valerian had official status in the United States for 150 years and was included in the *United States Pharmacopoeia* from 1820 to 1942 and the *National Formulary* from 1942 to 1950. More than 150 different drug products are marketed in Germany containing valerian or one of its active compounds. It has the added benefit of not being synergistic with alcohol. The content of its volatile oils varies among different species and ranges widely from 0.5 to 6.0 percent with the main constituent being bornyl acetate.[18,19]

Two major groups of psychoactive compounds have been studied in depth. These are the iridoids and the sesquiterpenoids. Japanese valerian contains kessyl glycol diacetate (KGD), which is felt to be an active ingredient and works on the central nervous system. This compound was found to have anxiolytic effects similar to those of diazepam and antidepressant effects, the latter possibly due to blockage of monoamine uptake.[20]

Santos found that valerian reduces the release of GABA by an exchange process, although its mode of action in vivo is still undetermined.[21] Purportedly the high concentrations of glutamine in the valerian extracts could also explain the sedative properties of valerian. As glutamine crosses the blood-brain barrier, it appears that glutamine can be taken up by nerve terminals and subsequently metabolized to GABA in GABAergic neurons thus causing some of the relaxing effects of valerian. There is also a possibility that the

GABA present in valerian could be responsible for the relaxant activity found in the peripheral tissues. Leuschner confirmed that a commercially available valerian root extract had significant sedative properties in animal studies.[22] Evaluation of valerian extract revealed pronounced sedative properties in mice with respect to a reduction in motility and an increase in the thiopental-induced sleeping time. A direct comparison with diazepam and chlorproma-zine revealed that valerian extract had moderate sedative activity. In another double-blinded study, 48 healthy volunteers were placed in stressful social situations involving mental arithmetic calculations. They were distributed into the following four treatment conditions at random:

- placebo
- valerian (100 mg extract of valerian)
- propranolol (20 mg)
- valerian (100 mg)-propranolol (20 mg) combination

Results showed that valerian root was effective in decreasing the feelings of somatic arousal when subjects were placed in stressful situations.[23]

Valerian root also improves the quality of sleep, which is often disrupted in PMS. Valerian produced a decrease in subjective latency sleep scores and significantly improved subjective sleep quality, especially in people who considered themselves poor sleepers.[24,25] These sleep studies, along with many others using subjective ratings as well as laboratory-performed sleep EEGs, show that valerian was effective in improving the ease of falling asleep as well as the quality of that sleep.[26,27] The active compounds were thought to be valepotriates by some and sequiterpenes by others. These may be selective effects on non-REM sleep, especially in slow-wave sleep.[28]

Valerian is quite safe. In an overdose attempt, a patient ingested 40 to 50 470 mg capsules of valerian root, resulting in only minor side effects such as fatigue, abdominal cramping, and light-headedness.[29] The German Commis-sion E monographs have approved valerian as an anxiolytic and sleep agent.[18] It has also been used in combination with other herbs to help allevi-ate the agitated state associated with drug withdrawal.[30]

Hops

Hops *(Humulus lupulus)* also has a long history of being known as a mild sedative.[14,18] It is native to Europe, Asia, and North America and grows as a perennial vine. The sedative properties of hops were suspected when it was noticed that hop pickers tired easily, presumably as the result of absorption of resins through the skin.[11] One of its active compounds, a volatile alcohol 2-methyl-3-buten-2-ol, was shown to have sedative effects that occurred within two minutes and then decreased over a two-hour time period.[31] Hops may be used synergistically with valerian but alone, it is considered to be a milder sedative than valerian.[19]

Hops has also been known to relieve abdominal cramping. Hops has been shown to contain phytoestrogens and was a known cause of dysfunctional uterine bleeding (DUB) through skin absorption of the resins in girls who worked in the fields picking hops.[19] Fresh hops or extracts should be used since most of this herb's potency is lost when stored due to instability when exposed to light and air. To date there are no contraindications or recognized side effects, but if fresh extracts are used, DUB is possible.

Passion Flower

Passion flower *(Passiflora incarnata)* has been used as an anxiolytic and sedative agent and was on the *National Formulary* from 1916 to 1936.[11] It is a milder herb and therefore is a very useful supportive drug in many herbal teas.[17,19] Several animal studies have demonstrated its sedative effects.[16,32] It is approved by the German Commission E as a treatment for nervous unrest although the FDA disallowed its use in OTC sedatives in 1978 due to lack of proven effectiveness.[16]

St. John's Wort

Some patients with PMS complain of more symptoms of depression than those relating to anxiety or nervous tension. For those, there is a wealth of information supporting the beneficial effects of St. John's wort *(Hypericum perforatum)* for the treatment of mild to moderate depression.[11,16,18,19] At the strength of 0.3 percent hypericin, it has been found to be as effective as fluoxetine (Prozac), amitriptyline (Elavil, Endep) and nortriptyline (Pamelor) but without many of the associated side effects (e.g., xerostomia, mydriasis, constipation).[33] St. John's wort was felt to be such an important herb that the *Journal of Geriatric Psychiatry and Neurology* devoted an entire supplement to the benefits of this herbal compound.[34] It is also approved in the German Commission E monograph for the treatment of depressive states.[18] St. John's wort is also recommended for the depression that may accompany menopause. Photosensitiviy is a potential side effect of this herbal treatment.[9,16,17]

Diuretics

Many herbs have been used to relieve fluid retention. As with all folk remedies, we do not always know what we think we know, as demonstrated in a paper by Dat. He studied four traditional Vietnamese herbs known for their diuretic properties and found that none of them was more effective than placebo.[35]

Dandelion *(Taraxacum officinalis)* is one of the oldest herbs used as a diuretic.[36] Animal studies suggest dandelion is one of the most effective diuretics (see discussion in Chapter 8 regarding aquaretic versus diuretic aspects). Test animals sometimes lost as much as 25 percent of their body weight. Obviously this amount of water loss is not recommended in humans but demonstrates the potential of this herb.[37] It was comparable to furosemide (Lasix) and superior to the most potent diuretic herb, juniper. It is recommended by the German Commission E monographs. It is contraindicated in persons with obstruction of the bile duct system or with gallstones.[18] It is also worth noting that dandelion contains a high percentage of potassium.[17,18] Concomitant use with potassium supplements, ACE inhibitors, and potassium-sparing agents (e.g., traimaterene) may be ill-advised.

Juniper *(Juniperus communis)* has long been known for its diuretic properties. It is native to Europe, northern Asia, and North America.[12] There is wide variation of the essential volatile oils and to date over 70 components have been identified.[18] The diuretic effect was thought to be due to the compound terpinen-4-ol which, in contrast to other terpenes, is not known to be nephrotoxic.[11,18] Some oils contain other terpene hydrocarbons such as pinene in the range of 55:1 and can be nephrotoxic, as demonstrated by glomeruli hyperemia.[16] Therefore this herb cannot be recommended unless the manufacturer lists the terpene hydrocarbon to terpinene-4-ol ratio (e.g., 3:1) and even with this, its use must be cautioned and limited to short periods (four weeks). It is contraindicated in patients with any type of kidney disease as well as in pregnancy and should be in avoided in patients taking known nephrotoxic drugs (e.g., aminoglycosides, amphotericin B, foscarnet).[11,17-19,38]

Parsley is probably the most commonly known diuretic herb.[14] Derived from the plant *Petroselinum crispum,* it contains two to seven percent of two principal volatile oils, myristic and apiol, which are thought to contribute to much of its diuretic properties. These compounds can also cause uterine contractions and apiol was once used as an abortifacient, so special precautions for use in pregnancy are in order.[11,16-19] Its volatile oils are too potent to be recommended.

One of the most effective herbs used as a diuretic is goldenrod *(Solidago species)*. Animal studies have demonstrated significant diuretic properties although, as with most herbs, the exact compound has not been isolated.[16,19] This herb is endorsed by the German Commission E (as a diuretic) since toxicity and contraindications have not been reported.

Buchu *(Barosma folium)* consists of dried leaves from a South African plant of the Rutaceae family and has been recommended for over 135 years.[11,12,17,18] It has a mild diuretic effect due to its volatile oils, flavonoids, and terpenes (terpinene-4-ol), which are also present in juniper berries.[18] It is considered a very safe herb although not recommended in pregnancy.[39] It is approved as a diuretic by the German Commission E.

Corn silk from *Zea mays* has a diuretic effect thought to be due to its relatively high potassium content. In animal studies, corn silk was found to have significant diuretic activity.[17,18,38]

CASE STUDY 2: MENSTRUAL DISORDERS

A 28-eight-year-old woman presents with dysmenorrhea and menometrorrhagia. She has been evaluated to rule out other causes such as infection, uterine fibroids, or endometriosis. She has experienced gastric upset secondary to NSAID use. She is interested in natural alternatives.

Discussion

Herbal Treatments

Primary dysmenorrhea is prostaglandin-induced myometrial contractions originating in the endometrium. There is a 300 percent increase in the prostaglandin levels from the follicular phase to the luteal phase with a secondary increase during menstruation.[10] Dysfunctional uterine bleeding is a varied complex of menstrual patterns generally relating to anovulation.[10]

Chaste tree *(Vitex agnus-castus)* is found in Europe and grows as a shrub reaching nine to 17 feet tall. *Vitex* is the ancient Latin name. The species name comes from *agnus,* "lamb," and *castus* meaning "chaste." Studies in Germany indicated that extracts of the seed can help regulate menometrorrhagia.

Milewicz studied the effects of *Vitex agnus-castus* extract in 52 patients who had a luteal phase defect.[40] These patients also had mild hyperprolactinemia. He found that after three months, the short luteal phases were normalized and that the deficits in luteal progesterone synthesis were eliminated. Also, two patients in the *Vitex* group subsequently conceived during the study, indicating its potential use in the treatment of infertile patients with luteal phase defects and mild hyperprolactinemia.[40] This has been confirmed by other studies showing that *Vitex* increases luteinizing hormone production, shifting the ratio of estrogens to progestins and hence addressing a corpus luteum hormone effect.[11,19,38] This demonstrated the usefulness of *Vitex* in treating menstrual disorders due to a corpus luteum insufficiency.

The mode of action of *Vitex* is due to its dopaminergic properties. It therefore has the ability to inhibit the secretion of prolactin by the pituitary gland by binding to the dopamine receptor.[41] This was determined by measuring the effect of *agnus-castus* extract on the prolactin levels in cultured rat pituitary cells under basal and TRH stimulation conditions. Significant inhibition of prolactin secretion was found and this prolactin inhibition was found to be blocked by adding a dopamine receptor antagonist (haloperidol). *Vitex* also has diuretic effects that are helpful in patients with fluid retention.

In another study, powdered *Vitex agnus-castus* was tested against a placebo in a double-blind randomized controlled trial with 217 volunteers self-diagnosed with PMS. No difference was found in patients being treated with *Vitex* compared with a placebo except in one symptom ("feeling jittery or restless").[42] This study was criticized for treating patients for only three months as opposed to the recommended six months.[43] There was a report of one infertile patient whose use of a *Vitex*-containing compound resulted in abnormal ovarian hormonal measurements (elevated FSH, LH, and estradiol levels) and symptoms suggestive of a mild ovarian hyperstimulation syndrome. The authors cautioned against using hormonally active herbs to restore normal ovarian function.[44] The German Commission E has recommended the use of *Vitex* or chaste tree berry for a variety of menstrual discomforts.

Raspberry *(Rubus idaeus)* teas and extracts are well known as treatments for dysmenorrhea and to promote easier labor.[16,38,39,45] There are a few older studies in animals that show raspberry extracts cause uterine relaxation.[46] Other studies indicate that the effects are isolated in the muscle of a pregnant uterus.[47] The studies were done 40 to 50 years ago and are very crude by today's standards thus limiting the strength of the findings.[11,16] Although it is not recommended by the German Commission E monographs, it is considered safe and without side effects.[18]

Other herbs found to have uterine muscle antispasmodic effects are cramp bark *(Viburnum opulus)* and black haw *(Viburnum prunifolium)*. The active principles of these herbs have yet to be entirely identified.[17-19,48]

Black cohosh *(Cimicifuga racemosa)* consists of dried rhizomes and has long been used as a female tonic since it was first introduced by the American Indians. Early studies could not demonstrate any effects on menstruation in test animals.[16] Other studies showed that the herb contains compounds that bind to estrogen receptors and cause a selective reduction in luteinizing hormone in ovariectomized rats.[49] Although, studies confirm that black cohosh is effective in treating PMS and dysmenorrhea in humans, its use is still popular. German Commission E has found black cohosh to be effective for the treatment of PMS and dysmenorrhea.[11,16] It is felt that it should be avoided in early pregnancy[17,38] but may be used in the last four to six weeks of pregnancy as a uterine preparatory agent.[38,39]

Another herb not to be confused with black cohosh is blue cohosh *(Caulophyllum thalictroides).* It is one of the oldest American herbal plants and derives its name from its dark blue fruits. It is known as an inducer of menstruation as well as labor.[38,39] One of its compounds, the alkaloid methylcytisine, has action that closely mimics nicotine although only $1/25$th as toxic.[11] It can cause uterine contractions thus inducing menstruation as well as causing hypertension.[16,17] Its oxytocic effects are felt to be due to caulosaponin. This compound constricts coronary blood vessels as well as causing intestinal spasms in animal studies.[50,51] Although speculative, these properties could antagonize the desired pharmacologic effects of vasodilators (e.g., isosorbide) and antispasmodics (e.g., dycyclomine). As with many of the studies in herbal medicine, these studies are 40 to 50 years old and indicates an enormous need for ongoing research with contemporary methodology. Therefore, this herb cannot be recommended.

Dong quai *(Radix Angelicae sinensis)* has been used for more than 2,000 years and Xiao in 558 A.D. purportedly stated it helped regulate the menstrual cycle as well offering relief from menstrual pain.[52] Animal studies demonstrate increased uterine contractions.[53] The contractive rhythm of the smooth muscle changed from fast, irregular, and weak to stronger, slower, and more regular patterns. Some feel that this may be the basis for the use of dong quai in dysmenorrhea.[52] Other studies suggest this herb increases sexual activity in female animals.[52]

Traditional Chinese medicine recommends injections of 10 percent dong quai extract into the acupuncture points associated with relief of chronic pelvic pain, menstrual disorders, hypertension, and herpes zoster. Although dong quai has been used for thousands of years and is one of the most popular herbs for female conditions,[38,39] there are very few studies demonstrating effectiveness in humans.[11]

Grapefruit juice increases the bioavailability of ethinyl estradiol, as demonstrated in a study of 13 healthy volunteers.[54] It was found that 100 ml of grapefruit juice could increase the peak concentration of ethinyl estradiol by 137 percent ($p = 0.0088$). This could possibly cause breakthrough bleeding in patients using birth control pills who are on fruit juice cleansing diets.[54] This reinforces the importance of a practitioner inquiring about dietary and alternative therapies, as they may be the cause of seemingly unrelated symptoms.

CASE STUDY 3: MENSTRUAL MIGRAINES

A 24-year-old female presents with a history of migraine headaches for the past five years that are cyclic and occur just prior to the time of menses. She has used propranolol as prophylaxis but could not tolerate the side effects. She now treats the migraines with narcotics or sumatriptan succinate (Imitrex). She is requesting information on herbal prophylaxis.

Discussion

Feverfew

A subgroup of women exist who have exacerbations of headaches in relation to their menstrual cycle. It is felt that the decrease in progesterone may be the precipitating factor of migraine headaches for these patients.

Feverfew *(Tanacetum parthenium)* has been used as a medicinal plant as far back as the ancient Greek herbal text *De Materia Medica* by Pedanius Dioscorides, a Greek army surgeon under Nero. The name feverfew is a corruption of the old English name *febrifuga,* which is derived from the Latin term *febrifugia.* This word relates to one of its claims of exhibiting antipyretic properties.[55] In the eighteenth century, herbalist John Hill stated that feverfew "exceeds whatever else is known" in the treatment of headaches. A number of British publications have reported on this herb over the past few years, but it has gone unnoticed in the United States, at least in terms of scientific research.[56]

Feverfew has been used to reduce the number and severity of migraine attacks and its active ingredient is felt to be parthenolide.[57-59] Feverfew contains sesquiterpene lactones with a methylenebutyrolactone unit, which have been shown to inhibit prostaglandin biosynthesis, thus giving feverfew its anti-inflammatory activity.[55,60] It is unknown if its effects are additive or synergistic with nonsteroidal anti-inflammatory drugs (NSAIDs) (e.g., ibuprofen, diclofenac, indomethacin, sulindac).

Other research has shown its effects on the inhibition of platelet activity as well as platelet 5-HT (serotonin) secretion by as much as 50 percent.[61] Caution should be exercised when used concomitantly with allopathic drugs known to affect platelet activity (e.g., sulfinpyrazone) or serotonin (e.g., fluoxetine, paroxetine). It is felt that serotonin plays a significant role in the pathogenesis of migraine headaches.[57,61] This is also the basis of the newer medications for the treatment of migraines such as sumatriptan succinate (Imitrex), which is a selective agonist for 5-HT.[62] It is unknown if a drug-herb interaction exists for these medications.

Feverfew is also rich in sesquiterpene lactones. Several newer compounds of this group have been isolated which are spasmolytic in that they render the smooth muscle less responsive to endogenous substances such as norepinephrine, acetylcholine, bradykinin, prostaglandins, histamine, and serotonin in a noncompetitive manner. The antagonist properties work through inhibition of the influx of extracellular calcium into the vascular smooth-muscle cells.[63] Would patients taking both feverfew and an ACE inhibitor (e.g., enalapril, lisinopril) be less likely to experience cough secondary to inhibition of bradykinase? Would a pregnant woman taking feverfew be less responsive to cervical ripening with dinoprostone (ProstinE2), a prostaglandin? Would a patient taking both feverfew and amitripyline experience less anticholinergic side effects (e.g., xerostoma, mydriasis, urinary retention) secondary to amitripytline? These questions remained unexplored and unanswered.

In another study, feverfew was found to prevent the initial step of the release of arachidonic acid substrate from platelet phospholipids and the formation of thromboxane as well as the production of prostaglandin biosynthesis.[60,64] Antipyretic and antiplatelet activities were purportedly due to a phospholipase inhibitor that prevents the release of arachidonic acid. Since arachidonic acid is the precursor to prostaglandins and leukiotrienes, this may explain the many activities attributed to feverfew.

The minimum level of of 0.2 percent parthenolide in feverfew has been set by the Canadian government. At this level, the Canadian health authorities have given feverfew a Drug Identification Number (DIN), allowing it to be prescribed for migraine prevention.[16,65] One study showed that most of the North American products have less than 0.1 percent of parthenolide.[66] The percentage of parthenolide is higher in feverfew grown in the UK and Germany compared with that grown in Mexico or Yugoslavia, which contain only scant amounts of parthenolide.[66] The parthenolide content is higher in the flowering tops than in leaves, stalks, and roots. The content of parthenolide decreases, as is the case with many herbs, over time and when exposed to light.[66,67] Feverfew can induce a widespread inflammation of the oral mucosa and tongue.[68]

CASE STUDY 4: NAUSEA AND VOMITING IN PREGNANCY

A 19-year-old female, G1P0 is ten weeks pregnant and presents with complaints of nausea most of the day that results in several episodes of vomiting daily. This has become worse over the past ten days and she has had a five-pound weight loss. Specific gravity of her urine is 1.20

and she is not spilling ketones. She has not tried any treatments and although she understands it is a normal symptom of pregnancy, she would like some relief.

Discussion

Ginger Root

Vomiting is a common occurrence during pregnancy and the incidence varies from 60 to 80 percent. Because vomiting is so common in pregnancy, it has been accepted as an unfortunate but natural discomfort. The term morning sickness is used to describe the most common form and refers to nausea and vomiting starting early in pregnancy. The symptoms are usually mild and resolve between the thirteenth and eighteenth week.[19]

Ginger root is officially known by the scientific Latin name *Zingiber officinale.* The genus name *zingiber* was given to the plant based on the ancient Sanskrit name *shringavera* meaning "horn shaped." Despite the name, it is actually not a root but a rhizome, which is described as a horizontally growing stem. It has been used in Asia for over 4,000 years as a food, spice, and medicine. Some of the best commercial varieties come from Jamaica although 80 percent of today's imports come from China. The composition of the essential oils varies tremendously depending on country of origin and the nonvolatile components including gingerols and shogoal. This may explain some of the conflicting findings among the itinerant studies that examined the role of ginger root as a postoperative antiemetic.[69,70]

Ginger root was noted in an 1881 book, *The Mystery of Medicine,*[12] as a treatment for sea sickness. Grontved, 100 years later, found ginger root was indeed effective in reducing vomiting and sweating among naval cadets at sea for the first time.[71] It has also been studied as an antiemetic and several studies have shown that it is effective in many medical scenarios involving animals and humans. In animal studies, known emetics were given and the latency period was recorded after administering ginger extracts. Ginger was shown to produce a prolongation of emetic latency by 154 percent in these animal studies.[72]

Phillips studied 120 women undergoing outpatient laparoscopy and found ginger root (1 gram) was as effective in reducing nausea and vomiting as metoclopramide (Reglan). The need for postoperative antiemetics was significantly reduced by ginger but not metoclopramide.[73] In another study to test ginger's antiemetic effect, women undergoing major gynecological surgery were given either ginger or metoclopramide.[74] Results were similar. These studies were contradicted by Arfeen, who found that ginger root (0.5 to 1.0 gram) did not decrease nausea and vomiting in patients undergoing laparoscopic surgery.[70] Myers studied the effects of ginger root (1.5 grams) before ingestion of 8-MOP (psoralen), finding this caused a reduction in nausea by approximately 30 percent. Psoralen typically causes nausea within one hour of ingestion.[75] Ginger does not have any extrapyramidal or sedative properties; hence it was concluded that ginger root was an excellent antiemetic.

Mowrey showed that ginger was more effective than dimenhydrinate (Dramamine) in reducing motion sickness. It was demonstrated that ginger exacted its effect on the gastrointestinal tract (GIT) as opposed to the central nervous system (CNS).[76] Holtmann found ginger did not affect the nystagmus response, thus also supporting the theory that ginger acts at the level of the GIT.[77] It is felt that the antiemetic effect of ginger on the GIT is not based on increased gastric emptying rates.[78] Conflicting studies did find that some constituents of ginger actually enhance gastrointestinal motility when mice were given ginger followed by a charcoal meal. Thirty minutes later the mice were killed and the distance the charcoal meal traveled through the bowel was measured, thus showing an advancement that was superior to that of metoclopramide.[79] The use of gingerol has also been suggested as a treatment for motion sickness in weightless conditions such as those found in the space shuttle or space station.[80] As with many of these herbs, another study found that ginger root did not reduce the associated motion sickness in 28 human test subjects nor alter gastric motility.[81]

Ginger root has also been used in combination with ginkgo biloba as an antiemetic.[82] It was felt that since ginger root was a potent antagonist at the 5-HT receptor and ginkgo biloba extracts are indirect serotorun antagonists, these two herbs could work in a synergistic manner. This has been shown to be valid based on several animal studies.

Fischer-Rasmussen found that when ginger root (250 mg four times daily) was administered to pregnant patients, the women subjectively preferred the ginger root treatment over a placebo (double-blind randomized crossover trial).[83] Fischer-Rasmussen and colleagues felt that the studies related to the mutagenic effect of certain strains of *E. coli* were not applicable since the studies in question only tested the extract gingerol. The whole root and its other components are felt to be strongly antimutagenic.[84] The mutagenesis concern followed studies by Nakamura, who found that gingerol was mutagenic in certain strains of *E. coli* but subsequently demonstrated ginger juice, taken as a whole, contained antimutagenic components against gingerol and in fact suppressed spontaneous mutations.[85]

Other studies have shown certain components, such as gingerol and shoganol, as well as high concentrations (2 to 4 percent) of ginger extracts were mutagenic in growing roots of onions and in some strains of salmonella.[86,87] There are important questions about the significance of this data for humans. I am reminded that the effective birth control depot-medroxyprogesterone acetate was kept off the U.S. market for 20 years because studies in the 1950s showed that it might have caused breast tumors in beagles (a species prone to mammary dysplasia).[88]

Another concern is raised by Backon, who felt that ginger root may affect the testosterone-binding receptor sites in the fetus, possibly affecting sex differentiation in the fetal brain.[89] Backon has completed a significant amount of study on the therapeutic effects of ginger root and advises cautious use in pregnancy since as a potent thromboxane synthetase inhibitor, ginger may, in theory, affect testosterone-receptor binding in the fetus, thus possibly affecting sex steroid differentiation of the fetal brain. This caution has been discounted by other researchers in the field who feel there is no clinical or experimental data supporting this concern.[90]

Based on these studies, the Commission E of the German Federal Health Agency issued an exclusion stating ginger root should not be given for morning sickness.[18] This is in spite of the fact that there are no reports or scientific literature showing ginger root causes miscarriages or birth defects.

Niebly considered ginger effective in the treatment of hyperemesis and also recommended vitamin B6 at a dose of 25 mg twice daily.[91] Other studies have found that vitamin B6 25 mg three times daily was effective in reducing the complaints of nausea and vomiting.[92,93] Vitamin B6 has been reported in the literature since 1942 and has been incorporated into several antiemetic preparations in the past (Bendectin).[94-96]

CASE STUDY 5: LACTATION

A 23-year-old woman, G2P1, reports that after her last delivery she did not have enough breast milk and had to supplement her infant with formula. She has recently delivered another child and wants to prevent the decrease in breast milk that occurred after her last delivery. What herbal remedies might she try?

Discussion

Prolactin is the principal hormone involved in breast milk production. The hormonal event for the initiation of milk production is the rapid reduction of estrogen and progesterone after delivery. Breast engorgement and milk production begin three to four days after progesterone and estrogen have cleared. Suckling stimulates an increase in prolactin, which is important in starting milk production. Prolactin also sustains the secretion of casein, fatty acids, lactose, and secretion volume.[10]

To increase breast milk production in nursing mothers, *Vitex* or chaste tree berry has been used.[19,38] Purportedly, two to four weeks are required for this herb to take effect but it can be taken for weeks or months to help maintain adequate breast milk production. This is one of the contradictions found in the study of herbal medicine. On one hand, it has been reported that *Vitex* is useful in restoring normal menstrual patterns in women with mild hyperprolactinemia by reducing prolactin levels.[19] Yet, in the area of breast feeding, it is considered effective in increasing the production of breast milk. Bromocriptine (Parlodel) was used in the past to suppress lactation.[10] Since the secretion of prolactin is important in the initiation of lactation but less important in maintaining lactation, there may be some other mechanism for *Vitex*'s effect on breast milk production.

Raspberries have been recommended to increase breast milk production although scientific data is sparse.[38,39]

Sage *(Salvia perforatum)* has long been reported to stop breast milk production.[11,17,18,38,39] Although it is reported in many books, I could not find literature to support this claim. I have been using it in my practice for years and feel it offers excellent results. This is one of those areas in which a patient has to decide an issue based on historical but unscientific data.

Jasmine flowers lightly taped to the breasts have been shown to significantly reduce prolactin levels in women wishing to suppress lactation. The possible mechanism may be through olfactory stimulation.[97]

Depending on the source, there are herbs that are not recommended for use during pregnancy.[98] Although this list may be contested, it is felt that pregnant women should avoid the following herbs: black cohosh, blue cohosh, bloodroot, cayenne, dong quai, fumaria, helonias, hydrastis, juniper, kelp, mistletoe, mugwort, pennyroyal, and pokeroot. These herbs may be related to early miscarriages, but more study is needed.[11,17,38,39,98]

CASE STUDY 6: MENOPAUSE

A 53-year-old female presents with complaints of hot flashes, mood swings, vaginal dryness, and sleeplessness. She wants to take the lowest dose of synthetic hormones, which have been shown to be cardioprotective, and then supplement with natural estrogens as the need arises. Is this a legitimate approach?

Discussion

Menopause occurs in the United States between the ages of 48 and 55 years with a median age of 51 years. The age of menopause has not changed significantly during the course of recorded history. It is a set of symptoms initiated as the ovarian production of estrogen begins to decrease. The symptoms most frequency related to estrogen loss are menstrual irregularities, vasomotor instability (hot flashes), psychological symptoms (e.g., depression, anxiety), atrophic conditions, insomnia, low libido, and palpitations. The severity of these symptoms varies widely among women. It is also known that estrogen is beneficial in reducing the risk of strokes, heart attacks, fractures related to osteoporosis, colon cancer, and possibly Alzheimer's disease.[10]

Based on anthropological studies, during the time of the Neanderthals approximately 70,000 years ago, only two out of ten persons who survived childhood and adolescence could expect to reach the age of 30, with only 1 percent surviving to the age of 50.[99] By the late seventeenth century, an affluent woman might be expected to live to the age of 38. The average age of death in England between 1891 and 1900 was only 47.8 years. Even as late as 1950, the life expectancy worldwide was only 38 to 43 years and even lower when developed countries are excluded. The average life span in Guinea is still only 30 to 35 years.[100-104]

Menopause is unique to higher primates and particularly to humans. This is because our species has been able to modify its environment and change many factors that affect longevity. These data are presented to advance the idea that menopause is a biological anomaly. In the course of human evolution, which occurred over millions of years, there was no biological species advantage to maintain ovarian function into the later years because as a whole only a small percentage of the population lived past age 40. It makes teleological sense that if a hormone was beneficial to a woman age 30 that it would then be beneficial at age 60.

Phytoestrogens are naturally occurring substances found in foods and are defined as plant compounds that are functionally similar to estradiol.[19] They consist of several classes including isoflavones, coumestones, lignans, and resorcyclic acid lactones, with the first two being the major groups.[105-106] The plant lignan and isoflavonoid glycosides are converted by intestinal bacteria to compounds with estrogenic activity.[107] These are very weak estrogens when compared to estradiol. Over 500 plant species contain phytoestrogens. Some of the more common examples of these herbs are dong quai *(Angelica sinesis),* red clover *(Trifolium praeteus),* alfalfa *(Medicago sativa),* licorice root *(Glycyrrhiza glabra),* black cohosh *(Cimicifuga racemosa),* and soybeans *(Glycine max).*[108] To date, there are no reports of adverse effects in humans.

Isoflavone is a synthetic phytoestrogen extract. It has been shown to maintain bone density in women taking gonadotropin-releasing hormone agonists.[109] Vertebral bone density and total body bone mineral were measured by energy X-ray absorptiometry every three months during the study as well fasting urinary excretion of hydroxyproline, which is a measure of bone resorption. Another synthetic phytoestrogen based on zearalenone was shown to be effective in treating hot flashes and dyspareunia as well as increasing vaginal wall maturation.[110-112]

Since 1931 it has been known that soy contains two potent estrogenic isoflavonoid phytoestrogens (up to 100 to 300 mg and 100 mg, respectively), daidzein and genistein.[113] After ingestion of soy protein, intestinal flora can convert the soy isoflavone to equol, which has more potent estrogenic activity.[114] Many studies have shown that these phytoestrogens bind to estrogen receptors and have weak estrogenic activity. The most well-known estrogenic effect is red clover disease, which caused an epidemic of infertility that almost destroyed the sheep breeding industry in southwest Australia in the 1940s. Studies of soy protein show that a diet supplemented with soy flour can improve a patient's lipid profile by decreasing cholesterol, LDL cholesterol, and antitriglycerides as well as decreasing the incidence of hot flashes.[115] It is felt that the phytoestrogens found in certain products account for 60 to 70 percent of these effects. In a study where animals were fed soy protein with or without the phytoestrogens removed, it was found that phytoestrogens exerted the favorable effect on plasma lipid proteins. The phytoestrogens genistein and daidzein were found to reduce LDL, VLDL, and cholesterol while increasing the high-density lipoprotein concentration.[116] These changes were more pronounced in female than male test animals.

Estrogen replacement therapy decreases the relative risk of coronary heart disease (CHD) by 35 to 50 percent.[117,118] Unfortunately there are no good studies showing a direct correlation between reduced risk of stroke and heart attacks and the use of phytoestrogens, although preliminary studies are promising.

Wilcox and others demonstrated that patients using the phytoestrogens in soy flour and linseed showed an increase in vaginal maturation consistent with adequate estrogen levels.[110,111,114] These findings were not seen with red clover.[112] The soy flour findings were not replicated by Murkies.[115] There was a minimal decrease in the FSH level and no change in the LH ratio and vaginal maturation when using these phytoestrogens.

Oral ingestion of the phytoestrogen genistein from soy was effective in low doses (1.0 mg/day) in maintaining trabecular bone loss but high doses had no retentive effect on bone tissue.[119] This effect was similar to conjugated estrogens. Anderson suggests a biphasic response, which has also been found for isoflavone. The dominant effect of phytoestrogen at moderate to high doses (3.2 to 10 mg/day) is interference with normal cell function of body tissue.[119] Another phytoestrogen, coumestrol, has been shown to inhibit bone resorption and at the same time stimulate bone mineralization in animal studies.[120] KCA-098 is a synthetic analogue of coumestrol that inhibits bone resorption while it stimulates bone mineralization in organ cultures of fetal rat and chick embryonic bones. It lacks the weak estrogenic activity of its parent compound, coumestrol, making it a potential for women where estrogen is contraindicated.[121]

Diets high in isoflavonoid excretion, which is a measure of dietary intake, seems to confer some protection against breast cancer in animal and human studies.[113] Genistein has an inhibitory effect on tyrosine kinase, which seemingly plays an important role in cell proliferation and transformation. This enzyme has been associated with the oncogene products of the retroviral src gene family and the ability of this virus to transform cells. Tyrosine kinase activity is also associated with breast cancer oncogene expression. Genistein, as well as other isoflavonoids, has been shown to be antiproliferative with regard to breast cancer cells and acts to inhibit mammary tumor progression in rats.[110]

Black cohosh extract *(Cimicifuga racemosa)* produced a significant decrease in LH but not in FSH levels in ovariectomized rats ($p < 0.01$).[46] One hundred and ten menopausal women with climacteric symptoms experienced significant symptom reduction ($p < 0.05$).[46] FSH levels remained elevated (mean 62 mU/ml).[46] This lack of reduction in menopausal hormone markers concurs with studies.[122,123] This herb was also shown to help with vaginal atrophy accompanying menopause secondary to its estrogenic type compounds.[19,49,124] As with many herbal treatments, the effect is slow and develops over months. Three endocrine-active components have been identified in black cohosh with one identified as formononetine (an isoflavone).[123] It was shown that this compound is a competitor for estrogen in receptor assays, but failed to reduce the serum levels of lutenizing hormone in orphorectomized rats.[123]

In 1936, Japanese researchers discovered glycoside saponins in the Mexican yam (Dioscorea). The primary steroid saponin, diosgenin, can be converted to progesterone through chemical processing.[19] Yams do not contain estrogens or progesterones as is commonly touted in marketing advertisements.[125] The human body cannot convert diosgenin into progesterone[126] although progesterone can be delivered through the skin by transdermal patches, creams, and compounds.

CASE STUDY 7: MEMORY LOSS

A 72-year-old female in good general health wants to know if there is anything she can take to help with her memory. She finds her forgetfulness very frustrating. She also complains of ringing in her ears and cannot tolerate other medications she has tried for tinnitus.

Discussion

Ginkgo Biloba

Fossils of ginkgo trees date back as far as 250 million years. These trees are known for their longevity and specimens have been known to live more than 1,000 years. They were saved from extinction by Chinese monks over 800 years ago.[127]

Ginkgo biloba has been recommended for problems related to memory loss and retention typically found in the elderly.[11,16,19] One hundred fifty-six patients with degenerative dementia of Alzheimer's type and multi-infarct dementia were given ginkgo biloba extract in a prospective, randomized double-blind placebo-controlled, multicenter study over a 24-week period. Psychopathological assessment, attention, memory, and behavioral assessment of daily life activities were studied. The frequency of therapy responders in the two treatment groups differed significantly in favor of the ginkgo biloba extract group. This well-designed study demonstrated clinical efficacy of ginkgo biloba extract for Alzheimer's type dementia.[128] Although increased brain activity was seen after a single dose, the most dramatic changes did not appear for six months.[127]

Additionally, ginkgo biloba extract has decreased glucose utilization in the frontal parietal somatosensory cortex, nucleus accumbens, cerebellum, and pons, which may assist in explaining how it improves mental and physical conditions in the elderly.[129] Furthermore, ginkgo biloba extract EGB 761, containing 24 percent ginkgo-flavone glycosides and 6 percent terpenoids (as a measure of standardization), has been found to have memory-enhancing ability as well as neuroprotective effects.[11,16,130] Allain found that ginkgo biloba extract improved psychometric testing performance in patients with slight memory improvements.[131] This showed that ginkgo biloba extract has pharmacological effects on the basic components of human memory. Ginkgo biloba can reduce the negative effect of learning as the result of stress. These effects are most pronounced on older subjects or test animals.[132] Gingko biloba has also improved the retention of learned behavior.[133] The study concluded that ginkgo biloba is beneficial and ranks as one of the best cognition-enhancing drugs. The German Commission E has recently approved ginkgo biloba extract as a treatment for dementia symptoms.[127] It is unknown if ginkgo biloba will have a beneficial effect in countering the amnesic effects of benzodiazepines (e.g., lorazepam, diazepam).

Ginkgo biloba reportedly improves cerebral insufficiency associated with aging. Problems include but are not limited to difficulties in concentration and memory, confusion, fatigue, and tinnitus.[134] These symptoms have been associated with a decrease in cerebral circulation. As in all areas of scientific study, some studies are good and some are poor. The majority of studies showed a positive effect and Kleijnen and Knipchied concluded that based on the data, they would be willing to take this herb themselves.[134]

In a study of patients with permanent, severe tinnitus (PST), ginkgo biloba extract had no effect.[135] The paper went on to discuss that in this type of patient, PST results from many etiologies. The source may be located in the middle ear, in the cochlea, in the acoustic nerve, or in more central auditory pathways. Therefore it is not surprising that an herbal treatment or any drug treatment would be less than effective when tested in a population with many disease entities for the same symptoms. It is unknown if ginkgo would delay or alter the presentation of aspirin-induced tinnitus.

In a review of how drug treatment affects vestibular compensation, ginkgo biloba was found to accelerate compensation for symptoms caused by unilateral vestibular deafferentation as a result of the destruction of vestibulus receptor cells in animals.[136] The theorized mechanism is a direct effect on the vestibular nuclei. Other animal studies have indicated that ginkgo biloba extracts protect the neurons against oxidative stress induced by hydrogen peroxide.[137-139] It would be interesting to know if ginkgo would afford similar protection against neuronal oxidative stress induced by neuroleptics (e.g., chlorpromazine, haloperidol).

During menopause, Shen demonstrated that ginkgo biloba extract was cardioprotecive on myocardial ischemia repercussion injury. The study suggested antioxidant properties protect the heart on a cellular level.[137,140] Jassens found that ginkgo biloba extract was protective against hypoxia-induced damage in endothelial cells. He found that the extract slows the natural decrease in ATP, thus preventing the normal rise in lactate production.[141] Other animal studies showed that ginkgo biloba extracts were as effective as aspirin in prevention of thrombosis.[142]

Ginkgo biloba has also been shown to increase walking distance in patients with intermittent claudication, implying an anti-ischemic action that may be useful in treating peripheral arterial disease.[19,143] Comparative data with pentoxifylline (Trental) are lacking.

Ginkgo biloba is not without side effects. A 33-year-old Korean woman experienced bilateral subdural hematomas after ingestion of 120 mg ginkgo biloba daily. It was postulated this may have been due to inhibition of platelet

activating factors from ginkgo biloba.[144] Hence caution should be exercised in predisposed patients whose vascular integrity may already have been interrupted (e.g., by stroke).
See Table 15.1 for a summary of herbs reviewed in this chapter.

TABLE 15.1. Summary

Valerian	May be used for PMS; is not synergistic with alcohol; may contain GABA, accounting for its relaxant effects; improves sleep.
Hops	May be used for PMS; considered to be a milder sedative than valerian; contains phytoestrogens.
Passion flower	Anxiolytic and sedative used for PMS.
St. John's wort	0.3 percent hypericin as effective as traditional antidepressants (e.g., fluoxetine); may cause photosensitivity.
Diuretics	Questionable efficacy for use in PMS; dandelion contains high amounts of potassium; juniper contraindicated in renal disease and pregnancy; parsley should be avoided in pregnancy.
Chaste tree	May be used to help regulate menometrorrhagia; may normalize luteal phase defects; dopaminergic properties; may increase breast milk production.
Raspberry	May cause uterine relaxation; not recommended by German Commission E.
Black cohosh	May reduce LH; German Commission E found it effective for PMS and dysmenorrhea; should be avoided in early pregnancy.
Blue cohash	Methylcytisine induces menstruation and labor; not recommended.
Grapefruit juice	Increases bioavailability of ethinyl estradiol by 137 percent.
Ginger	*Zingiber officinale* may reduce nausea and vomiting of morning sickness; comparable to metoclopramide in antiemetic activity; direct effect on GIT; mutagenesis potential unresolved.
Sage	May decrease or stop breast milk production.
Phytoestrogens	May possess estrogenic activity (e.g., dong quai, red clover, alfalfa, licorice root, black cohosh, and soybeans).
Jasmine flower	Reduces prolactin levels, decreasing breast milk production.
Dong quai	Purportedly regulates menstrual cycle and relieves menstrual pain; need studies demonstrating effectiveness in humans.

REFERENCES

1. Runganga A. The use of herbal and other agents to enhance sexual experience. *Soc Sci Med* 1992;35:1037-1042.

2. Van Asdall W. A new medicinal plant from Amazonian Ecuador. *J Ethnopharmacol* 1983;9:315-517.

3. Singh Y. Folk medicine in Tonga. A study of the use of herbal medicines for obstetric and gynecological conditions and disorders. *J Ethnopharmacoll* 1984;12: 305-329.

4. Puyvelde L. Rwandese herbal remedies used against gonorrhea. *J Ethnopharmacol* 1983;8:279-286.

5. Peters H. *Pictorial History of Ancient Pharmacy.* Chicago, G.P. Engelhard and Company, 1906.

6. Dubick M. Historical perspectives on the use of herbal preparations to promote health. *Am Inst Nutrition* 1986;1348-1354.

7. Baker J. Midwifery and herbs. *Midwifery Today* 1993;26:29-31.

8. Bunce K. The use of herbs in midwifery. *J Nurse-Midwifery* 1987;32: 255-259.

9. Freeman E. PMS: New treatments that really work. *Contemporary OB/GYN* 1996;41:25-44.

10. Speroff L. *Clinical Gynecologic Endocrinology and Infertility,* Fourth Edition. Baltimore, Williams and Wilkins. 1989.

11. Tyler V. *The Honest Herbal.* Philadelphia, George F. Stickley, 1982.

12. Byrn ML. *The Mystery of Medicine.* New York, M. Lafayette Byrn, MD, 1881.

13. Dickson J. Mark Jameson's physic plants. A Sixteenth-Century Garden. *Gynaecology* (Glasgow) 1987;32:60-62.

14. Comrie J. *Black's Medical Cyclopedia.* New York, Macmillan, 1926.

15. Houghton P. The biological activity of valerian and related plants. *J Ethnopharmacol* 1988;22:121-142.

16. Tyler V. *Herbs of Choice.* Binghamton, NY, The Haworth Press, 1994.

17. Mabey R. *The New Age Herbalist.* New York, Macmillan, 1988.

18. Bisset N. *Herbal Drugs and Phytopharmaceutical.* Stuttgart, Scientific Publishers, 1996.

19. Weiss R. *Herbal Medicine.* Beaconsfield Publishers Ltd., Beaconsfield, England.

20. Sakamoto T. Psychotropic effects of Japanese valerian root extract. *Chem Pharm Bull* 1992;40:758-761.

21. Santos M. The amount of GABA present in aqueous extracts of valerian is sufficient to account for [3H]GABA release in synaptosomes. *Planta Medica* 1994;60:475-476.

22. Leuschner J. Characterization of the central nervous depressant activity of commercially available valerian root extract. *Arzneim-Forsch/Drug Research* 1993;43:638-641.

23. Kohnen R. The effects of valerian, propranolol, and their combinations on activation, performance, and mood of healthy volunteers under social stress conditions. *Pharmacopsychiatry* 1988;21:447-448.

24. Leathwood P. Aqueous extract of valerian root improves sleep quality in man. *Pharmacol Biochem Behav* 1982;17:65-71.

25. Leathwood P. Quantifying the effects of mild sedatives. *J Psychiatric Re* 1982;17:115-122.

26. Balderer G. Effect of valerian on human sleep. *Psychopharmacology* 1985; 87:406-409.

27. Lindwall O. Double blind study of a valerian preparation. *Pharmacol Biochem Behav* 1989;32:1065-1066.

28. Schulz H. The effect of valerian extract on sleep polygraphy in poor sleepers: A pilot study. *Pharmacopsychiatry* 1994;27:147-151.

29. Willey L. Valerian overdose: A case report. *Vet Human Toxicol* 1995;37(4): 364-365.

30. Nebelkopf E. Herbal therapy in the treatment of drug use. *International J Addictions* 1987;22(8):695-717.

31. Wohlfart R. The sedative-hypnotic principle of hops. *Planta Medica* 1983; 48:120-123.

32. Speroni E. Neuropharmacological activity of extracts from *Passiflora incarta. Planta Medica* 1988;54:448-491.

33. Murray M. St. John's wort for depression. *Health Counselor* 1995;7(4): 36-38.

34. Jenike M. (ed.) Hypericum: A novel antidepressant. *J Geriatric Psychiatry and Neurology* 1994; Vol. 7, Supplement: October.

35. Dat D. Studies on the individual and combined diuretic effects of four Vietnamese traditional herbal remedies. *J Ethnopharmacol* 1992;36:225-231.

36. Mitchell R. Herbal medicine. *Virginia Medical* 1984;12:752-756.

37. Racz-Kotilla E. The action of *Taraxacum officinale* extracts on the body weight and diuresis of laboratory animals. *Planta Medica* 1974;26:212-217.

38. McIntyre A. *The Complete Woman's Herbal.* New York, Henry Holt Company, 1994.

39. Weed S. *Wise Woman Herbal for the Childbearing Year.* New York, Ash Tree Publishing, 1986.

40. Milewicz A. *Vitex agnus castus* extract in the treatment of luteal phase defect due to latent hyperprolactinemia. *Arzeim-Forsch/Drug Res* 1993;43:752-756.

41. Sliutz G. *Agnus castus* extracts inhibit prolactin secretion of rat pituitary cells. *Horm Metab Res* 1993;25:253-255.

42. Turner S. A double-blind clinical trial on a herbal remedy for premenstrual syndrome: A case study. *Complementary Therapies in Medicine* 1993;1:73-77.

43. Maciocia G. Letter to the editor. *Complementary Therapies in Medicine* 1993;1:221-223.

44. Cahill DJ. Multiple follicular development with herbal medicine. *Human Reproduction* 1996;9(8):1469-1470.

45. Stapleton H. Herbal medicines for disorders of pregnancy. *Modern Midwife* 1995;4:18-22.

46. Burn J. A principle in raspberry leaves which relaxes uterine muscle. *Lancet* 1942;7:6149-6151.

47. Bamford DS. Raspberry leaf tea: A new aspect to an old problem. *British Pharmacological Society* 1970;4:161P-162P.

48. Jarboe C. Uterine relaxant properties of *Viburnum. Nature* 1996;389(5064): 837.

49. Duker E. Effects of extracts from *Cimicifuga racemosa* on gonadotropins release in menopausal women and ovariectomized rats. *Planta Medica* 1991;57: 420-424.

50. Ferguson H. A pharmacological study of a crystalline glycoside of *Caulophyllum thalictroides. J Am Pharm Assoc* 1953;43:16-21.

51. Scott C. The pharmacological action of N-methylcystine. *J Pharmacol Experimental Therapeutics* 1943;79:334-339.

52. Zhu D. Dong quai. *Am J Chinese Med* 1987;15:117-125.

53. Harada M. Effects of Japanese *Angelica* root and peony root on uterine contraction in the rabbit in situ. *J Pharmacobiodyn* 1984;1(5):304-311.

54. Weber A. Can grapefruit juice influence ethinylestradiol bioavailability? *Contraception* 1996;53:41-47.

55. Groenewegen W. Progress in the medicinal chemistry of the herb feverfew. *Prog Medicinal Chem* 1992;29:217-239.

56. Tyler V. Herbal medicine in America. *Planta Medica* 1987;1:1-4.

57. Marles R. A bioassay for inhibition of serotonin release from bovine platelets. *J Natural Prod* 1992;55:1044-1056.

58. Johnson E. Efficacy of feverfew as prophylactic treatment of migraine. *Brit Med J Clin Res* 1985;291(6495):569-573.

59. Murphy J. Randomized double-blind placebo-controlled trial of feverfew in migraine prevention. *The Lancet ii* 1988;189-192.

60. Collier H. Extract of feverfew inhibits prostaglandin biosynthesis. *Lancet* 1980;10:922-923.

61. Knight D. Feverfew: Chemistry and biological activity. *Natural Products Report* 1995;12(3):271-276.

62. Skaer T. Therapeutic use of sumatriptan in the treatment of migraine. *Female Patient* 1995;20:19-28.

63. Diamond S. Herbal therapy for migraine. *Migraine* 1987;1:197-198.

64. Makheja A. The active principle in feverfew (letter). *Lancet* 1981;2(8254): 1054.

65. Kemper K. Seven herbs every pediatrician should know. *Contemporary Pediatrics* 1996;13:79-91.

66. Heptinstall S. Parthenolide content and bioactivity of feverfew (*Tanacetum parthenium* (L.) Schultz-Bip.) estimation of commercial and authenticated feverfew products. *Pharm Pharmacol* 1992;44:391-395.

67. Barsby R. Feverfew and vascular smooth muscle: Extracts from fresh and dried plants show opposing pharmacological profiles, dependent upon sesquiterpene lactone content. *Planta Medica* 1993;59:20-25.

68. Frost J. Herbalism: An overview of an ancient art. *Professional Nurse* 1992; 1:237-241.

69. Blumenthal M. Ginger: Pungent spice and popular medicine. *Let's Live* 1994; 12:41.

70. Arfeen Z. A double blind randomized controlled trial of ginger for the prevention of postoperative nausea and vomiting. *Anaesth Intens Care* 1995;23:449-452.

71. Grontved A. Ginger root against seasickness. *Acta Otolaryngol* 1988;105: 45-49.

72. Kawai T. Anti-emetic principles of *Magnolia obovata* bark and *Zingiber officinale* rhizome. *Plant Medica* 1994;60:17-20.

73. Phillips S. *Zingiber officinale* (ginger)—an antiemetic for day case surgery. *Anesthesia* 1993;48:715-717.

74. Bone M. Ginger root—a new antiemetic: The effect of ginger root on postoperative nausea and vomiting after major gynecological surgery. *Anaesthesia* 1990; 45:669-671.

75. Meyer K. *Zingiber officinale* (ginger) used to prevent 8-MOP associated nausea. *Dermatology Nursing* 1995;7:242-244.

76. Mowrey D. Motion sickness, ginger, and psychophysics. *Lancet* 1982;1: 655-657.

77. Holtmann S. The anti-motion sickness mechanism of ginger. *Acta Otolaryngol* 1989;108:168-174.

78. Phillips S. *Zingiber officinale* does not affect gastric emptying rate. *Anesthesia* 1993;48:393-395.

79. Yamahara J. Gastrointestinal motility enhancing effect of ginger and its active constituents. *Chem Pharm Bull* 1990;38:430-431.

80. Timsit C. These vestibular problems out of gravity. *Ann Oto-Laryng* 1986; 103:235-243.

81. Stewart J. Effects of ginger on motion sickness susceptibility and gastric function. *Pharmacology* 1991;42:111-120.

82. Frisch C. Blockade of lithium chloride-induced conditioned place aversion as a test for antiemetic agents: Comparison of metroclopramide with combined extracts of *Zingiber officinale* and *Ginkgo biloba*. *Pharmacol Biochem Behav* 1995;52:321-327.

83. Fischer-Rasmussen W. Ginger treatment of hyperemesis gravidarum. *Eur J Obstet Gynecol Reproductive Biol* 1990;38:19-24.

84. Nakamura H. Mutagen and anti-mutagen in ginger, *Zingiber officinale*. *Mutation Res* 1982;103:119-126.

85. Nakamura H. The active part of the [6]-gingerol molecule in mutagenisis. *Mutation Res* 1983;122:87-94.

86. Nagabhushan M. Mutagenicity of gingerol and shogoal and antimutagenicity of zingerone in Salmonella/microsome assay. *Cancer Letters* 1987;36:221-233.

87. Abraham S. Mutagenic potential of the condiments, ginger and turmeric. *Cytologia* 1976;41:591-595.

88. Connell E. DMPA: A saga of drug approval in the United States. *Female Patient* 1993;18:56-61.

89. Backon J. Letter to the editor. *Eur J Obstet Gynecol Reproductive Biol* 1991; 42:163-164.

90. Fischer-Rasmussen W. Letter to the editor—reply. *Eur J Obstet Gynecol Reproductive Biol* 1991;42:163-164.

91. Niebyl J. Drug therapy during pregnancy. *Curr Opin Obstet Gynecol* 1992; 4:43-47.

92. Sahakian V. Vitamin B6 is effective therapy for nausea and vomiting of pregnancy: A randomized, double-blind placebo-controlled study. *Obstet Gynecol* 1991;78:33-36.

93. Erick M. Vitamin B-6 and ginger root in morning sickness. *J Am Diet Assoc* 1995;95(4):416.

94. Willis R. Clinical observations in treatment of nausea and vomiting in pregnancy with Vitamins B1 and B6. *Am J Obstet Gynecol* 1942;44:265-271.

95. Weinstein B. Clinical experience with pyridoxine hydrochloride in treatment of nausea and vomiting of pregnancy. *American Journal of Obstet Gynecol* 1943;46:283-285.

96. Weinstein B. Oral administration of pyridoxine hydrochloride in the treatment of nausea and vomiting of pregnancy. *American Journal of Obstet Gynecol* 1944;47:389-394.

97. Shrivastav P. Suppression of puerperal lactation using jasmine flowers *(Jasminum Sambac). Aust NZ J Ostet Gynecol* 1988;28:6871.

98. Trevelyan J. Herbal medicine. *Nursing Times* 1993;89(43):36-38.

99. Hall D. *The Biomedical Basis of Gerontology.* Wright-PSG, London, 1984: 53-76.

100. Fries J. *Vitality and Aging.* New York, W.H. Freeman, 1981;74-77.

101. Cassel C. *Geriatric Medicine.* New York, Springer-Verlag, 1984;13-21.

102. Finch C. *Handbook of the Biology of Aging.* New York, Van Nostrand Reinhold, 1985;27-44.

103. Andres R. *Principles of Geriatric Medicine.* New York, McGraw-Hill, 1985:22-29.

104. Golub S. *Health Needs of Women as They Age.* New York, The Haworth Press, 1988;4-7.

105. Sheehan D. The case for expanded phytoestrogen research. *Pro Soc Experi Biol Med* 1995;1:3-5.

106. Knight D. A review of the clinical effects of phytoestrogens. *Obstet Gynecol* 1996;87:897-904.

107. Adlercreutz H. Phytoestrogens: Epidemiology and a possible role in cancer protection. *Envir Health Perspectives.* 1995;103(supplement 7):103-112.

108. Costello C. Estrogenic substances from plants: *Glycyrrhiza. J Am Pharm Assoc* 1950;39:177-180.

109. Gambacciani M. Ipriflavone prevents the bone mass reduction in premenopausal women treated with gonadotropin hormone-releasing hormone agonists. *Bone Mineral* 1994;26:19-26.

110. Nilsson K. The vaginal epithelium in the postmenopause—cytology, histology and pH as methods of assessment. *J Climacteric Postmenopause* 1995;21:51-56.

111. Price K. Naturally occurring oestrogens in foods—A review. *Food Additives Contaminants* 1985;2:73-106.

112. Wilcox G. Oestrogenic effects of plant foods in postmenopausal women. *Br Med J* 1990;301:905-906.

113. Adlercreutz H. Phytoestrogens: Epidemiology and a possible role in cancer protection. *Envir Health Perspectives* 1995;103:103-112.

114. Baird D. Dietary intervention study to assess estrogenicity of dietary soy among postmenopausal women. *J Clin Endocrinol Metabolism* 1995;80(5):1685-1690.

115. Murkies A. Dietary flour supplementation decreases post-menopausal hot flashes: Effect of soy and wheat. *Maturitas* 1995;21(3):189-195.

116. Anthony M. Soybean isoflavones improve cardiovascular risk factors without affecting the reproductive system of peripubertal rhesus monkeys. *J Nutrition* 1996;126:43-50.

117. Grady D. Hormone therapy to prevent disease and prolong life in postmenopausal women. *Ann Internal Med* 1992;117:1016-1037.

118. Meir J. Estrogen: What protection against heart disease? *Contemporary OB/GYN* 1992;37:13-30.

119. Anderson W. Orally dosed genistein from soy and prevention of callcellous bone loss in two ovariectomized rat models. *Am Inst Nutr* 1995;799S.

120. Tsutsumi N. Effect of coumestrol on bone metabolism in organ culture. *Biol Pharmaceutical Bull* 1995;18:1012-1015.

121. Kawashima K. Effect of KCA-098 on the function of osteoblast-like cells and the formation of TRAP-positive multinucleated cells in a mouse bone marrow cell population. *Biochem Pharmacol* 1996;51:133-139.

122. Jarry H. Studies on the endocrine effects of the contents of *Cimicifuga racemosa:* 1. Influence on the serum concentration of pituitary hormones in ovariectomized rats. *Planta Medica* 1985;46:46-49.

123. Jarry H. Studies on the endocrine effects of the contents of *Cimicifuga racemosa*: 2. *In vitro* binding of compounds to estrogen receptors. *Planta Medica* 1985;46:316-319.

124. Lehmann-Willenbrock V. Clinical and endocrinologic examinations about therapy of climacteric symptoms following hysterectomy with remaining ovaries. *Zent Bl Gynakol* 1988;110:611-618.

125. Mowery D. *The Scientific Validation of Herbal Medicine.* New Canaan, CT, Keats Publishing, 1986:111-112.

126. Challem J. Natural progesterone. *Natural Health* 1997;27:124.

127. Turan I. Natural substance in psychiatry (ginkgo biloba in dementia). *Psychopharmacol Bull* 1995;31:147-158.

128. Kanowski S. Proof of efficacy of the *Ginkgo biloba* special extract Egb 761 in outpatients suffering from mild to moderate primary degenerative dementia of the Alzheimer type or multi-infarct dementia. *Pharmacopsychiatry* 1996;29:47-56.

129. Duverger D. Effects of repeated treatments with an extract of ginkgo biloba (Egb 761) on cerebral glucose utilization in the rat: An antoradiographic study. *Gen Pharmac* 1995;26:1375-1383.

130. Smith P. The neuroprotective properties of the Ginkgo biloba leaf: A review of the possible relationship to platelet-activating factor (PAF). *J Ethnopharmacol* 1996;50:131-139.

131. Allain H. Effect of two doses of ginkgo biloba extracts (Egb 761) on the dual coding test in elderly subjects. *Clinical Therapeutics* 1993;3:549-558.

132. Rapin J. Demonstration of the "anti-stress" activity of an extract of ginkgo biloba (Egb 761) using discrimination learning task. *Gen Pharmac* 1994;25:1009-1016.

133. Petkov V. Memory effects of standardized extracts of *Panax ginseng* (G115), *Ginkgo biloba* (GK 501) and their combination Gincosan (PHL-00701). *Planta Medica* 1993;59-106-114.

134. Kleijnen J. *Ginkgo biloba* for cerebral insufficiency. *Brit J Clin Pharmacol* 1992;34:352-356.

135. Holgers K. *Ginkgo biloba* extract for the treatment of tinnitus. *Audiology* 1994;33:85-92.

136. Smith P. Can vestibular compensation be enhanced by drug treatment? *J Vestibular Res* 1994;4:169-179.

137. Maitra I. Peroxyl radical scavenging activity of *Ginkgo biloba* extract Egb 761. *Biochem Pharmacol* 1995;49:1649-1655.

138. Joyeux M. Comparative antilipoperoxidant, antinecrotic and scavenging properties of terpenes and biflavones from *Ginkgo* and some flavonoids. *Planta Medica* 1995;61:126-129.

139. Oyama Y. *Ginkgo biloba* extract protects brain neurons against oxidative stress induce by hydrogen peroxide. *Brain Res* 1996;712:349-352.

140. Shen J. Efficiency of *Ginkgo biloba* extract (Egb 761) in antioxidant protection against myocardial ischemia and reperfusion injury. *Biochemistry Mol Biol International* 1995;35:125-134.

141. Jassens D. Protection of hypoxia-induced ATP decrease in endothelial cells by ginkgo biloba extract and bilobalide. *Biochemical Pharmacol* 1995;50:991-999.

142. Belougne E. Experimental thrombosis model induced by laser beam. Application of aspirin and an extract of *Ginkgo biloba*: Egb 761. *Thrombosis Res* 1996;82:453-458.

143. Mouren X. Study of the antischemic action of Egb 761 in the treatment of peripheral arterial occlusive disease by Tc P02 determination. *Angiology* 1994;45:413-417.

144. Rowin J. Spontaneous bilateral subdural hematomas associated with chronic *Ginkgo biloba* ingestion. *Neurology* 1996;46:1175-1776.

Chapter 16

Specific Toxicologic Considerations of Selected Herbal Products

Lucinda G. Miller, PharmD, BCPS
Wallace J. Murray, PhD

INTRODUCTION

Not all major drug-herb interactions fell within the categories developed for this textbook. Hence, we have undertaken to review a potpourri of selected herbal products with known or potential interactions or adverse sequelae that should be known to the practicing clinician. For interactions that are not included in this chapter or elsewhere in the textbook, the reader is directed to tap his or her own expertise in clinical matters, pharmacology, and the many general herb textbooks. Such an approach should allow the clinician to adeptly ascertain the causal relationship, if any, between adverse sequelae and drug/herb therapy. As always, the reader is encouraged to help sort through this burgeoning area with submissions of case reports and other data relevant to the medical literature.

CASE STUDY 1: SHANKHAPUSHPI

JV is a 38-year-old man with a 22-year history of tonic-clonic seizures. He has been controlled with phenytoin 400 mg/ day with an average blood level of 11 mg/dl during this time. JV is in a motor vehicle accident (MVA) and arrives at the emergency room (ER) stating the MVA was preceded by a blackout, but JV suspects he had a seizure. Ambulance attendants concur, stating JV appeared postictal when they arrived at the scene. When you question JV regarding possible causes for this seizure, it becomes apparent that he has been compliant with his phenytoin and has not started any other medications, either prescription or over-the-counter, nor drugs of abuse (additionally his tox screen is negative in the ER). When you question him regarding any herbal medications, he admits that he recently began Shankhapushpi. His phenytoin level now is 6 mg/dl in the ER. How do you interpret JV's phenytoin level and breakthrough seizure in the context of his herb use?

Discussion

Shankapushpi (SRC) is an Ayurvedic preparation marketed as a nonalcoholic antiepileptic syrup.[1] It is a combination of six plants:

1. *Convolvulus pluricaulis* Chois.; leaves
2. *Centella asiatica* Urban; whole plant
3. *Nardostachys jatamansi* DC; rhizome
4. *Nepeta hinostana* Haines; whole plant
5. *Nepeta elliptica* Royle; whole plant
6. *Onosma bracteatum* Wall; leaves and flowers

The first three ingredients, specifically, have been associated with anticonvulsant activity.[2-4] In the recommended dose of one teaspoonful three times daily, it has been associated with loss of seizure control and a decrease in phenytoin levels in two patients.[1] Phenytoin plasma levels 30 and 60 minutes after a single dose of SRC were not altered, but phenytoin levels were significantly lower following five days of administration of SRC.[1] Induction of hepatic microsomal enzyme induction by SRC has been proposed but bear in mind that most hepatic enzymes are maximally stimulated already by phenytoin.[1,5] It is questionable if SRC could significantly further stimulate these enzymes; hence further study is needed to elucidate the underlying mechanism of action. However, prudence dictates avoidance of SRC in patients adequately stabilized with phenytoin, as concomitant administration may result in loss of seizure control.

CASE STUDY 2: GOSSYPOL

AS is a 25-year-old male of Asian descent. He reports having begun use of gossypol as an antifertility drug one month ago. He now presents to the family medicine clinic with muscle weakness, fatigue, and malaise. His potassium level in the clinic is 3.2 mEq/L. Would you advise potassium supplementation or triamterene for this patient?

Discussion

Gossypol is a male contraceptive known to lower serum potassium.[6] Although not approved in the United States as a contraceptive, it is available in China. Triamterene, acting directly on the distal renal tubule of the nephron, blocks excretion of potassium.[7] Triamterene is often used with hydrochlorothiazide for hypertension (e.g., Dyazide). Potassium serum levels in patients administered gossypol versus triamterene 50 mg/day were not significantly different (serum potassium levels decreased 0.062 mEq/l and 0.11 mEq/l, respectively).[8] Additionally, when compared to gossypol plus potassium 1.5 g daily, again serum potassium levels were unaffected (serum potassium levels decreased 0.056 mEq/l).[8] However, this has been disputed in other studies where potassium supplementation was effective.[9,10] A general decline in potassium levels, which may attain a hypokalemic state, may occur with gossypol use and this cannot be consistently prevented with the use of potassium supplementation or triamterene. It will be necessary to understand the underlying mechanism of gossypol-induced potassium loss before treatment or prevention strategies can be devised. AS should be advised to avoid drugs that can also cause hypokalemia, which would exaggerate gossypol's effects (e.g., hydrochlorothiazide).

CASE STUDY 3: NSAIDs

AS sustained an ankle injury while jogging and is self-medicating with ibuprofen approaching doses of 1,800 mg/day. He now complains of anorexia, nausea, and weight loss of three pounds. Is this being caused by gossypol, ibuprofen, or both?

Discussion

Nonsteroidal anti-inflammatory drugs (NSAIDs) are well known for causing gastrointestinal distress.[11,12] Even though low-dose ibuprofen appears to be associated with the least risk, when taken in higher doses, such as AS is, for long enough periods of time, any NSAID can cause gastrointestinal side effects. Of additional concern for AS is the concomitant intake of gossypol. Gossypol has been associated with tissue congestion, mucosal sloughing, mucosal necrosis, and hemorrhage of the intestinal wall.[13] This can result in anorexia and weight loss. While enteric-coated preparations of gossypol have been tried, both the systemic side effects and the antifertility activity were diminished.[10] AS would be well-advised to avoid concomitant use of drugs known to irritate the gastrointestinal tract such as NSAIDs (e.g., naproxen, fenoprofen, indomethacin, diclofenac).

CASE STUDY 4: ANEMIA

One and one-half years later, AS is again seen in the clinic, referred from the blood bank. He was not allowed to donate blood as he was found to be anemic. AS reports continued fatigue now accompanied by dizziness. He has continued gossypol use. In the clinic today, you find his iron level to be 40 mcg/dl (normal: 50 to 160 mcg/dl) with a hemoglobin of 8 g/dl (normal 14 to 18 g/dl). What is the cause and do you recommend iron supplementation?

Discussion

Gossypol is the most likely cause of AS's iron-deficiency anemia. Gossypol chelates iron in the gastrointestinal tract and in the liver.[14] Additionally, gossypol inhibits oxygen release from hemoglobin, which is probably contributing to AS's symptoms of fatigue and dizziness.[14] While iron replenishment would seem the logical course, it is unknown how much iron will be needed before gossypol's chelation ability is overwhelmed. Furthermore, AS should not continue gossypol use beyond two years in order to avoid permanent infertility.[14] Hence, AS is approaching the end of the duration of reversible usefulness of gossypol and should be advised to employ alternative contraceptives. In so doing, continued iron deficiency can be resolved and intermediate supplementation can be instituted as necessary. AS should be advised to avoid other herbs known to inhibit iron absorption such as burdock, huckleberries, red raspberries, and yarrow.

CASE STUDY 5: HAWTHORN

KK is a 62-year-old man diagnosed with congestive heart failure. His general internist placed him on digoxin 0.25 mg/day with a resulting serum level of 1.0 ng/ml (normal: 0.8 to 2.0 ng/ml). KK begins hawthorn after consulting with an herbalist and reports less edema and improved exercise tolerance. Are there any known or potential interactions between hawthorn and digoxin?

Discussion

Hawthorn berries *(Crataegus oxyacanthia)* are considered a nutritional tonic for the heart.[15] It has also been advocated for atherosclerosis, angina, rheumatism, liver problems, and congestive heart disease.[15] Studies have shown hawthorn to dilate blood vessels away from the heart, lowering blood pressure and reducing the heart's work load.[16,17] Purportedly, hawthorn can potentiate the action of digoxin.[15] No data exists, however, to refute or substantiate this claim. It is unknown if the interaction is pharmacokinetic or pharmacodynamic in nature. Given the paucity of data, at best, one can advise caution with concomitant use and to obtain digoxin serum levels judiciously to avoid toxicity with this narrow therapeutic window drug.

CASE STUDY 6: ELEVATED DIGOXIN LEVEL

At KK's next routine office visit three months later he states he is feeling fine but his digoxin serum level is 2.5 ng/ml. KK is not taking any other medications and has normal renal and hepatic function. KK however denies anorexia, nausea, vomiting, diarrhea, headache, weakness, drowsiness or visual disturbances (specifically blurred yellow vision with a halo effect). His heart rate is normal as is his EKG. He is not taking any other medications. What herbs should you question him about that may have this effect on digoxin levels?

Discussion

KK has an elevated digoxin level but does not have any symptoms suggestive of digoxin toxicity. Anorexia, nausea, vomiting or diarrhea, headache, weakness, drowsiness or visual disturbances (specifically blurred yellow vision with a halo effect) would be expected with an elevated digoxin level. Ventricular tachycardia, unifocal and multiform premature ventricular contractions, AV dissociation and accelerated junctional (nodal) rhythm also occur in digoxin toxicity but are absent in KK. Nonspecific arrhythmias have been estimated to occur in 80 to 90 percent of patients with digoxin toxicity and may be the only manifestation of the toxicity.[18] Neither does KK have abnormal renal or hepatic function, which has been demonstrated to affect digoxin levels.[19,20] A considerable number of drugs interact with digoxin such as erythromycin, quinidine, alprazolam, amiodarone, calcium channel blockers, captopril, and propafenone but KK is not taking any of these medications.[21-24] Hence drug-drug interactions would not account for KK's elevated digoxin levels. The following herbs reputedly contain cardiac glycosides and hence could possibly interact with digoxin:[25]

- *Adonis vernalis* (adonis, false hellebore, pheasant's eye)
- *Convallaria majalis* (lily of the valley)
- *Cytisus scoparius* (broom)
- *Digitalis lanata* (yellow foxglove)
- *Digitalis purpurea* (purple foxglove)
- Kyushin (Chinese medicine)
- *Leonurus cardiaca* L. (motherwort)
- *Scilla maritima* (white squill)
- *Scrophularia nodosa* L. (figwort)
- *Stropanthus kombe* (strophanthus)

Of these, kyushin is perhaps the best documented in its ability to interfere with digoxin immunoassays. Kyushin contains chan-su, the dried venom of Chinese toad (*Bufo bufo gargarizans* Cantor), known to have digoxin-like activity.[26] The usual dose of kyushin of two tablets three times a day resulted in a digoxin level of 0.4 ng/ml in half a day.[27] One tablet of kyushin has digoxin-like immunoreactivity equivalent to 1.5 to 72 mcg digoxin de-pending on the cross-reactivity of the antibody used in the immunoassay (DuPont Aca V analyzer, Enzymun-Test, Boehringer Mannheim).[27] In this report, the patient taking 0.25 mg digoxin concomitantly with kyushin had a digoxin level of 2.5 ng/ml with no signs or symptoms of digoxin intoxication. Hence, it is possible that while kyushin elevates digoxin levels, this may not correlate with pharmacodynamic potency equivalent to that of digoxin.

CASE STUDY 7: COUMARIN DERIVATIVES

DM is a 45-year-old woman who is using red clover as an herbal remedy for her psoriasis. She takes the liquid extract (1:1 in 25 percent alcohol) 1.5 to 3.0 ml three times daily. Her psoriasis has worsened so she doubled the dose of the extract. She also developed deep venous thromboembolism, was hospitalized, and was treated with heparin. She was discharged on warfarin 10 mg daily. Two days later she complains of bleeding gums and easy bruising on her extremities. Her PT and INR were within the desired range at discharge. How do you explain this?

Discussion

Red clover *(Trifolium pratense)* is used herbally as a dermatologic agent for chronic skin diseases such as eczema and psoriasis. It is also used for whooping cough and as an expectorant. Red clover contains coumarin derivatives, specifically coumarin and medicagol. Hence, it possesses the potential ability to augment warfarin's anticoagulant effect and may account for DM's bleeding gums and easy bruising. A new PT and INR should be obtained for DM. Other herbs containing coumarin derivatives are listed in Table 16.1.

Anticoagulant activity has also been ascribed to brown seaweed although further information documenting the exact nature of this activity is not available.[28] Clinicians should observe caution with concomitant use of warfarin with any of the above-listed herbal medicinals. It is unknown if their effect when given concomitantly is additive, synergistic, or clinically significant. An astute clinician will obtain frequent PT/INRs for patients taking warfarin and the above herbals.

From a nutraceutical viewpoint, broccoli and other foods with a high vitamin K content should be eaten in moderation while a patient is on an anticoagulant. The vitamin K content of some of the more common vegetables is listed below:[29]

- turnip greens   650 mcg/100 g
- broccoli   200 mcg/100 g
- lettuce   129 mcg/100 g
- cabbage   125 mcg/100 g
- spinach   89 mcg/100 g
- green beans   14 mcg/100 g
- potatoes   3 mcg/100 g

Patients ingesting excessive amounts of these vegetables may be perceived as demonstrating warfarin resistance. One such patient was seen in consultation for warfarin "allergy" and resistance who had been treated with heparin followed by warfarin for a pulmonary embolism.[30] Clinicians were unable to maintain her prothrombin time within the therapeutic range. It was discovered that she consumed 230 to 340 g of raw broccoli daily.

Adequate warfarin-mediated coagulation was achieved on a broccoli-free diet for this patient. The ability of vitamin K-rich foods and herbal teas to offset the anticoagulant effects of warfarin must not be overlooked when obtaining a thorough drug history.[31,32]

TABLE 16.1. Herbs Containing Coumarin Derivatives

Herbs containing coumarin derivatives	Comments
alfalfa	May reactivate quiescent SLE; possesses estrogenic activity.
angelica	Large doses may interfere with anticoagulant therapy; concern regarding carcinogenic risk of bergapten content.
aniseed	Large doses may interfere with anticoagulant and MAOI therapy; possesses estrogenic activity.
arnica	Generally used in homeopathic remedies in such small amounts that coumarin content is probably inconsequential.
asafoetida	Large doses may interfere with anticoagulant therapy; related species cause hemorrhages in livestock.
celery	Furanocoumarin constituents may cause photosensitivity.
chamomile, German and Roman	Cross-sensitivity to ragweed; large doses may interfere with anticoagulant therapy.
fenugreek	Large doses may interfere with anticoagulant therapy; high mucilaginous fiber content of fenugreek may inhibit absorption of drugs ingested concomitantly.
horse chestnut	Contains coumarins aesculetin, fraxin, and scopolin (contained in leaves and bark); saponin content may irritate GIT.
melilot	Contains coumarins melilotoside and melilotin.
prickly ash, northern and southern	Anti-inflammatory activity is approximately twenty times less than indomethacin, thought to be mediated in part by inhibition of prostaglandin synthesis; possesses neuromuscular blocking properties.
quassia	Contains coumarin scopoletin; large doses may irritate GIT.

Herbs containing coumarin derivatives	Comments
red clover	Contains coumarin medicagol; possesses estrogenic activity.
sweet woodruff	Contains coumarin in glycoside form, which is freed by enzymatic action during drying process; coumarins not uniformly present in woodruff; unlikely to cause bleeding disorders following normal dietary intake.
tonka beans	Contains 1 to 3 percent coumarin by weight; some strains may contain up to 10 percent; contains coumarin unbelliferone.

CASE STUDY 8: GINKGO BILOBA AND WARFARIN

AR is a 58-year-old man who has experienced recurrent transient ischemic attacks and was placed on warfarin 10 mg/day by his internist. AR also appears to be suffering from some memory loss and, having consulted an herbalist, was recommended to begin ginkgo. He ingests 40 mg three times a day of ginkgo biloba extract. AR reports back to the internist complaining of epistaxis and easy bruising. Is there a potential drug-herb interaction between ginkgo and warfarin?

Discussion

Ginkgo biloba extract (GBE) has been shown to be effective for chronic cerebral insufficiency in 112 patients averaging 70.5 years with significant regression of short-term memory problems, vigilance, and mood disturbances.[33] No drug-herb interactions were noted in these patients, some of whom were also taking cardiac glycosides and antidiabetic medications. Mild adverse reactions associated with ginkgo include gastrointestinal upset and headache.[34] However, GBE has been shown to reduce the clotting time of blood, leading to concern regarding concomitant use with anticoagulants.[35] While this potential interaction has not yet been documented clinically, practitioners should be advised of the possibility and exercise vigilance if given concomitantly.

CASE STUDY 9: KELP AND LEVOTHYROXINE

DL is a 39-year-old woman experiencing weight gain, fatigue, lethargy, and cold intolerance. She visits her local health food store and is advised to begin kelp liquid extract (1:1 in 25 percent alcohol) 4 to 8 ml three times daily to facilitate weight loss. She does lose five pounds and is less fatigued but at the urging of her husband has sought the advice of her internist. He diagnoses hypothyroidism and begins her on levothyroxine 0.125 mg/day. Is there any problem with concomitant administration of levothyroxine with kelp?

Discussion

Kelp generically refers to seaweed species including *Laminaria, Macrocystitis, Nereocystis,* and *Fucus.* It has been used as an antiobesity agent presumably by supplying iodine, hence increasing thyroid hormone production with consequent increased metabolism and removal of fat. Some kelp products contain 0.7 mg iodine per tablet.[37] This product, however, is not without side effects. Hyperthyroidism has been reported in a 72-year-old woman after ingestion of a commercial kelp product for six months.[37] Worsening of preexisting acne and development of new acne-iform eruptions have also been reported with kelp use but will resolve after discontinuation of use.[38] Variable iodine content and arsenic contamination complicate kelp use as well. Even different samples of the same kelp product varied in iodine content, which was at times was present in unsafe levels.[39] Arsenic content ranged from 16 to 58 mcg/g product.[40,41] Kelp and related seaweed products also will typically contain sodium in quantities sufficient to be avoided in hypertensive patients and others who must limit their sodium intake. Additionally, the potassium iodide content may result in hypersensitivity reactions in sensitive patients.[42]

Concomitant use of kelp with levothyroxine could result in excessive replacement resulting in typical symptoms of hyperthyroidism including but not limited to weight loss, sweating, and frequent soft stools. At the very least, it will be difficult to monitor DL's hypothyroidism with thyroid function tests due to the confounding variable of iodine ingested in variable amounts from the kelp product. Using any thyroid hormone-related product to control body weight is inadvisable and should be discouraged. Given this patient's concomitant condition of hypothyroidism, the patient should be advised to avoid kelp use.

CASE STUDY 10: INK CAP MUSHROOM

JR is a 52-year-old man who is the chief executive officer of a Fortune 500 company. He is a mushroom aficionado, and after one of his excursions with his friends sat down to a mushroom and wine-tasting party. After a while he began to experience nausea, vomiting, sweating, facial flushing, throbbing headache, and tachycardia. One of his friends recognizes ink cap *(Coprinus atramentarius)* as one of the mushrooms collected. Could ink cap be responsible for this reaction? What herbal medicinals can cause the same effect?

Discussion

Ingestion of ink cap *(Coprinus atramentarius)* with alcohol gives rise to symptoms resembling those of the alcohol-disulfiram syndrome.[43] Coprine, an unusual amino acid component of ink cap, is metabolized by the body to form cyclopropanone hydrate, which interferes with the function of liver acetaldehyde dehydrogenase.

Coprine   Cyclopropanone hydrate

As acetaldehyde blood concentrations rise flushing, palpitations, dyspnea, hyperventilation, and tachycardia occur within one-half to two hours following ingestion of mushroom and alcohol. Vomiting and diarrhea are usually absent. Recovery is generally spontaneous and uncomplicated, though severe cases may require gastric lavage and symptomatic care.

Kudzu, a fast-growing vine native to Asia, now proliferates in the southern United States. In China extracts of kudzu have been used in the management of alcoholism.[44] Isoflavones in kudzu have been found to be potent inhibitors of alcohol and aldehyde dehydrogenases with much the same profile as the allopathic medicinal disulfiram.

CASE STUDY 11: SALICYLATES

ER is a 24-year-old woman who presents to her gynecologist with menometrorrhagia. She also reports epistaxis and melena in the past three months. She reports nausea and anorexia and appears lethargic. She has a history of juvenile rheumatoid arthritis, which she states is now in remission. She is not taking aspirin, nonsteroidal anti-inflammatory drugs or any other medications. Her hemoglobin was 11.5 g/dl (normal: 12 to 16 g/dl) and her hematocrit was 35 percent (normal: 37 to 47 percent). Gastroscopy indicated bleeding gastric erosions. Her physician feels her symptoms are consistent with mild salicylism. Which herbs could be implicated?

Discussion

White willow *(Salix alba)*, other willow species, and poplar *(Populus tremuloides)* are trees whose bark has an appreciable content of salicylates. The bark of both trees are used for their anti-inflammatory, antirheumatic, and antipyretic effects. The principal salicylate constituent of willow is salicin. Salicin is hydrolyzed by the acid of the stomach to saligenin and glucose. Once absorbed, saligenin is probably metabolically converted to salicylic acid, which is responsible for the anti-inflammatory, antirheumatic, and antipyretic effects. Salicin lacks the carboxylic acid and phenol functional groups and so is not irritating to the GI tract as are salicylic acid or aspirin.[45]

Salicin → $C_6H_{12}O_6$ + Saligenin $\xrightarrow{[O]}$ Salicylic Acid

Meadowsweet *(Filipendula ulmara)*, an herbal medicine used traditionally for atonic dyspepsia, has salicylates as part of its volatile oil fraction (salicylaldehyde, forming 70 percent of the volatile oil, methyl salicylate and salicin).[46] Thus, the precautions usually recommended for salicylates should pertain to the use of meadowsweet as well.

See Table 16.2 for a summary of this chapter's material.

TABLE 16.2. Summary

Shankhapushpi	An Ayurvedic preparation has decreased phenytoin levels resulting in seizures.
Gossypol	Causes hypokalemia; should not be used concomitantly with hydrochlorothiazide; may irriate GIT, hence should not be used with other GI irritants (e.g., NSAIDs); chelates iron enough to cause anemia.
Hawthorn	Purported to have vasodilatory properties; ill-advised to use with other cardiac drugs (e.g., digoxin).
Kyushin	May interfere with digoxin assays; other herbs may contain cardiac glycosides (e.g., false hellebore, lily of the valley, motherwort), which may interfere with digoxin both pharmacodynamically and pharmacokinetically.
Red clover	Contains coumarin derivatives with potential ability to augment warfarin's anticoagulant effect; many other herbs purportedly contain coumarion derivatives as well (e.g., alfalfa, fenugreek, tonka beans).
Ginkgo biloba	Has reduced blood clotting time; should be avoided in patients with coagulatin disorders and those requiring anticoagulant therapy.
Kelp	Some kelp products contain 0.7 mg iodine/tablets; may also contain arsenic; salt content enough to be problematic in hypertensive patients; avoid concomitant use with thyroid replacement therapies (e.g., levothyroxine).
Ink cap	May induce disulfiram-type reaction if taken concomitantly with alcohol or alcohol-containing products; also true of kudzu.
White willow	Contains appreciable salicylate content; may encounter additive effects if used concomitantly with other salicylates.

REFERENCES

1. Dandekar UP, Chandra RS, Dalvi SS. Analysis of a clinically important interaction between phenytoin and Shankhapushpi, an Ayurvedic preparation. *J Ethnopharmacol* 1992;35:285-288.

2. Arora RB. Pharmacological actions of Jatamansi. In: Arora RB, Ed., *Nardostachys Jatamansi: A Chemical, Pharmacological and Clinical Appraisal.* Indian Council of Medical Research, Delhi, 1965;36-37.

3. Zaheer H, Prasad B, Chopra RN, Deshprabhu SB. *Centella asiatica.* In: Sastri BN, Ed., *Wealth of India, Publication and Information Directorate,* North Delhi, Council of Scientific and Industrial Research, 1966;2:116-118.

4. Satyavati GV. *Convolvulus Pluricaulis.* In: Satyavati GV, Raina MK, Sharma M, Eds., *Medicinal Plants of India,* Volume I. Delhi, 1976;1:276.

5. Miller LG. Cigarettes and drug therapy: Pharmacokinetic and pharmacodynamic considerations. *Clin Pharm* 1990;9:125-135.

6. Liu GZ, Lyle KC, Cao L. Clinical trial of gossypol as a male contraceptive drug. Part I. Efficacy study. *Fertil Steril* 1987;48:459-461.

7. McEvoy GK, Ed., *AHFS Drug Information,* Bethesda, MD: American Society of Health-System Pharmacists, 1996;1935.

8. Liu GZ, Ch'iu-Hinton K, Cao J, Zhu C, Li B. Effects of K salt or a potassium blocker on gossypol-related hypokalemia. *Contraception* 1988;37:111-117.

9. Wu DF. An overview of the clinical pharmacology and therapeutic potential of gossypol as a male contraceptive agent and in gynecological disease. *Drugs* 1989;38:333-341.

10. Qian SZ, Wang ZG. Gossypol: A potential antifertility agent for males. *Ann Rev Pharmacol Toxicol* 1984;24:329-360.

11. Miller LG, Prichard JG. Selecting nonsteroidal anti-inflammatory drugs: Pharmacologic and clinical considerations. *J Am Board Fam Practice* 1989;2:257-271.

12. Henry D, Lim LL, Rodriquez LA, et. al., Meta-analysis: Low-dose ibuprofen has the lowest gastrointestinal risk of any NSAID. *BMJ* 1996;312:1563-1566.

13. Waller DP, Zaveveld LJD, Farnsworth NR. Gossypol: Pharmacology and current status as a male contraceptive. In: Wagner H, Hikino H, Farnsworth NR, Ed., *Economic and Medicinal Plant Research.* London: Academic Press, 1985;87-112.

14. Woerdenbag HJ. Gossypol. In: DeSmet PAGM, Keller K, Hansel R, Chandler RF, Eds., *Adverse Effects of Herbal Drugs,* Berlin: Springer-Verlag, 1993;2:195-208.

15. Mowery DB. Heart. In: Mowery DB, Ed., *The Scientific Validation of Herbal Medicine,* New Canaan, CT: Keats Publishing, Inc., 1986;135-143.

16. Ullsperger R. Preliminary communication concerning a coronary vessel dilating principle from hawthorn. *Pharmazie* 1951;6:141-144.

17. Hammerl H, Kranzl C, Pichler O, Studlar M. Clinical and experimental investigations on metabolism with an extract of Crataegus. *Aerztliche Forschung* 1967;21:261-270.

18. Kelly R, Smith T. Recognition and management of digitalis toxicity. *Am J Cardiol* 1992;69:180G.

19. Graves SW, Brown B, Valdes R. An endogenous digoxin-like substance in patients with renal impairment. *Ann Intern Med* 1983;99:604-608.

20. Rosenkranz B, Frolich JC. Falsely elevated digoxin concentrations in patients with liver disease. *Ther Drug Monit* 1985;7:202-206.

21. Maragno I, Gianotti C, Tropeano PF, et al., Verapamil-induced changes in digoxin kinetics in cirrhosis. *Eur J Clin Pharmacol* 1987;32:309-311.

22. Nademanee K, Kannan R, Hendrickson J, Ookhtens M, Kay I, Singh BN. Amiodarone-digoxin interaction: Clinical significance, time course of development, potential pharmacokinetic mechanisms and therapeutic implications. *JACC* 1984;4:111-116.

23. North DS, Mattern AL, Hiser WW. The influence of diltiazem hydrochloride on trough serum digoxin concentrations. *Drug Intell Clin Pharm* 1986;20:500-503.

24. Fichtl B, Doering W. The quinidine-digoxin interaction in perspective. *Clin Pharmacokinet* 1983;8:137-154.

25. D'Arcy PF. Adverse reactions and interactions with herbal medicines. *Adverse Drug React Toxicol Rev* 1993;12:147-162.

26. Suga T. Chemistry and pharmacology of Chan-su, Taisha. *Chin Med* 1973; Suppl 10:762-773.

27. Fushimi R, Tachi J, Amino N, Miyai K. Chinese medicine interfering with digoxin immunoassays. *Lancet* 1989;i:339.

28. Whistler RL, Ed. *Industrial Gums,* Second edition. New York: Academic Press, 1973;13.

29. Oren B, Shvartzman P. Unsuspected source of vitamin K in patients treated with anticoagulants: A case report. *Fam Pract* 1989;6:151-152.

30. Kempin SJ. Warfarin resistance caused by broccoli. *N Engl J Med* 1983; 317:1229-1230.

31. Wells PS, Holbrook AM, Crowther NR, Hirsh J. Interactions of warfarin with drugs and food. *Ann Intern Med* 1994;121:676-683.

32. Hogan RP. Hemorrhagic diathesis caused by drinking an herbal tea. *JAMA* 1983;249:2679-2680.

33. Vorberg G. Ginkgo biloba extract: A long-term study on chronic cerebral insufficiency in geriatric patients. *Clin Trials J* 1985;22:149-157.

34. Pizzorno JE, Murray MT. *A Textbook of Natural Medicine.* Seattle, WA: John Bastyr College Publications, 1985.

35. Tyler VE. Ginkgo. In: *The Honest Herbal,* Binghamton, NY: The Haworth Press, 1993;149-151.

36. Bisset NG, Ed., *Max Wichtl's Herbal Drugs and Phytopharmaceuticals: A Handbook for Practice on a Scientific Basis.* Boca Raton, FL: CRC Press 1989: 212-213.

37. Shilo S, Hirsch HJ. Iodine-induced hyperthyroidism in a patient with a normal thyroid gland. *Postgrad Med J* 1986;62:661-662.

38. Harrell BL, Rudolph AH. Kelp diet: A cause of acneiform eruption. *Arch Dermatol* 1976;112:560.

39. Norman JA. Human intake of arsenic and iodine from seaweed-based food supplements and health food available in the UK. *Food Additives Contaminants* 1987;5:103-109.

40. Walkiw O, Douglas DE. Health food supplements prepared from kelp—a source of elevated urinary arsenic. *Can Med Assoc J* 1974;111:1301-1302.

41. Walkiw O, Douglas DE. Health food supplements prepared from kelp—a source of elevated urinary arsenic. *Clin Toxicol* 1975;8:325-331.

42. Tyler VE. Kelp. In: In: *The Honest Herbal,* Binghamton, NY: The Haworth Press, 1993;189-191.

43. Tyler VE, Brady LR, Robbers JE. *Pharmacognosy,* Ninth Edition, Baltimore, MD: Lea and Febiger, 1988;453-454.

44. Hagemann RC, Ed., *Lawrence Review of Natural Products,* St. Louis: Facts and Comparisons, 1996

45. Meier B et al. Pharmaceutical aspects of the use of willows in herbal remedies. *Planta Med* 1988;54:559-560.

46. Barnaulov OD et al. Chemical composition and primary evaluation of the properties of preparations from *Filipendula ulmaria* (L.) Maxim flowers. *Rastit Resur* 1977;13:661-669.

NOTICE TO THE READERS FROM THE EDITORS

After reading this book, the reader is most likely left wondering why standardization, adequate safety, and efficacy regulations are not in place for herbal medicinals in the United States. The following chapter by Mark Blumenthal of the American Botanical Council and Loren Israelsen of LDI Group succinctly outlines the history of herbal regulations to date, resulting in the Dietary Supplement Health and Education Act of 1994 (DSHEA). Certainly, it would be considered inappropriate for such legislation (i.e., DSHEA) to be applied to prescription and over-the-counter drugs. Yet, this is allowed for herbal medicinals. This chapter does not necessarily represent the view of the editors or other chapter authors. It does provide the reader with a flavor of how contentious this issue has become.

Chapter 17

The History of Herbs
in the United States:
Legal and Regulatory Perspectives

Mark Blumenthal
Loren D. Israelsen, JD

INTRODUCTION

A review of the history of the regulation of herbs in the United States reveals that, unlike some other industrialized nations (e.g., Germany, France), there are no specific laws or policies that deal exclusively with herbs and botanical products. Prior to the passage of the DSHEA—landmark legislation passed as a result of widespread consumer concern about continued availability of herbs, vitamins, and related products—herbs were variously regulated as drugs (both prescription and nonprescription), food additives, and foods. Though traditionally used as drugs, herbal products are generally unable to pass the stringent requirements imposed by the FDA for new drugs. Thus, they have been sold as foods without medical claims.

The relationship of the herb industry with the FDA has been difficult in the past twenty-five years. This has been characterized as being due to at least three factors: (1) The FDA has known very little about herbs and related botanical products; (2) the pattern of usage for many herbs is often derived from other cultures where there has been a "health" use that does not fit into the conventional Western view of these matters; and (3) the industry itself has created some of the problems, being led in the early years by people who knew very little about the FDA and the laws it enforced, thus often causing "needless confrontations."[1] In the opinion of a former FDA attorney:

the import detentions of herbal products instituted by FDA, the warning letters issued, and the lawsuits, directed at both products and companies, have been disproportionate to the size of this industry. Many seem to have been brought not because of any genuine need to protect public health or pocketbook but rather to advance novel legal arguments in order to simply harass this industry either into submission or extinction. The food additive provisions of the Food, Drugs and Cosmetic Act (FDCA) have been an especially abused tool.[1]

DEFINITION OF HERB

There is no provision that specifically defines the word "herb" in any federal legislation or FDA regulations. The current legislation that governs the marketing and sale of herbal products in the United States is DSHEA, where herbs are classed as "dietary supplements." In this law dietary supplements are defined as either a vitamin, a mineral, "an herb or other botanical," an amino acid, "a dietary substance for use by man to supplement the diet by increasing the total dietary intake," or "a concentrate, metabolite, constituent, extract, or combination of any ingredient described" previously.[2] Although DSHEA deals with herbs and botanicals, they are not specifically defined in the law.

Herbs can be defined generally in commerce as a plant, plant part, or extract thereof used for flavor, fragrance, or medicinal purposes. This definition, adopted by the Herb Trade Association around 1976, represents a practical, commercial reality. This definition is broader than the definition of herb used in botany, which refers to a plant whose stem dies back in winter, compared to a shrub or tree—plants whose stems or trunks maintain their general erectness and shape throughout the year. In pharmacy and pharmacognosy (the study of drugs of natural origin), the term herb refers to the aerial or aboveground part of a plant. This definition is especially useful when defining a plant used in medicine to distinguish it from other plant parts that may also be used as medicines, such as the root, rhizome, bark, leaf, flower, seed, or fruit.

The World Health Organization (WHO) has provided a more exact definition of "herbal medicines"[3]:

> Finished, labelled medicinal products that contain as active ingredients aerial or underground part or parts of plants, or other plant material, or combinations thereof, whether in crude state or as plant preparations. Plant material includes juices, gums, fatty oils, essential oils, and any other substances of this nature. Herbal medicines may contain excipi-

ents in addition to the active ingredients. Medicines containing plant material combined with chemically defined active substances, including chemically defined, isolated constituents of plants, are not considered to be herbal medicines. (p. 17)

This latter definition distinguishes an herbal medicine from a "plant-derived drug"—a single isolated chemical constituent of the plant, such as atropine from belladonna leaves *(Atropa belladonna)*, colchicine from the bulb of the autumn crocus *(Colchicum autumnale)*, quinine from the bark of the cinchona tree *(Cinchona* spp.), and reserpine from Indian snakeroot *(Rauwolfia serpentina)*. Herbs and herbal medicines (recently referred to as phytomedicines) contain the complex chemistry of the whole plants or plant parts used as the remedy as compared to single drugs derived from plants. As stated, there is no such distinction or definition in federal statutes.

EARLY LAWS REGULATING
FOODS AND DRUGS IN THE UNITED STATES

The laws affecting the sale of foods and medicines in the United States derive from colonial times. As early as 1652 the Massachusetts Bay Colony began to regulate potential fraud by standardizing the sizes of bread loaves. The state of Massachusetts passed the first comprehensive law dealing with food adulteration and safety, the Act Against Selling Unwholesome Provisions of 1875. Concern over protecting the public from misbranding and adulteration was reflected by passage of the Food and Drug Act of 1906, the first national legislation intended to deal with such issues.[4] Although this law was founded on good intentions, it did not carry adequate means of regulation and enforcement. Thus, after the sulfanilamide tragedy of 1937 (when a sulfa drug containing an unsafe additive similar to automobile antifreeze killed over 100 people), public outrage prompted Congress to pass the Food, Drug, and Cosmetic Act of 1938 (FDCA), which is still the primary body of legislation dealing with foods and drugs, as amended periodically.[5] The FDCA gave the FDA new authority and powers of criminal prosecution, seizure, and injunction.[6]

HERBS AS DRUGS IN THE USP

Initially, most medicinal herbs were considered remedies and traditional medicines in the United States. These included herbs brought over from Europe by colonists as well as the native botanicals used by North American Indians. The first edition of the *United States Pharmacopoeia* (USP), published in 1820, contained at least 207 botanical substances officially recognized as drugs. Herbal drugs included common foods such as prunes *(Prunus domestica)* and raisins *(Vitis vinifera)*, plus spices such as black pepper *(Piper nigrum)*, cinnamon *(Cinnamomum zeylanicum)*, cloves *(Eugenia caryophillata* syn. *Syzygium aromaticum)*, garlic *(Allium sativum)*, and ginger *(Zingiber officinale)*, as well as other relatively well-known medicinal herbs such as hops *(Humulus lupulus)*, licorice *(Glycyrrhiza glabra)*, peppermint *(Mentha piperita)*, senna *(Cassia senna)*, and valerian root *(Valeriana officinalis)*, among many others.[7]

By 1936, the number of vegetable-based ingredients that were still official had dwindled to seventy-nine. When the twenty-second revision was published in 1990, the number had dropped to only twenty-six vegetable ingredients. Those still official include aloe *(Aloe vera* and related species), belladonna leaf *(Atropa belladonna)*, foxglove leaf *(Digitalis purpurea)*, cascara sagrada *(Rhamnus purshiana)*, and castor *(Ricinus communis)*. Belladonna and foxglove, though officially recognized as drugs, are not sold commercially as herbal medicines or "dietary supplements" due to their relative toxicity.

1938 FOOD, DRUG, AND COSMETIC ACT

Definition of Drug

The FDCA defines "drug" as[5]

(a) articles recognized in the official United States Pharmacopoeia, official Homeopathic Pharmacopoeia of the United States, or official National Formulary [now part of the USP], . . . and (b) articles *intended for use* in the diagnosis, treatment, or prevention of disease in man or other animals; and (c) articles *(other than food) intended to affect the structure or function* of the body of man or other animals. . . . (p. 551, emphasis added)

Intended Use

Inasmuch as most herbs that were formerly official in the USP were deleted due to lack of use by 1936, when the FDCA was passed in 1938 most herbs in general use by the public in the United States no longer enjoyed official status as USP drugs. From a regulatory perspective herbs were in a regulatory "twilight zone"—being used for health purposes but no longer recognized as medicines. The key concept used by FDA and the courts in the intervening years has been "intended use."[6]

> Courts have classified as "drugs" many products not ordinarily thought of as drugs due to the manufacturer's or seller's intended use of the products. Examples include mineral water, honey, and vitamin and mineral capsules. The United States Supreme Court has explicitly determined that Congress intended a broader definition of drug than the ordinary medical one for the purposes of the FDCA. (p. 551)

Thus, intended use can be determined by review of labels, advertising, and promotional claims whether directly tied to the product or distributed separately. Accordingly, until passage of DSHEA herbs and herbal preparations, when sold as foods, could not make any direct or indirect claims for therapeutic or preventive health effects, lest they be considered misbranded or unapproved drugs.

The FDCA contained no provision to define the effectiveness of a drug. FDA was responsible for monitoring the drug safety and it incorporated[6] "a notion of effectiveness into its safety determination. Since no drug is absolutely safe, safety decisions were based on a comparison of benefits to risks. The burden was on the government to prove lack of safety" (p. 579).

1962 HARRIS-KEFAUVER AMENDMENT

After the thalidomide tragedy of 1961 in which children in Europe were born with birth defects attributed to the use of a new synthetic, nonherbal sedative, Congress responded with the 1962 Drug Amendments.[8] "Ironically, the thalidomide disaster was caused by a lack of safety, not effectiveness. Thalidomide was recognized as an effective sedative, but the FDA had withheld registration of thalidomide due to safety concerns. The new effectiveness criteria would not have changed the status of thalidomide in the United States"[6] (pp. 579-580). The new requirements of 1962 now shifted the burden of proof of proving safety and effectiveness to the manufacturer of a new drug.

As a result, the modern New Drug Application (NDA) was created. In order to protect the public against unsafe drugs (e.g., thalidomide), FDA now requires a stringent premarket approval process to market a substance as a new drug. This process is time-consuming (average about four to seven years or more) and costly (estimates range from $150 to 350 million per drug). Such huge costs require that a company obtain exclusive market rights in order to justify such a large capital investment. Such exclusivity is available from a patent. Most herbs and herbal products are not patentable. Hence, there is little financial incentive for large pharmaceutical firms to conduct the type of research necessary to achieve NDA status.

OVER-THE-COUNTER DRUG REVIEW

Over-the-counter (OTC) medicines are available without a physician's prescription and are generally used for minor, self-diagnosable, self-treatable, and self-limiting conditions. Such conditions include upset stomach, colds and flus, sore muscles, runny nose, headache, constipation, and so on. Many of the ingredients (both herbal and nonherbal) used in OTC drugs have been sold since the turn of the nineteenth century and have never been proven effective by modern scientific methods. They remained on the market for many years and, prior to 1972, were not required to prove efficacy or submit NDAs to maintain their market status.

From 1972 to the present, FDA has been conducting a massive review of all ingredients used in nonprescription (OTC) medicines. One result of this review was the creation of the OTC monographs. Under this system, various expert advisory panels reviewed data on active ingredients in various thera-peutic classes of medicines to determine the ingredient's safety and efficacy. If the ingredient was determined to be generally recognized as safe and effective (GRASE), it was designated as a Category I ingredient. If the panel's review found evidence that the drug was unsafe or ineffective, the expert panel would recommend the ingredient be classed as Category II (unsafe and/or ineffective) and the ingredient would be banned from use in any OTC drug. If the expert panels could not determine safety and efficacy due to lack of adequate information, the ingredient would be classed as Category III. Eventually, when final rules for a particular monograph are published in the *Federal Register,* all Category III ingredients would automat-ically default to Category II and would thus be banned from use in nonpre-scription drugs. This was deemed necessary on the premise that the govern-ment must protect the public from unsafe and/or ineffective drug ingredients and thus cannot allow the sale of substances whose safety and/or efficacy is uncertain (due to lack of adequate information).

If an ingredient receives a Category I designation in an OTC monograph, this is tantamount to approval for safety and efficacy under an NDA. Drugs approved in OTC monographs are not considered "new drugs" and therefore do not require and NDA for marketing. The approval as GRASE:[6]

was intended to be an exception to the new drug approval procedures. Thus, a drug generally recognized as safe and effective is *not* a new drug and arguably should *not* need to meet the strict new drug approval procedures. Ironically, the FDA's interpretation of GRASE and its incorporation into the OTC monograph system has effectively resulted in identical standards for new drugs with NDA status and for GRASE drugs with OTC monograph status. The standard is "safe and effective" as judged by the FDA's own expert panels, based on data submissions by industry applicants. The process of gaining OTC status, therefore, may be as difficult for herbal products as gaining NDA approval. (p. 555)

The inadequacies of this regulatory system with respect to botanicals and other relatively common substances were highlighted in 1989 when the FDA advisory panel on OTC stimulant laxatives ruled that prunes were Category III; panel members were not provided any new human clinical studies that confirmed the safety and efficacy of prunes as a laxative ingredient.[9] Up to that time, some OTC laxatives contained prune powder or prune juice concentrate. When the stimulant laxative monograph was finally published in November 1990, prunes defaulted to Category II and were thus banned. Prunes and prune juice are still allowed to be sold as foods, where the labels of these products do not contain any laxative claims. Fortunately, most American consumers are familiar with the well-known pharmacological effects of prunes and prune juice and thus do not need indications, warnings, and other elements of drug labeling on prune products.

The banning of prunes as a laxative drug ingredient was only part of the story. In the November 7, 1990 publication of final rules for 21 categories of drugs, FDA banned 258 ingredients that were not found to be safe and/or effective.[9] Of these, at least 85 were of herbal or vegetable origin. The OTC review process is done by of experts qualified by training to evaluate drug products. These are usually physicians and pharmacists, trained in the areas of conventional pharmaceuticals; the opinions of persons not considered experts are not included. The conventional pharmaceutical drugs almost invariably contain one single chemical entity (monosubstance). Herbs, on the other hand, always contain multiple chemical constituents, usually at relatively low levels (polysubstance). Thus, the bias of expert panel members is often skewed toward the conventional drug ingredients and away from herbal products. In addition, the herb industry did not submit new clinical studies to the FDA for consideration during this review process. This was due primarily to the small size of the herb industry at that time and the individual companies' general lack of adequate capital to finance the type of studies needed.[9]

EAPC Petitions

To participate in the OTC review process for certain key European phyto-medicines (herbal medicines), a group of European and American companies working through an organization called the European-American Phytomedi-cines Coalition (EAPC) filed a petition with the FDA to open the OTC review to old drugs from Europe that have been sold for a material time and to a material extent.[10,11]

A predicate of the OTC monograph review process in 1972 was that all ingredients included in the process were regarded as old drugs. Old drugs were treated more leniently than new drugs that required an NDA, because old drugs had been on the market in the United States for a material time and to a material extent. The FDA took the position that such status extended only to old drug ingredients sold only in the United States. The EAPC petition attempted to extend this policy to phytomedicines sold in selected Western countries for a material time (at least five years) and to a material extent (at least 10 million doses) in countries that have a well-developed system of pharmacovigilance (adverse reaction reporting system). Thus, the safety of these European phytomedicines was well established by common use in countries where reliable epidemiological data was available.[10]

The EAPC petition was filed July 24, 1992. By fall 1997, more than five years after the filing, the agency had not yet responded. This lack of timely response has given some herbal advocates the impression that the agency (at least those in the drug division (Center for Drug Evaluation and Research, CDER) is really not interested in developing an appropriate mechanism for evaluating herbs as nonprescription drugs, despite occasional statements from some FDA officials that herbs are essentially drugs and should be regulated as such.

In 1994 and 1995, in order to add some substance to the above-referenced petition, the EAPC filed petitions to amend the nighttime sleep-aid mono-graph to include valerian root *(Valeriana officinalis)*[12] and the antiemetic monograph to include the popular herb and spice ginger *(Zingiber offici-nale)*.[13] Both petitions cited the widespread safe and effective use of these common botanical products in Europe as OTC medications, without evidence of adverse reaction reports in countries where pharmacovigilance is routinely established and practiced. Both petitions documented the safety of the two ingredients as well as the efficacy as determined by human clinical trials and registrations as medicines in various Western European countries.[14] To date (fall 1997) FDA has not responded to these two petitions. Thus, prospects appeared dim for obtaining OTC drug status for herbs whose safety and efficacy to treat minor, self-limiting conditions has been well established by both scientific data and empirical use.

The GRAS List and Food Additives

An important number of botanicals were included in the 1958 publication of the GRAS list, a list of botanical ingredients that were deemed "Generally Recognized As Safe." This list was prepared by the Flavor and Extract Manufacturers Association (FEMA), an industry group that had reviewed the relative safety of botanicals as flavorings for alcoholic beverages.

According to the FDCA, a food is adulterated if it "contains any food additive which is unsafe"[5] (p. 500). A food additive is defined as "any substance the intended use of which results or may reasonably . . . result . . . in its becoming a component or otherwise affecting the characteristic of any food" (p. 561). Food additives are presumed to be unsafe unless proven safe; the burden of premarket approval of safety is on the seller or proponent of the ingredient.[6]

In 1958 Congress passed the so-called Delaney Amendment, which gave FDA the power to regulate food additives. This was passed in response to growing concern about the number of chemical ingredients being added to food for technical purposes (preservatives, stabilizers, etc.). Under Delaney, no food could be marketed if it contained an additive that had not been approved by FDA for use in foods.

The first application of Delaney giving food additive status to an herbal product occurred in the Seelect Tea Sassafras case *(United States v. Seelect Tea)*. Research in the late 1950s indicated that safrole, a primary compound in the oil of sassafras, caused cancer in laboratory animals. In 1960 FDA was successful in persuading soft drink manufacturers to abandon the use of oil of sassafras as the primary flavoring in root beer. In the late 1970s FDA seized a shipment of sassafras *(Sassafras albidum)* at the Seelect Tea company, claiming that the herb was a food additive containing a carcinogenic substance that was banned under the Delaney Clause. After several years of legal maneuvering, the company claimed that the herb was no longer fit for human consumption by virtue of its age; the material was destroyed, thus leaving FDA's action against sassafras extant and basically unchallenged.

The Proxmire Amendment

In response to consumer opposition to an apparent attempt by FDA to limit the potencies or combinations of vitamins and minerals, Congress passed what became known as the Rogers-Proxmire Amendment of 1976.[15] While not naming botanicals specifically (the herb industry was in its infancy in 1976 and had not yet developed to the point where its influence in the dietary supplement industry would produce such specific language in industry regulatory initiatives), the amendment defines the scope of foods to which it applies as including foods "supplying a vitamin, mineral, *or other ingredient* [emphasis ours]) for use by man to supplement his diet or by increasing his total dietary intake"[15] (p. 567). Medicinal herbs were deemed to be represented in "other ingredients" and were thus presumed to be given statutory safety under the amendment, despite the fact that they were not specifically stipulated. It was not until 1994 that herbs became specifically exempted from FDA regulation as drugs or food additives with the passage of the DSHEA.

"UNSAFE HERBS" AND "HERBS OF UNDEFINED SAFETY" LISTS

In the mid-1970s FDA began instituting a series of policies concerned with the relative safety of the increasing amount of herbal products being imported into and sold in the United States. As has been stated previously, the agency took the approach that many botanical products were food additives that were deemed unsafe unless proven safe by the importer or seller according to a formal food additive petition. At that time and subsequently, this approach was deemed by industry as an abuse of FDA authority. The issue of food additive status for herbs was remedied in 1994 by passage of DSHEA, which stipulated that FDA could no longer regulate herbs in this manner.

In 1975, in what in retrospect was a misguided attempt to warn industry and the public about the potential adverse effects of unsafe herbs, the FDA banned twenty-seven herbs from commerce by publishing a list of toxic plants and unsafe herbs which it considered too toxic for general sale. This was initially based on an internal memorandum, dated November 19, 1975, from Richard Hollingsworth of the FDA's Division of Toxicology to Curtis Cokar, Division of Regulatory Guidance.[16] Titled "Safe and Unsafe Herbs for Use in Herbal Teas," the memo became de facto FDA policy and was later published as Compliance Policy Guideline (CPG) 7117.04 on October 1, 1980.[17] The memo contained lists of "unsafe" herbs, herbs of "undefined safety," and safe herbs (GRAS or regulated flavors). As a result of the Fmali decision (discussed in the next section) it was subsequently rescinded on July 1, 1986 when FDA abandoned attempts to regulate herbs based on their safety as determined by review of data based solely on use in the United States and publication on such lists. The agency announced that the safety of herbs would be reviewed on a case-by-case basis.[18]

The list of "unsafe" herbs was criticized by botanical experts who pointed out basic errors in taxonomy and other problems. For example, the list contains well-known toxic plants such as hemlock *(Conium maculatum)* and deadly nightshade *(Atropa belladonna)*—herbs that were not sold in commerce in the United States. It also listed St. John's wort *(Hypericum perforatum)*, an herb that achieved phenomenal popularity in the United States in the second half of 1997 due to media stories reporting on clinical studies in Europe which confirm its safety and efficacy as a remedy for mild to moderate depression. St. John's wort had been added to the unsafe herbs list because it is listed in books on poisonous plants as a plant toxic to range livestock that eat large quantities of the herb (known in the Pacific Northwest as Klamath weed) and develop photosensitivity. There virtually no evidence to support such toxicity for reasonable doses in humans, who cannot consume the amounts ingested by sheep and cattle.[19,20]

The FDA also compiled the list of "Herbs of Undefined Safety," a list of herbs whose safety the agency was unable to determine at the time. Included in this list were arrowroot *(Maranta arundinacea),* a common item found in millions of American kitchens, used as a thickener for sauces and gravies, and catnip *(Nepeta cataria),* a relatively mild-acting herb found in various teas, as well as numerous other botanicals in common use at the time, often as household food ingredients.

One of the most controversial actions by FDA in the herbal arena pertains to agency attempts to classify the revered Asian herb ginseng *(Panax ginseng)* as an unsafe food additive. In the late 1970s FDA questioned the inherent safety of commercial ginseng products being imported from Korea and China. This was formalized when FDA issued Import Alert 66-02.[21] This action challenged the GRAS status of ginseng products by suggesting that ginseng was only safe as a water infusion (i.e., as an herbal tea) and that ginseng in any other form was considered unsafe a priori. "The import alert was intended primarily to preclude ingestion of ginseng other than as a water infusion."[22]

For several years after this alert was issued, importers of Chinese or Korean ginseng products labeled them in the country of origin as "ginseng tea capsules" (for products containing dried ginseng powder in gelatin capsules) or "ginseng tea extract" (for hydroalcoholic or semiliquid concentrated extracts, e.g., tinctures and related products). The inherent absurdity of this policy was patently obvious to most observers of the scene during that time and appears to be irrational in retrospect twenty years hence. There were few, if any, substantiated reports of adverse reactions to ginseng products at that time to justify this policy.

In addition to ginseng, FDA also published import alerts on other botanical products, including flaxseed oil/linseed oil *(Linum usitatissimum,* 26-02) and oil of evening primrose (aka EPO, *Oenothera biennis,* 66-04). FDA also enacted Import Bulletins on selfheal flower (*Prunella vulgaris,* 31-B01), Trichosanthis (*Trichosanthes kirilowii,* 54-B06), and the popular stimulant, decongestant herb ma huang or ephedra (*Ephedra sinica,* 66-B62). In most of these cases, FDA's position was that these botanicals were food additives and were thus considered unsafe until their safety was proven by the seller or importer. All the above import alerts, import bulletins, and compliance policy guidelines were lifted by FDA (60FR19579, April 19, 1995) as a consequence of DSHEA, which stipulated that herbs and all other dietary supplements were to be regulated as food additives and were not to be treated as unsafe and removed from the market unless FDA had evidence that the botanical posed a significant hazard to public health (see more about DSHEA in a later section).

FDA LEGAL CASES AND IMPORT ALERTS

Fmali v. Heckler

One of the landmark decisions in the food additive area of regulating herbs occurred in *Fmali v. Heckler,*[23] in which the Fmali Co. of Santa Cruz, California filed an action against the Secretary of Health and Human Services (Margaret Heckler) after FDA seized shipments of a product Fmali was importing from China. The product contained the traditional Chinese fruit schisandra *(Schisandra sinensis),* which the FDA claimed was an unapproved food additive, thus implying that it was unafe. *Fmali* argued that the material was a food. Foods are considered GRAS.

Many foods are grandfathered from FDA oversight as food additives because they were sold in the U.S. market prior to January 1, 1958, when FDA received authority from Congress to regulate additives. An ingredient could be considered GRAS (i.e., safe under conditions for its intended use) through a formal petition to the FDA based on scientific procedures including evaluations by experts qualified by training, or based on the ingredient's *experience based on common use in food.* In the Fmali case the Ninth Circuit court agreed that the FDA had been too narrow in its interpretation of the common use in food exemption by applying a standard of experience only within the United States. The court held that the language of the food additive statute did not limit common use to the United States.[23] One reviewer[6] has written that "The *Fmali* decision has allowed for the continued marketing of exotic traditional medicinal herbal teas and multiple herb preparations as foods, free from FDA 'food additive' challenges" (p. 565). It exempted any single herb in a multiherb formula from food additive status if the safety of the ingredient is demonstrated by use in food prior to 1958.

Black Currant Oil Case

The case of FDA against Traco labs was a watershed decision in the ongoing struggle between the FDA and the herb industry. FDA had become concerned about the proliferation of herbal products containing high amounts of gamma linolenic acid (GLA), an ingredient found in oil of evening primrose seed and black currant seed oil. FDA decided that instead of taking action against each company for what it considered unsubstantiated claims, it would be more cost effective to cut off the source of supply of the ingredients at the port of entry. FDA thus invoked its authority to regulate food additives by declaring black currant seed oil a food additive that had not gone through the premarket approval process. FDA seized and attempted to condemn two drums of the oil being imported by Traco Labs, Inc. in 1991 in a case that was later viewed by the herb industry and the courts as an abuse of the agency's authority.[24]

The agency's position was that because BCO (black currant oil) was being added to a soft gelatin capsule, it was a "food additive"—the gelatin capsule being the "food"—and was therefore unsafe by definition. The agency was unable to produce any evidence of adverse reactions to BCO or evidence that the material posed a public health hazard. The District Court ruled that there was no precedent that a pure substance should be a food additive solely because it is added to a gelatin capsule and determined that BCO was not a food additive. FDA subsequently appealed the case to the Circuit Court of Appeals. The court heard FDA's argument that BCO, if sold in a bottle to be ingested by the spoonful, was a food and thus safe; however, when added to the gelatin capsule, it became a food additive and was thus presumed to be unsafe. The Circuit Court found this logic to be an "Alice-in-Wonderland approach" and ruled in favor of Traco. FDA subsequently attempted to appeal the case to the U.S. Supreme Court but the U.S. Solicitor General (the federal official who argues the government's cases before the Supreme Court) would not take the case.[25]

In a related case *(United States v. 29 Cartons),*[26] FDA attempted to regulate BCO as an unsafe food additive because it was intended to be encapsulated into gelatin capsules. In this case the court concluded that FDA's position constituted a "logical and linguistic stretching" of the distinction between foods and food additives, which was contrary to the overriding goal of the FDA, which is to protect human health. The court concluded that BCO was a food and that FDA had improperly seized the product as an unsafe food additive.[6]

Evening Primrose Oil Case

Although FDA was unsuccessful in regulating BCO as a food additive, it was successful in the case of evening primrose oil (EPO). The oil of evening primrose *(Oenothera biennis)* also contains GLA and is used by consumers and some health practitioners for a variety of nutritional and health purposes. In 1990 FDA had issued an import alert on EPO on the basis that it was an unapproved food additive. In *United States v. 45/194 Kg. Drums of Pure Vegetable Oil (Efamol, Ltd),*[28] FDA was successful in getting the court to uphold food additive status for EPO since the purpose of the oil was to be blended with vitamin E oil; thus, it did not meet the single ingredient criteria of the BCO cases.

Stevia Import Alert

FDA continued to attempt to regulate some herbs under food additive provisions, as was the case of stevia. In 1991 FDA issued an import alert to ban the importation of the herb stevia *(Stevia rebaudiana),* a botanical with a naturally sweet taste that had been used as an ingredient in some herbal teas for its flavor rather than for any pharmacological actions.[29,30] Attempts by the American Herbal Products Association to support the safety of stevia with a comprehensive peer-reviewed safety review conducted by the Herb Research Foundation and Professor Douglas Kinghorn, a world-renowned expert on plant-derived sweeteners, were dismissed by FDA. Despite overwhelming evidence of the safety of stevia and little or no evidence of adverse reactions by users in the United States or in other countries, FDA has still maintained the import alert on this botanical. However, in 1995 FDA dropped the ban on stevia imported *for use as a dietary supplement,* pursuant to provisions of DSHEA (see below); however, stevia still cannot be imported for use as a flavoring ingredient or sweetener.[31,32]

NUTRITION LABELING AND EDUCATION ACT OF 1990

In 1990 the 101st Congress passed the Nutrition Labeling and Education Act of 1990 (NLEA), a law that stipulated changes in the labeling of conventional foods and dietary supplements.[33] One aspect of NLEA was the recognition by Congress that food and diet have a relationship to health and that certain *health claims* should be allowed on conventional food products as well as dietary supplements. Health claims may be loosely defined as a statement regarding the correlation of the consumption of a particular food with the prevention of a major illness or condition. NLEA requires FDA preapproval of health claims according to a standard of "significant scientific agreement." However, FDA stipulated various requirements for herbs and other dietary supplements in order for them to qualify for consideration for health claims to the extent that it became apparent to industry that FDA was intentionally attempting to preclude the ability for herb products to carry health claims.[34]

BOTANICAL INGREDIENT REVIEW

As part of the public comment on NLEA the American Herbal Products Association (AHPA) submitted a document prepared for it by the Herb Research Foundation (HRF) proposing a detailed peer-reviewed system to evaluate the safety and health benefits of botanical dietary supplements that some manufacturers might have submitted to FDA for consideration for a health claim. The proposal, called the Botanical Ingredient Review (BIR),[35] was modeled on a similar process called the Cosmetic Ingredient Review (CIR), in which the cosmetics industry pays for a team of independent academic scientists who review the safety of proposed new cosmetic ingredients. FDA historically has accepted the recommendations of the CIR expert panel.

The BIR proposal recognized that FDA did not have the internal scientific expertise to evaluate the safety of herbal products and that the political climate at the time encouraged reduction of the size of the federal government. The BIR proposed the evaluation of botanicals and stipulated that the recommendations of the BIR expert panel would be authoritative—that is, that if FDA did not agree, the agency would be required to justify its actions. This stipulation was deemed necessary in light of previous experience with the agency on matters such as the stevia import alert when a peer-reviewed safety evaluation by the world's foremost expert on the subject was still deemed inadequate documentation of safety by FDA. The BIR proposal recognized FDA's long-standing bias against herbs.

In November 1991, FDA summarily dismissed the BIR proposal when it published proposed rules on NLEA,[36] saying "Suggestions that the agency delegate the primary responsibility for evaluating the validity of claims for herbs to industry committees are not consistent with this agency's responsibility" (p. 60540). With the agency appearing to be intractable with regard to meaningful scientific dialog with industry, and with the FDA proposing more limiting regulations in 1992, herb and other dietary supplement industry leaders approached various members of Congress to seek legislative relief. Several years later this resulted in the eventual proposal of several pieces of legislation and the eventual passage of DSHEA.

DIETARY SUPPLEMENT HEALTH AND EDUCATION ACT OF 1994

In 1993 Senator Orrin Hatch introduced legislation that contained some of the elements of the Health Freedom Act of 1992 but also incorporated many additional aspects that reflected concerns of other congress-persons from the previous year's debate on the Health Freedom Act. The Dietary Supplement Health and Education Act of 1994 (DSHEA) (S. 784) was cosponsored by Senator Tom Harkin (D-IA). A similar version (H.R. 1709) was introduced into the House of Representatives by Representative Bill Richardson (D-NM). The resulting legislation was often referred to as the Hatch-Harkin-Richardson Bill.[2]

The bill received widespread support from consumers of both political parties as well as the natural food, dietary supplement, and herb industries. Some observers have claimed that consumers sent over two million letters, faxes, and phone calls to Congress in support of this bill. Passed by both houses of Congress and signed into law in October 1994, DSHEA has become the most important piece of legislation defining the legal status of herbs as dietary supplements. A key statement of the law is:[2]

> Although the Federal Government should take swift action against products that are unsafe or adulterated, the Federal Government should not take any actions to impose unreasonable regulatory barriers limiting or slowing the flow of safe products and accurate information to consumers. (p. 4326)

Because DSHEA constitutes the single most important piece of legislation addressing the sale of herbs and related botanical products in the United States, a review of the law follows.

Definition of Dietary Supplements

Section 3 creates for the first time a legal definition for dietary supplements as vitamins, minerals, herbs or other botanicals, amino acids, and other "dietary substances for use by man to supplement the diet by increasing total dietary intake," including "a concentrate, metabolite, constituent, extract, or combination" of these ingredients.

This section also states that when an ingredient is first marketed as a dietary supplement and is later approved as a new drug, it can continue to be sold as a supplement unless the Secretary of Health and Human Services (HHS) rules that it is unsafe to do so. This would allow a substance to stay on the market as a dietary supplement if it is already on the market and is subsequently the subject of a new drug application (NDA).

Section 3 also prohibits the FDA from regulating dietary supplements as food additives. This provision was added to the bill after testimony in Congressional hearings detailed previous abuses by FDA in attempting to remove herbal products from the market under provisions authorizing FDA to protect the public from unsafe food additives (see the black currant oil case previously discussed).

Safety Burden of Proof Shifts to FDA

Section 4 contains a significant provision that the burden of proof that a product is adulterated or unsafe rests on the FDA. The law developed a new safety standard whereby a product that presents a significant or unreasonable risk of illness or injury under the conditions of use on the label will be deemed unsafe. The law also grants the Secretary of HHS emergency powers to remove a supplement from the market if it is deemed to pose an imminent hazard to health. However, the government must then promptly convene proceedings to review the evidence justifying such action.

Dietary Supplement Claims

Section 5, the so-called "third party literature" provision, permits for the first time information from books and scientific literature to be used in connection with the sale of dietary supplements. This is permitted so long as the information is not false or misleading, does not promote a particular manufacturer or brand, presents a balanced view of the scientific literature, is physically displayed in a retail store, and does not have any other information appended to it, including the name of the manufacturer or a particular product. The literature must be presented in its entirety unless it is an abstract of a peer-reviewed scientific publication prepared by the author or editors of that publication. The law also allows retailers to continue to sell books and publications as part of their normal business. The FDA would bear the burden of proof that such literature or information is false and misleading.

Statements of Nutritional Support

Section 6 allows claims regarding a dietary supplement's effects on the structure and function of the body or well-being. A postmarket notification system is established in which a manufacturer must notify FDA within thirty days of marketing a product with such a claim. The manufacturer must document that such claims are truthful and not misleading. The label must contain the following disclaimer: "This statement has not been evaluated by the Food and Drug Administration. This product is not intended to diagnose, treat, cure or prevent any disease." Therapeutic claims (i.e., drug claims, claims dealing with treatment of symptoms or diseases) are not allowed.

New Label Requirements

Section 7 requires that the term "dietary supplement" appear on the label. (This provision was later amended in the final regulations to allow terms like "herbal supplement.") Each ingredient must be labeled by name and quantity, including, for herbs, the Latin name and plant part. Statements or representations of quality standards including purity, disintegration, and composition are also addressed. This section also amends the nutrition labeling and nutrient content claims under final regulations issued under NLEA. The protection granted to vitamins and minerals in section 411 of the FDCA (the Proxmire amendment, see above) are extended to all dietary supplements, thereby assuring that these substances cannot be treated as drugs by FDA solely due to their potency or combinations.

New Dietary Ingredients

Section 8 deals with the sale of new dietary ingredients present in the food supply as an article of food in a chemically unaltered form. FDA can consider a new dietary ingredient unsafe if it is sold in a form that is chemically altered from the form as found in the food supply unless the manufacturer notifies the agency seventy-five days prior to introduction of the ingredient. Such notice must include the information upon which the manufacturer has relied to conclude that the substance is safe, including any references to published articles on the ingredient. FDA is to keep information for 90 days and then make it available to the public unless it is confidential. A manufacturer also can petition FDA to issue a regulation prescribing conditions under which a new ingredient can be safely marketed, in which case FDA has 180 days to respond. New dietary ingredients are defined as those first marketed in the United States after October 15, 1994.

Good Manufacturing Practices

Section 9 provides that the Secretary of HHS can issue regulations prescribing good manufacturing practices (GMPs) for dietary supplements which are based on food GMPs, not drug GMPs. This includes sanitation and quality control measures, as well as numerous other aspects of the manufacturing process, and the possibility of expiration dating where deemed necessary. One of the customary criticisms of the herb and dietary supplement industries has been that some manufacturers do not produce their products in accordance with GMPs. The degree of GMP in these industries has been variable, with some manufacturers voluntarily conforming to more stringent pharmaceutical GMPs, while others use only GMPs for conventional foods, as previously required by law. Subsequent to passage of DSHEA, members of the dietary supplement industries proposed GMPs for supplements to FDA in accordance with the provisions of DSHEA for the agency's review and possible approval.[37] FDA published these industry proposals with a few modifications as proposed regulations in February 1997.[38]

Conforming Amendments

Section 10 ensures that a product will not be treated as a drug if statements of nutritional support, warnings, and directions for conditions of use are included on the label. This provision is significant as in prior years FDA had issued warning letters to manufacturers for simply providing a recommended dosage range on a bottle of garlic pills; FDA claimed that the product was misbranded because the use of the term "dosage" implied therapeutic activity for the product. Further, many manufacturers feared that putting specific warnings on products might result in FDA's treating the product as a drug. DSHEA now allowed manufacturers to fully warn consumers about potential adverse side effects of products, conditions in which the product may be contraindicated, and related types of special warnings—language that heretofore was usually found only on on approved drug labels—without such language constituting drug labeling.

Withdrawal of Regulations

Section 11 required that the Secretary of HHS declare null and void the advance notice of proposed rulemaking (ANPR) issued June 18, 1993 (based on the so-called "Dykstra Report" in which the FDA noted that botanicals have medicinal properties and should be regulated accordingly). In the ANPR, the agency proposed methods for possible regulation of botanicals and vitamins as drugs.[39] This proposed regulation and the report upon which it was based played a crucial role in consumer and industry Congressional testimony asserting that FDA's agenda was one of curtailing consumer access to herb and other dietary supplements. Despite FDA protests to the contrary, the language of the ANPR was clear evidence that the agency in fact was proposing regulations that would have limited access to botanicals by classifying them as drugs.

Establishment of the Commission on Dietary Supplement Labels

Section 12 of DSHEA provides for the establishment of a seven-member Presidential commission charged with the mission of conducting a two-year study and issue a report with its findings on the regulation of label claims and statements for supplements, and the evaluation of these claims, including the use of literature employed in the sale of supplements. The law stipulated that at least one of the commissioners must have expertise in the area of "pharmacognosy [the science of drugs of natural origin, usually from plants], medical botany, traditional herbal medicine, or other related sciences"[2] (p. 4331). (The composition of the commission resulted in the appointment of two commissioners with such qualifications.) Upon issuance of the commission's report (published in late November, 1997), HHS was allowed two years to issue regulations on the report. A summary of the relevant points of the commission's report is listed below.

Office of Dietary Supplements

Finally, Section 13 authorized $5 million to establish the Office of Dietary Supplements (ODS) at the National Institutes of Health (NIH) to collect, compile, conduct, and coordinate scientific research on dietary supplements. The office is to act as the principal advisor on supplements (including herbs) to the Secretary of HHS, NIH, Centers for Disease Control, and the FDA. By creating this new office, the locus of research and possible influence in policy decisions was removed from FDA to another branch of government; this provision followed from testimony indicating a longstanding antisupplement and antiherbal bias at FDA which, according to Congress, precluded the ability of FDA to coordinate and review research on botanicals in a fair and unbiased manner.

President's Comments

In assessing the purpose of DSHEA, President Clinton acknowledged that the act helped to correct some policy and regulatory problems when he wrote:[40]

> With perhaps the best of intentions agencies of the government charged with protecting the food supply and the rights of consumers have paradoxically limited the information to make healthful choices in an area that means a great deal to over 100 million people. . . . In an era of greater consciousness among people about the impact of what they eat and how they live, indeed how long they live, it is appropriate that we have finally reformed the way Government treats consumers and these supplements in a way that encourages good health.

Safety Concerns

Subsequent to passage of DSHEA the agency made numerous public statements that the new law had impaired its ability to protect the American public from unsafe products sold as dietary supplements. The agency was referring to Section 4, in which the burden of proof was shifted to FDA to prove that a product is unsafe after the agency has removed it from the market.

In fact, despite criticism to the contrary, DSHEA actually increases FDA's authority to remove potentially harmful products from the market. DSHEA adds a new provision to the FDC Act that provides that a dietary supplement shall be deemed to be "adulterated" if it presents, or it contains a dietary ingredient that presents "a significant or unreasonable risk of illness or injury under . . . conditions of use recommended or suggested in labeling, or . . . if no conditions of use are suggested or recommended in the labeling, under ordinary conditions of use." This provision gives FDA broad authority to act against any dietary supplement that is dangerous or otherwise unsafe for human consumption. Indeed, it should be noted that this provision does not require proof that a product will harm anyone; instead, it is sufficient for FDA to take regulatory action if a product simply presents a "significant or unreasonable risk" of illness or injury.[41]

COMMISSION ON DIETARY SUPPLEMENT LABELS

As established by DSHEA, the Commission on Dietary Supplement Labels (CDSL) received input from the public over an eighteen-month period, and after holding nine open meetings with testimony from hundreds of interested persons, issued its report to the President, the Congress and Secretary of HHS in November 1997. In DSHEA Congress mandated that the recommendations of CDSL be published as proposed rules, which could become regulations after public comment and any necessary revisions. The commission chose to limit the items in its report that could be considered proposed rules, making three kinds of statements: (1) findings—conclusions reached by the commission; (2) policy guidance—advice to agencies, groups, or individuals not meant as recommended regulatory changes; and (3) recommendations—proposals to Congress or governmental agencies, usually FDA, intended for action.[42]

The commission made no formal recommendations but made the following suggestions (policy guidance) regarding safety:[43]

1. The supplement industry must accept the responsibility of assuring the safety of dietary supplements and take actions to meet expectations expressed in DSHEA that supplements are and will continue to be safe for use by the public.
2. The CDSL urged the FDA, industry, scientists, and consumer groups to cooperate in the development of postmarketing surveillance systems so that adverse reactions can be reported and corrected quickly. The report cites examples of how other nations employ such reporting systems, including Australia, England, France, and the World Health Organization (WHO) monitoring center in Sweden.
3. The commission urged manufacturers to include appropriate warnings on labels, as permitted by DSHEA.
4. CDSL urged the FDA to take swift enforcement action to address safety issues such as those posed by "products containing ephedrine alkaloids."
5. Federal and state agencies are responsible for enforcement actions and may need to be given additional resources to develop the evidence, "in the context of their overall health priorities."

Regarding statements of nutritional support and "structure/function" claims for supplements (including botanicals), the commission offered the following policy guidelines (not regulatory proposals) in developing and evaluating these claims:[43]

1. "Statements of nutritional support should provide useful information to consumers about the intended use of a product" (p. 38).
2. "Statements of nutritional support should be supported by scientifically valid evidence substantiating that the statements are truthful and not misleading" (p. 38).
3. "Statements indicating the role of a nutrient or dietary ingredient in affecting the structure or function of humans may be made when the statements do not suggest disease prevention or treatment" (p. 38).
4. The terms "stimulate," "maintain," "support," "regulate," or "promote" can be appropriate when the statements do not suggest disease prevention or treatment or use for a serious health condition.
5. "Statements should not be made for products to 'restore' normal or 'correct' abnormal function when abnormality implies the presence of disease" (p. 38). The report cites a claim to "restore" normal blood pressure as an example, if the abnormality implies hypertension.
6. These statements should be distinct from NLEA health claims and should not "state or imply a link between a supplement and prevention of a specific disease or health-related condition" (p. 39).
7. These statements are not drug claims and should not refer to specific diseases, disorders, or classes of diseases and should not use the terms "diagnose," "treat," "prevent," "cure," or "mitigate"—words that are listed in the FDC Act as part of the definition of "drug."

Although the CDSL report deals with all classes of dietary supplements (e.g., vitamins, minerals, herbs, etc.) the commission made some specific recommendations regarding botanicals. The commission recognized the deficiency in the current regulatory system insofar as therapeutic (i.e., druglike) actions of herbs are not considered nor allowed. The commission suggested that for botanical products that cannot meet FDA OTC review requirements, "more study is needed regarding the establishment of some alternative system for regulating botanicals that are used for purposes other than to supplement the diet" (p. 57). The study should include "the types of disclaimers that might apply and the appropriateness of such a system within the U.S. regulatory framework. Such a comprehensive study would go beyond the mandate of this commission, which is limited to dietary supplement uses of these products" (p. 57). These are important words that can provide the basis for major progress for proper labeling of therapeutic claims for herbs. The commission concluded that "a comprehensive evaluation of regulatory systems used in other countries for botanical remedies is needed."[43]

CDSL Recommendations on Botanicals

1. "The Commission recognizes that, under DSHEA, botanical products should continue to be marketed as dietary supplements when properly labeled."
2. "The Commission strongly recommends that FDA promptly establish an OTC botanical products panel to consider petitions from manufacturers for preventive and therapeutic uses of such products"[43] (p. 57).

The CDSL recognized that herbs should be reviewed as OTC drug ingredients, in addition to their status as dietary supplements. "Botanicals have always been included as potential candidates for OTC status. The Commission is not recommending a new category of OTC drugs, but believes that a dedicated OTC panel on botanicals would facilitate the review of OTC claims"[43] (p. 57).

The commission also suggested that the industry consider establishing an expert advisory committee on supplements "to provide scientific review of label statements and claims and to provide guidance to the industry regarding the safety, benefit, and appropriate labeling of specific products" (p. 57). This is an important suggestion and echoes the proposal for a Botanical Ingredient Review expert panel initially proposed by the Herb Research Foundation and the American Herbal Products Association in 1991 in public comments on NLEA. Now the CDSL has suggested a similar system, with the additional mission of reviewing not only benefits and efficacy, but also the safety of these products.[42]

INDUSTRY SELF-REGULATION INITIATIVES

No review of the legal and regulatory history of herbs in the United States would be complete without a brief mention of some of the initiatives toward self-regulation undertaken by the herb industry in the past twenty years. Starting in the late 1970s, the now-defunct Herb Trade Association was instrumental in clearing the health food market of a fraudulently labeled product called Wild American Ginseng or Wild Red Desert Ginseng. The product was made from an herb called Canaigre or Tanner's Dock *(Rumex hymenosepalus)*, a botanical native to the desert Southwest. The herb is not botanically, chemically, or pharmacologically related to the true ginseng root *(Panax quinquefolius)*, an herb native to eastern America.[44]

In 1983 the American Herbal Products Association (AHPA) was formed to develop infrastructure for the growing herb industry. AHPA produced a code of ethics designed to assist member companies with proper identification of botanical materials, adherence to proper GMPs, concern about herb safety, and compliance with honest labeling and advertising practices.

In 1991 AHPA submitted the Botanical Ingredient Review (BIR) to the FDA in response to the NLEA (discussed earlier). This constitutes a major attempt by the industry at developing an external panel of experts to review the safety of botanicals sold in commerce.

Another important step toward self-regulation is the publication of *Herbs of Commerce* by AHPA in 1992.[45] This book lists about 550 herbs commonly sold in the United States with their preferred common name, any commercially acceptable appropriate synonym, and the proper Latin binomial scientific name corresponding to each common name. The purpose of *Herbs of Commerce* was to help establish a uniform common nomenclature for names used on herbal products. This is useful to consumers, industry, regulators, health professionals, and others in helping to eliminate confusion in the marketplace.

AHPA has also been active in the self-regulation of safety issues. In January 1992 the organization issued policy statements on the sale of comfrey *(Symphytum officinale)*, in which the organization recommended a voluntary withdrawal of all comfrey products designed for ingestion due to increasing concern about the potential hepatotoxic effects caused by the pyrrolizidine alkaloids in the root and leaf. Comfrey sold for topical use was not affected. In March 1994 AHPA issued a statement on the controversial herb ma huang, also known as ephedra *(Ephedra sinica)*. AHPA recommended a warning label and a restriction of sales to anyone under eighteen. The age limit was later reduced to age thirteen.[46]

In 1997 AHPA produced the *Botanical Safety Handbook,* a compilation of safety data on about 600 of the most popular herbs sold in the U.S. market.[47] The handbook classifies the herbs according to four categories of safety, based on reviews of primary and secondary scientific literature. The four classes are:

Class 1: Herbs which can be safely consumed when used properly. Class 2: Herbs for which the following restrictions apply: 2a: For external use only, except under the supervision of an expert qualified in the appropriate use of this substance. 2b: Not to be used during pregnancy, except under the supervision of an expert qualified in the appropriate use of this substance. No other restrictions apply, unless noted. 2c: Not to be used while nursing, except under the supervision of an expert qualified in the appropriate use of this substance. No other restrictions apply, unless noted. 2d: Other specific use restrictions, as noted. Class 3: Herbs for which significant data exist to recommend the following labeling: "To be used only under the supervision of an expert qualified in the appropriate use of this substance." Labeling must include proper use information: dosage, contraindications, potential adverse effects and drug interactions, and any other relevant information related to the safe use of the substance. Class 4: Herbs for which insufficient data is available for classification. (pp. 4-5)

The publication of this safety data is based on the fact that DSHEA allows manufacturers to include directions for use and any special warnings including contraindications and potential side effects of an herbal product. AHPA has created a method to help make such warnings uniform on an industry-wide basis, thereby helping to bring rational labeling to herbal products with respect to their safety.

CONCLUSION

The present and future regulation of botanicals is now determined by their status as either a dietary supplement (for ingredients sold in the United States prior to October 14, 1994) or new dietary ingredients (for any herb introduced into the U.S. market subsequent to October 14, 1994). The 1998 publication of the second edition of the American Herbal Product Association's *Herbs of Commerce* acts as a form of de facto "grandfather" list of botanicals sold in the United States prior to October 14, 1994, the effective date stipulated in DSHEA. The estimated number of botanicals expected to be published in this list is about 1600.

Currently an estimated one-third of all adult Americans use herbal dietary supplement products according to a survey conducted by NBC News and *Prevention* magazine.[48] As the market for herbal products continues to grow in the United States at an unprecedented rate, the consumer demand for these products and their eventual use by a growing body of health professionals necessitates that appropriate regulatory mechanisms be initiated to review the quality, safety, and efficacy of these products in a manner that is rational and consistent.

REFERENCES

1. Pendergast, WR. 1994. FDA and the Herbal Industry: Problems, Antagonisms and a Possible Solution. *Food, Drug, Cosmetics and Medical Device Law Digest,* 11(1), Jan. Reprinted in *HerbalGram* 33:23-27.

2. 103d Congress. 1994. Dietary Supplement Health and Education Act of 1994. Pub. Law 103-417. 108 Stat. 4325. Oct. 25.

3. World Health Organization. 1991. *Guidelines for the Assessment of Herbal Medicines.* Geneva. (published in *HerbalGram* 28:13-20).

4. Food and Drug Actof 1906. Pub. Law 59-384. 34 Stat. 768.

5. Food, Drug and Cosmetic Act. 1938. 21 U.S. Code 321(g)(1).

6. Martin, S. 1992. Unlabelled "Drugs" as U.S. Health Policy: The Case for Allowing Health Claims on Medicinal Herb Labels; Canada Provides a Model for Reform. *Arizona Journal of International and Comparative Law* 9(2):545-592.

7. Boyle, W. 1991. *Official Herbs: Botanical Substances in the United States Pharmacopoeias 1820-1990.* East Palestine, OH: Buckeye Naturopathic Press.

8. Drug Amendments of 1962. Pub. Law 87-781, 76 Stat. 780 (1962).

9. Blumenthal, M. 1990. FDA Declares 258 OTC Ingredients Ineffective: Many Herbs Included. *HerbalGram* 23:32-35.

10. Pinco, RG. and LD. Israelsen, 1992. European-American Phytomedicines Coalition Citizen Petition to Amend FDA's OTC Drug Review Policy Regarding Foreign Ingredients. July 24.

11. Blumenthal, M. 1993. European/American Phytomedicines Group Moves to Expand FDA OTC Drug Policy. *HerbalGram* 28:36.

12. Pinco, RG. and LD. Israelsen. 1994. European-American Phytomedicines Coalition Citizen Petition to Amend FDA's Monograph on Nighttime Sleep-Aid Drug Products for Over-the-Counter ("OTC") Human Use to Include Valerian. June 27.

13. Pinco, RG. and LD. Israelsen. 1995. European-American Phytomedicines Coalition Citizen Petition to Amend FDA's Monograph on Antiemetic Drug Products for Over-the-Counter ("OTC") Human Use to Include Ginger. May 26.

14. Blumenthal, M. 1995. EAPC Files Petitions for OTC Drug Use for Valerian and Ginger. *HerbalGram* 35:19-21, 63.

15. 104th Congress 1976. Pub. Law 94-278. 90 Stat. 401 (1976). Codified at USC §350.

16. Hollingsworth, R. 1975. Memorandum to Curtis Cokar, Division of Regulatory Guidance: "Safe and Unsafe Herbs for Use in Herbal Teas." Food and Drug Administration, November 19.

17. Food and Drug Administration. 1980. Compliance Policy Guideline 7117.04. "Botanical Products for Use as Food." October 1. Amended.

18. Food and Drug Administration. 1986. Compliance Policy Guideline 7117.04. "Botanicals Products for Use as Food." July 1.

19. Blumenthal M, A Goldberg, J Gruenwald, T Hall, CW Riggins, RS Rister (eds.), S Klein and RS Rister (trans). In press. *The German Commission E Monographs: Therapeutic Monographs on Medicinal Plants for Human Use.* Austin, TX: American Botanical Council.

20. Upton, R. (ed.) 1997. St. John's Wort, *Hypericum perforatum:* Quality Control, Analytical and Therapeutic Monograph. Santa Cruz, CA: American Herbal Pharmacopoeia and Therapeutic Compendium. In *HerbalGram* 40.

21. Food and Drug Administration. 1980. Import Alert No. 66-02 (May 5).

22. Leger, ER. nd. Personal communication from ER Leger, Assistant to the Director, Division of Regulatory Guidance, Bureau of Foods, FDA to Jay H Geller.

23. *Fmali v. Heckler,* 715 F.2d 1385 (9th Cir. 1983).

24. *United States v. Two Plastic Drums . . . Black Currant Oil.* 984 F.2d 814 (7th Cir. 1993).

25. Blumenthal, M. 1993. Firm Wins Appeal in Black Currant Oil Case: Court Chides FDA's "Alice-in-Wonderland Approach." *HerbalGram* 29: 38-39.

26. *United States v. 29 Cartons of an Article of Food,* 792F. Supp. 139 (D. Mass. 1992).

27. Food and Drug Administration. 1990. Import Alert No. 66-04. (March 5).

28. *United States v. 45/194 Kg. Drums of Pure Vegetable Oil (Efamol, Ltd.),* C.D. Cal. No. CV-89-0073-MRP. Cited in Martin, 1992, p. 563.

29. Food and Drug Administration. 1991. Import Alert No. 45-06 (May 17).

30. Blumenthal, M. 1992. AHPA Petitions FDA for Approval of Stevia Leaf Sweetener. *HerbalGram* 26:22, 55.

31. Food and Drug Administration. 1995. Revision of Import Alert #45-06, "Automatic Detention of Stevia Leaves, Extract of Stevia Leaves, and Foods Containing Stevia." September 18.

32. Blumenthal, M. 1995. FDA Lifts Import Alert on Stevia: Herb Can Be Imported Only as Dietary Supplement; Future Use as a Sweetener is Still Unclear. *HerbalGram* 35:17-18.

33. 101st Congress. 1990. Nutrition Labeling and Education Act of 1990. Pub. Law 101-535. November 8.

34. American Herbal Products Association. 1993. Analysis of FDA's Proposed Preconditions for Health Claims as Applied to Garlic Dietary Supplements. August 16. Reprinted in *HerbalGram* 30:14-16.

35. American Herbal Products Association. 1991. Botanical Ingredient Review Proposal to the Food and Drug Administration, May 8. *HerbalGram* 25:32-37.

36. Food and Drug Administration. 1991. Proposed Rules on NLEA. Federal Register, p. 60540. November 27.

37. Blumenthal, M. 1996. FDA Accepts Supplement Industry GMP Proposal: New Good Manufacturing Practices Required Under DSHEA to be Published for Public Comment. *HerbalGram* 38:27-28.

38. Food and Drug Administration. 1997. Current Good Manufacturing Practice in Manufacturing, Packing, or Holding Dietary Supplements; Proposed Rule. *Federal Register* 62(25):5700-5709. February 6.

39. Food and Drug Administration. 1992. Dietary Supplement Task Force. Final Report.

40. Clinton, WJ. 1994. White House press release of November 13, quoted in Clinton Says Law Brings "Common Sense" to Supplement Regulation. *HerbalGram* 33:19.

41. McNamara, SH. 1996. FDA Has Adequate Power and Authority to Protect the Public from Unsafe Dietary Supplements. *HerbalGram* 38: 25-26.

42. McCaleb, RS and M Blumenthal. 1997. President's Commission on Dietary Supplement Labels Issues Final Report. *HerbalGram* 41:24-26, 57, 64.

43. Commission on Dietary Supplement Labels. 1997. Report to the President, Congress and the Secretary of HHS. Washington, D.C. November 24.

44. Blumenthal, M. n.d. *Report on Canaigre (Rumex hymenosepalus).* Austin, TX: Herb Trade Association.

45. Foster, S. (ed.) 1992. *Herbs of Commerce.* Austin, TX: American Herbal Products Association.

46. Blumenthal, M and P King. 1995. Ma Huang: Ancient Herb, Modern Medicine, Regulatory Dilemma. *HerbalGram* 34: 22-26,43,56-57.

47. McGuffin, M, C Hobbs, R Upton, and A Goldbert. 1997. *American Herbal Product Association's Botanical Safety Handbook.* Boca Raton, FL:CRC Press.

48. Johnston, B. 1997. One-Third of Nation's Adults Use Herbal Remedies: Market Estimated at $3.24 Billion. *HerbalGram* 40:49.

Index

Order Your Own Copy of
This Important Book for Your Personal Library!

HERBAL MEDICINALS
A Clinician's Guide

_____ in hardbound at $59.95 (ISBN: 0-7890-0466-6)

COST OF BOOKS_____

OUTSIDE USA/CANADA/
MEXICO: ADD 20%_____

POSTAGE & HANDLING_____
(US: $3.00 for first book & $1.25
for each additional book)
Outside US: $4.75 for first book
& $1.75 for each additional book)

SUBTOTAL_____

IN CANADA: ADD 7% GST_____

STATE TAX_____
(NY, OH & MN residents, please
add appropriate local sales tax)

FINAL TOTAL_____
(If paying in Canadian funds,
convert using the current
exchange rate. UNESCO
coupons welcome.)

☐ **BILL ME LATER:** ($5 service charge will be added)
(Bill-me option is good on US/Canada/Mexico orders only;
not good to jobbers, wholesalers, or subscription agencies.)

☐ Check here if billing address is different from
shipping address and attach purchase order and
billing address information.

Signature_____

☐ **PAYMENT ENCLOSED: $**_____

☐ **PLEASE CHARGE TO MY CREDIT CARD.**

☐ Visa   ☐ MasterCard   ☐ AmEx   ☐ Discover
☐ Diner's Club

Account #_____

Exp. Date_____

Signature_____

Prices in US dollars and subject to change without notice.

NAME _____

INSTITUTION _____

ADDRESS _____

CITY _____

STATE/ZIP _____

COUNTRY _____ COUNTY (NY residents only) _____

TEL _____ FAX _____

E-MAIL_____
May we use your e-mail address for confirmations and other types of information? ☐ Yes   ☐ No

Order From Your Local Bookstore or Directly From
The Haworth Press, Inc.
10 Alice Street, Binghamton, New York 13904-1580 • USA
TELEPHONE: 1-800-HAWORTH (1-800-429-6784) / Outside US/Canada: (607) 722-5857
FAX: 1-800-895-0582 / Outside US/Canada: (607) 772-6362
E-mail: getinfo@haworthpressinc.com
PLEASE PHOTOCOPY THIS FORM FOR YOUR PERSONAL USE.

BOF96